Radiopharmaceutical Chemistry

Radiopharmaceutical Chemistry

Editor: Tera Brinson

AMERICAN
MEDICAL PUBLISHERS
www.americanmedicalpublishers.com

AMERICAN
MEDICAL PUBLISHERS
www.americanmedicalpublishers.com

Cataloging-in-Publication Data

Radiopharmaceutical chemistry / edited by Tera Brinson.
p. cm.
Includes bibliographical references and index.
ISBN 979-8-88740-418-9
1. Radiopharmaceuticals. 2. Pharmaceutical chemistry. 3. Medical radiology.
4. Pharmacology. I. Brinson, Tera.
RS431.R34 R33 2023
616.075 75--dc23

American Medical Publishers,
41 Flatbush Avenue,
1st Floor, New York,
NY 11217, USA

ISBN 979-8-88740-418-9 (Hardback)

Contents

Preface

This book has been a concerted effort by a group of academicians, researchers and scientists, who have contributed their research works for the realization of the book. This book has materialized in the wake of emerging advancements and innovations in this field. Therefore, the need of the hour was to compile all the required researches and disseminate the knowledge to a broad spectrum of people comprising of students, researchers and specialists of the field.

Radiopharmaceutical chemistry is the field of chemistry that aims at exploring the role of radiopharmaceuticals or radiotracers in developing scientific and clinical tools for use in the medical field. Radiopharmaceuticals are radioactive agents used to diagnose or treat certain medical problems or diseases. They are used to examine blood flow to the brain, functioning of the liver, lungs, heart, or kidneys, assess bone growth, and confirm other diagnostic procedures. The dosages of radiopharmaceuticals that are used to diagnose medical problems vary depending on the patient and the type of test. Some radiopharmaceuticals are used in large quantities to treat certain types of cancer and other illnesses. In these cases, the radioactive material is absorbed into the cancerous area and destroys the affected tissue. Radiopharmaceutical therapy (RPT) has emerged as a safe and effective targeted approach for treating many types of cancer. RPT is a new treatment for cancer that offers several advantages over existing treatment approaches. Unlike radiation therapy, radiation is not delivered externally, but is delivered systemically or locally, similar to chemotherapy or biological targeted therapy. Radiopharmaceutical chemistry is an upcoming field of science that has undergone rapid development over the past few decades. Those in search of information to further their knowledge on this discipline as well as its applications will be greatly assisted by this book.

At the end of the preface, I would like to thank the authors for their brilliant chapters and the publisher for guiding us all-through the making of the book till its final stage. Also, I would like to thank my family for providing the support and encouragement throughout my academic career and research projects.

Editor

1

^{68}Ga-Based Radiopharmaceuticals: Production and Application Relationship

Irina Velikyan [1,2]

[1] Section of Nuclear Medicine and PET, Department of Surgical Sciences, Uppsala University, Uppsala SE-751 85, Sweden; E-Mail: irina.velikyan@akademiska.se

[2] PET Center, Center for Medical Imaging, Uppsala University Hospital, Uppsala SE-751 85, Sweden

Academic Editor: Svend Borup Jensen

Abstract: The contribution of ^{68}Ga to the promotion and expansion of clinical research and routine positron emission tomography (PET) for earlier better diagnostics and individualized medicine is considerable. The potential applications of ^{68}Ga-comprising imaging agents include targeted, pre-targeted and non-targeted imaging. This review discusses the key aspects of the production of ^{68}Ga and ^{68}Ga-based radiopharmaceuticals in the light of the impact of regulatory requirements and endpoint pre-clinical and clinical applications.

Keywords: positron emission tomography; ^{68}Ga; chemistry; receptor targeting; peptide; GMP; dosimetry

---

1. Introduction

Development and availability of radiopharmaceuticals is a key driving force of nuclear medicine establishment and expansion. The role of ^{68}Ga in the growth and worldwide spreading of clinical research and routine positron emission tomography (PET) has been proven considerable especially during last two decades. Some important features influencing such progress are the generator production of ^{68}Ga, availability of commercial generators, robust labeling chemistry diversity, and potential for personalized medicine and radiotheranostics [1–3]. Small compounds, biological macromolecules as well as nano- and micro-particles have been successfully labeled with ^{68}Ga, and the resulting agents demonstrated promising imaging capability pre-clinically and clinically [1,3–6]. In particular ^{68}Ga was used for the labeling of ligands targeted to specific protein expression products such as receptors, enzymes, and antigens; small effector or hapten molecules for pre-targeted imaging; and various compounds for imaging of general biologic properties and processes such as proliferation, apoptosis, hypoxia, glycolysis, and angiogenesis. ^{68}Ga is most often utilized in radiopharmaceuticals for oncology diagnostics, however its potential has also been demonstrated for imaging of myocardial perfusion, pulmonary perfusion and ventilation as well as inflammation and infection. Feasibility of non-invasive monitoring of transplantation and survival of beta cells in diabetes mellitus is one more growing application area [7–9].

PET in combination with targeted imaging agents allows tumor-type specific non-invasive diagnosis with precise delineation of tumors and metastases and thus disease staging. Moreover, quantification of receptor expression, uptake kinetics and pre-therapeutic dosimetry may allow more efficient and effective treatment selection and planning as well as monitoring response to the therapy and early detection of recurrent disease resulting in personalized medicine and, in particular, radiotheranostics (Figure 1). The primary aims of the individualized patient management are to optimize therapeutic response and avoid futile treatments, minimize risks and toxicity as well as reduce cost and patient distress. Clinical intra-patient studies with variable amount of administered ^{68}Ga-based imaging agents demonstrated significance of individualized patient management [10–12].

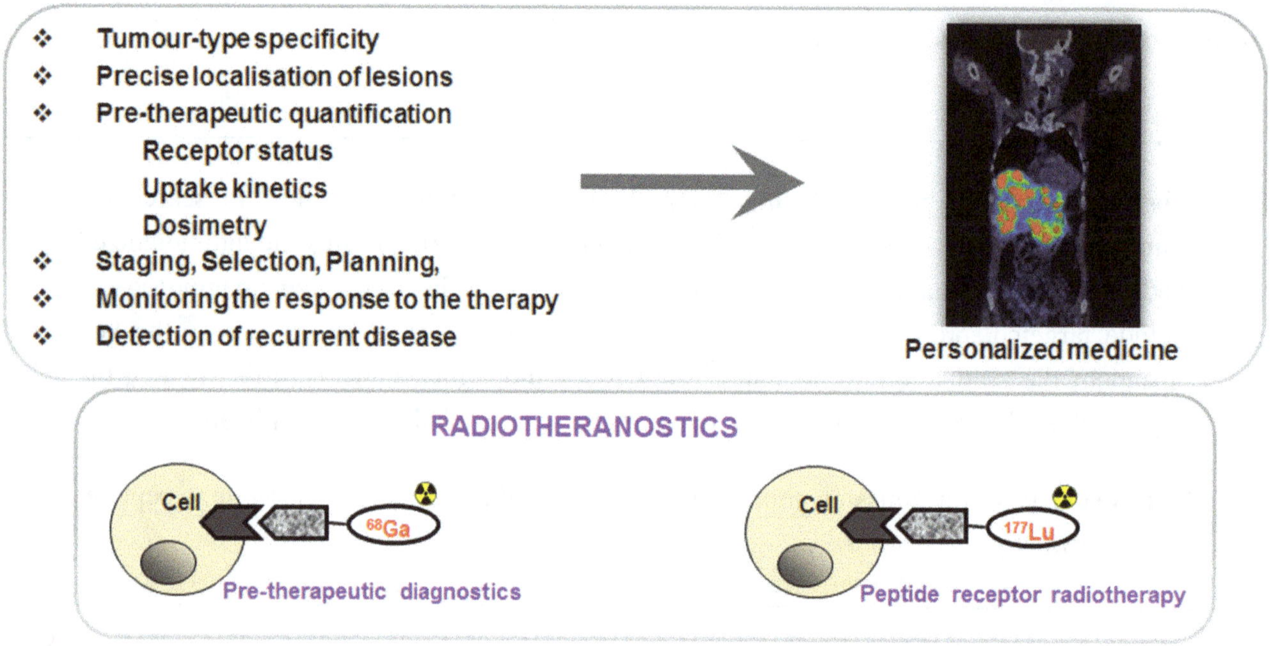

Figure 1. (Upper panel) Peptide receptor targeted imaging and radiotherapy provide personalized and thus more effective and efficient treatment of patients. (**Lower panel**) Drawing of the interaction of an agent, either imaging if labeled with ^{68}Ga (**left**) or radiotherapeutic if labeled with ^{177}Lu (**right**), with the cell receptor.

Such characteristics of ^{68}Ga as its availability from a generator system and amenability for kit type radiopharmaceutical preparation make this radionuclide as functional as ^{99m}Tc, but with additional advantages of higher sensitivity, resolution, quantification and dynamic scanning. Moreover, some therapeutic radionuclides resemble coordination chemistry of Ga(III) thus facilitating the radiotheranostic development wherein the pre-therapeutic imaging and radiotherapy are conducted with the same vector molecule exchanging the imaging and therapeutic radionuclides (Figure 1, lower panel).

A number of methods for ^{68}Ga-labeling have been developed allowing choice dependent on the application objectives and logistics. Production for the clinical use can be divided into three groups: manual good manufacturing practice (GMP) production; automated GMP manufacturing; and kit type preparation. This review presents such critical aspects of ^{68}Ga-radiopharmaceutical development as: generator production of ^{68}Ga and its subsequent handling; essential features of labeling chemistry in relation to the endpoint biological and clinical applications; important aspects of ^{68}Ga-radiopharmaceutical production process with respect to the regulatory issues.

2. Characteristics and Generator Production of ^{68}Ga

The advantages of ^{68}Ga have been presented in details previously and they are multiple with regard to both physical and chemical properties [1,3,4,6]. Those that are relevant to the aspects discussed in this review are summarized here. The high positron emission fraction (89%, E_{max}: 1899 keV, E_{mean}: 890 keV) and half-life of 68 min provide sufficient levels of radioactivity for high quality images while minimizing radiation dose to the patient and personnel. It requires short scanning time and allows repetitive examinations. In modern generators ^{68}Ga is obtained in ionic form compatible with subsequent highly reproducible and straightforward labeling chemistry. The only oxidation state stable at physiological pH is Ga(III) providing robust labeling chemistry with ligands that can fill the octahedral coordination sphere of Ga(III) with six coordination sites. The long shelf-life generator ($t_{½}$(^{68}Ge) = 270.95 d) is simple to use and a steady source of the radionuclide for medical centers without cyclotrons or remote from distribution site. Moreover, it is a source of the enrichment of radiopharmaceutical arsenal at centers equipped with cyclotrons. As compared to cyclotron it does not require: (i) special premises with radiation shielding constructions; (ii) consumption of energy; and (iii) highly qualified personnel for running and maintaining the equipment (Figure 2A).

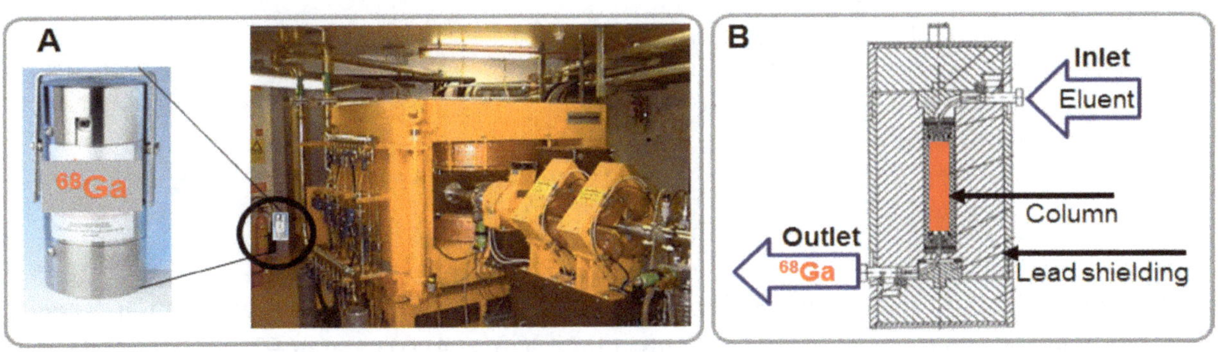

Figure 2. (**A**) Pictures of a ^{68}Ge/^{68}Ga generator and a cyclotron; (**B**) Schematic presentation of the cross section of a column-based generator.

A generator is a self-contained system housing a parent/daughter radionuclide mixture in equilibrium. Modern commercial generators consist of a small chromatographic column situated in a shielding container (Figure 2B). ^{68}Ge is produced in a high energy cyclotron from stable Ga-69 isotope (^{69}Ga(p,2n)^{68}Ge). Then, ^{68}Ge is immobilized on a column filled with inorganic, organic or mixed matrix where it spontaneously decays to ^{68}Ga (Equation (1)), which can then be extracted by an eluent. ^{68}Ga decays in its turn to stable Zn(II) (Equation (2)). Thus Ge, Ga, and Zn elements populate the generator and can be found in the eluate.

$$^{68}_{32}Ge + ^{0}_{-1}e \rightarrow ^{68}_{31}Ga + \nu \quad (1)$$

$$^{68}_{31}Ga \rightarrow ^{68}_{30}Zn + \beta^{+} + \nu; p \rightarrow n + \beta^{+} + \nu \quad (2)$$

The relation of ^{68}Ge decay and ^{68}Ga accumulation is described by secular equilibrium since the half-life of the ^{68}Ge is over 100 times longer than that of ^{68}Ga (Equation (3)).

$$\frac{t_{½}(^{68}_{32}Ge)}{t_{½}(^{68}_{31}Ga)} = 5762 \quad (3)$$

At the equilibrium, the radionuclides have equal radioactivities achieved at 14 h post elution (Figure 3). However, already 68 min post elution 50% of the maximum achievable radioactivity is accumulated and 4 h later it is over 91%. So, the tracer production can be performed every hour or up to three productions within one working day dependent on the generator loaded radioactivity (^{68}Ge) and the age of the generator. The graph depicts a theoretical plot of ^{68}Ga generation (Figure 3, red line). In reality, ^{68}Ga recovery from the generator chromatographic column is less than quantitative and the proportion of ^{68}Ga separated during the elution process to the theoretical value expected at the secular equilibrium is defined as elution efficiency (Figure 3, black line). The precise determination of ^{68}Ga half-life time still continues reporting 67.83 min [13], 67.71 min [14], and 67.85 min [15], but for the simplicity 68 min value is used in this illustrative graph (Figure 3). It can also be mentioned that the range of the half-life values covers 62–74 min in the specification of the European Pharmacopoeia monographs [16,17].

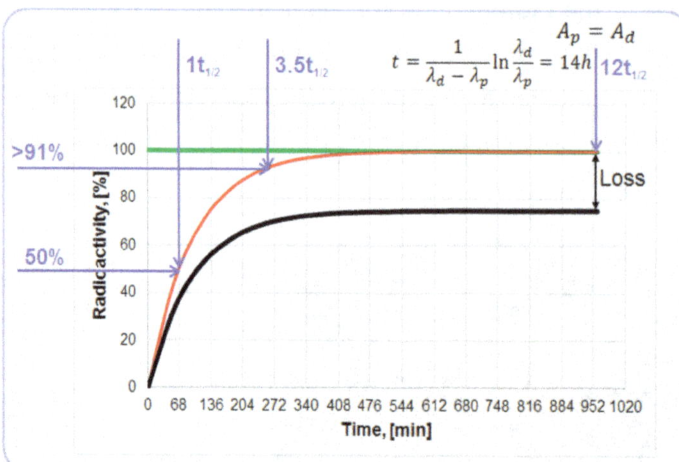

Figure 3. Graph of the secular equilibrium with ^{68}Ge decay and ^{68}Ga accumulation. The green line represents decay of ^{68}Ge described by $A_p(t) = A_p(0) * \exp(-\lambda_p t)$; the red line represents ingrowth of ^{68}Ga described by $A_d(t) = \frac{A_p(0)\lambda_d}{\lambda_d - \lambda_p}(\exp(-\lambda_p t) - \exp(-\lambda_d t))$; and the black line represents accumulation kinetics of ^{68}Ga with correction for hypothetical elution efficiency.

Commonly, modern ^{68}Ge/^{68}Ga generators demonstrate highly reproducible and robust performance, as, for example, ^{68}Ga elution yield for three generator units of various age presented in Figure 4A [18]. Elution yield has both ^{68}Ge-decay and elution efficiency components. The elution efficiency depends on the ^{68}Ge breakthrough and column matrix, and may drop in time course, however the ^{68}Ge-decay component is larger (Figure 4B).

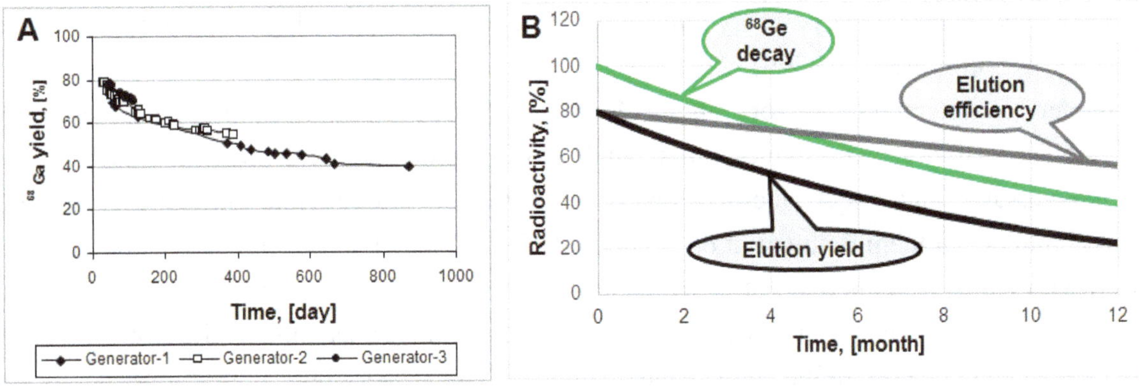

Figure 4. (**A**) ^{68}Ga elution yield for Generator-1 over 29 months, Generator-2 over 14 months and Generator-3 over three months; (**B**) Hypothetical graphs representing ^{68}Ge decay, elution efficiency and resulting non-decay corrected elution yield.

Historically, there have been two basic Ge-Ga separation methods: liquid–liquid extraction and column technology with various eluents (alkaline, acidic or complexing agents). The column technique is most widely used with various sorbents made of inorganic, organic or mixed materials (Table 1) [1,19].

Table 1. Various sorbents and respective eluents used in column based ^{68}Ge/^{68}Ga generators.

^{68}Ge/^{68}Ga Generator Column Matrix	
Inorganic (Eluent)	**Organic (Eluent)**
SnO_2 (1 M HCl)	*N*-methylglucamine (0.1 M HCl; 0.1 M NaOH; citrate; EDTA)
TiO_2 (0.1 M HCl)	Pyrogallol-formaldehyde (0.3 M HCl)
CeO_2 (0.02 M HCl)	Nanoceria-polyacrylonitrile (0.1 M HCl)
ZrO_2 (0.1 M HCl)	
Zr-Ti ceramic (0.5 M NaOH/KOH; 4 M HCl; acetate; citrate)	
Nano-zirconia (0.01 M HCl)	

The major parameters of a generator performance are: chemical separation specificity; radiation resistance and chemical stability of the column material; eluate sterility and apyrogenecity; ^{68}Ge breakthrough; eluent type; and elution profile. Most of the generators use acidic eluent since it provides cationic Ga(III) for the further direct chemistry. Inorganic column sorbents are used more widely as they are less sensitive to radiolysis. Development work continues in order to improve these characteristics and a number of commercial and in-house built generators have been introduced. Column matrixes that allow elution of ^{68}Ga using several different eluents dependent of the application have been developed. Organic resin with N-methylglucamine functional groups allows elution with HCl, NaOH, citrate and EDTA dependent on the subsequent synthesis and application [20]. Highly stable nanocrystalline Zr-Ti ceramic material was developed, and the respective generator elution and in-line eluate concentration/purification was automated [21]. The elution of ^{68}Ga could be performed using various eluents: basic, acidic or buffering (acetate, citrate). This generator also showed low ^{68}Ge breakthrough of $<10^{-3}$%, and the subsequent eluate purification not only further decreased ^{68}Ge content ($<10^{-6}$%) but also diminished cationic impurities. The narrow elution profile with 95% of ^{68}Ga in 2 mL volume was achieved in a generator with SnO_2 column sorbent [22]. A novel nanoceria-polyacrylonitrile-based generator provided high ^{68}Ga concentration eluate and low ^{68}Ge breakthrough (<10^{-5}%) [23].

The modern commercial generators rely on chromatographic separation and provide advantages such as long shelf-life of 1–2 year, stable column matrixes, cationic chemical form of ^{68}Ga(III) allowing subsequent versatile and direct labeling chemistry as well as reproducible and robust performance. There are a number of them with variation in the molarity of HCl eluent, metal cation content and ^{68}Ge breakthrough (Table 2). This diversity is a result of over six decade journey (Table 3) from the first liquid–liquid extraction generator system [24] and simple radiopharmaceuticals for clinical application such as ^{68}Ga-EDTA solution for the brain lesion imaging, ^{68}Ga-citrate for bone uptake imaging, ^{68}Ga-ferric oxide for bone marrow scanning, and ^{68}Ga-polymetaphosphates for kidney and liver scanning [25]. Further development was directed towards the generators providing cationic ^{68}Ga(III), and the first commercial one was introduced in late 1990s contributing to the blossom of the ^{68}Ga-PET together with the advent of somatostatin (SST) ligands. The first generator of pharmaceutical grade appeared on the market in 2014. More generators are on their way to the market and marketing authorization acquisition.

Table 2. Examples of commercial ^{68}Ge/^{68}Ga generators.

	Eckert & Ziegler Cyclotron Co. Ltd.	**Eckert & Ziegler IGG100 and IGG101 GMP; Pharm. Grade**	**I.D.B. Holland B.V.**	**Isotope Technologies Garching**
	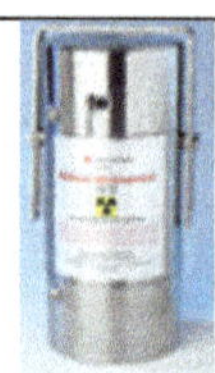	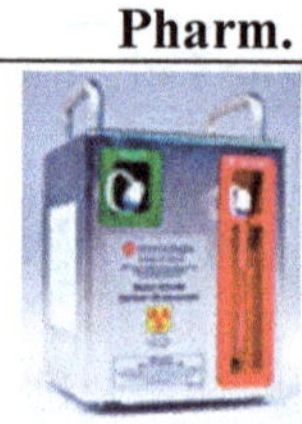 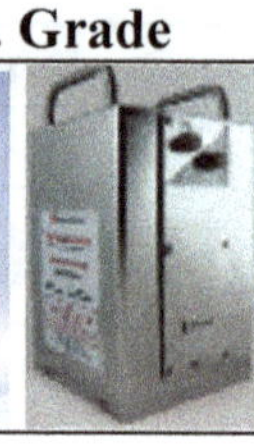	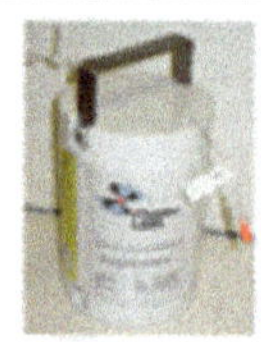	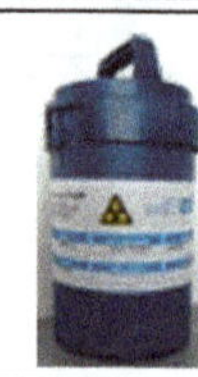
Column matrix	TiO_2	TiO_2	SnO_2	SiO_2/organic
Eluent	0.1 M HCl	0.1 M HCl	0.6 M HCl	0.05 M HCl
^{68}Ge breakthrough	<0.005%	<0.001%	~0.001%	<0.005%
Eluate volume	5 mL	5 mL	6 mL	4 mL
Chemical impurity	Ga: <1 µg/mCl Ni < 1µg/mCl	Fe: <10 µg/GBq Zn: <10 µg/GBq	<10 ppm (Ga, Ge, Zn, Ti, Sn, Fe, Al, Cu)	Only Zn from decay
Weight	11.7 kg	10 kg 14 kg	26 kg	16 kg

Table 3. Milestones of ^{68}Ge/^{68}Ga generator development.

Time Period	Milestone
1950–1970	First ^{68}Ge/^{68}Ga generator Clinical applications: ^{68}Ga-EDTA; ^{68}Ga-citrate; ^{68}Ga-colloid
1970–1980	Further development of ^{68}Ge/^{68}Ga generator: ^{68}Ga(III)
1990s	Commercial generator: ^{68}Ga(III)
2000s	Clinical use with advent of SST ligands
2011	GMP generators
2014	Marketing authorization

The ^{68}Ge/^{68}Ga generator meets criteria of an ideal generator in terms of: efficient separation of the daughter and parent elements due to their different chemical properties; physical half-life of parent allowing rapid daughter regrowth after generator elution; stable granddaughter with no radiation dose to the patient; long shelf-life; effective shielding of the generator, minimizing radiation dose to the user and expenses of hot cells; sterile and pyrogen-free output of the generator; as well as mild and versatile chemistry of the daughter ^{68}Ga amenable to automation and kit preparation. However, long shelf-life may raise concern with regard to radiolytic stability of column material, sterility of the eluate, and long-lived ^{68}Ge waste management. In addition, the volatility of $GeCl_4$ should be kept in mind and precautions to prevent the contamination of the surrounding must be taken. As the half-life of ^{68}Ge is over 100 d, it is classified as long-lived waste. The waste and storage expenses depend on radioactivity amount and container size. It would take 10 years for the loaded radioactivity of a commonly used 50 mCi generator to decay to the amount below 1 MBq (Figure 5) that would allow regular waste. In some European countries [26] according to the regulation, the eluate of the generator must contain <10 Bq/g of ^{68}Ge in order to be considered as regular waste. It has been suggested to solidify ^{68}Ge in order to decrease the concentration of ^{68}Ge in the bulky solution, so that the solution can be discarded as regular waste. The best-case scenario in terms of environment, sustainability and economy for the waste handling would be the re-cycling of costly ^{68}Ge by the manufacturers. This would provide a problem solution on the global level. It is known that the acidic environment is not favorable to the microbiological growth and it was confirmed by loading a ^{68}Ge/^{68}Ga generator column intentionally with various bacteria and fungi in exhaustive amounts and following their survival during two weeks [27]. The risk of incidental microbial contamination was found very low.

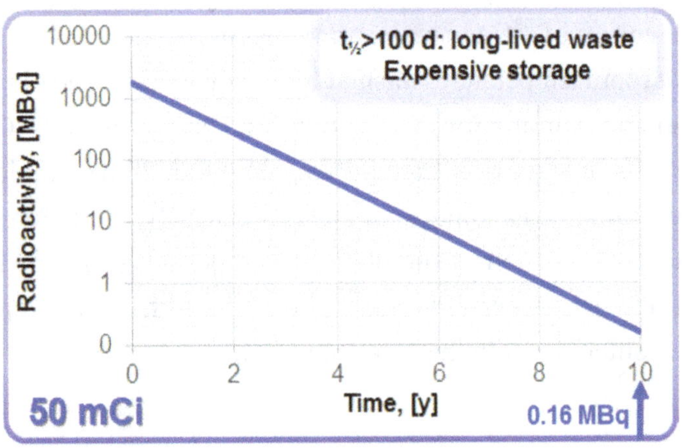

Figure 5. Decay of ^{68}Ge in a generator with loaded radioactivity of 50 mCi.

3. ^{68}Ge/^{68}Ga Generator Eluate Quality and Subsequent Labeling Chemistry

Quality and characteristics of the generator eluate including eluate volume, ^{68}Ga radioactivity concentration, HCl eluent molarity, and content of metal cationic impurities influence the efficiency of ^{68}Ga-labeling chemistry. Such aspects as pH, prevention of Ga(III) precipitation and colloid formation, radiolysis of vector molecules, competition of metal cations in the labeling chemistry are discussed in this section.

The disadvantages of the currently available generators are the large ^{68}Ga eluate volume and consequently low ^{68}Ga concentration; contamination of the eluate with long-lived parent nuclide ^{68}Ge; and also presence of cationic metal ion impurities that might compete with ^{68}Ga in the complexation reaction. The use of full generator eluate volume requires high ligand amount and long heating time resulting still in non-quantitative ^{68}Ga incorporation (Figures 6A and 7, Table 4) [18]. To overcome the drawbacks either eluate fractionation or eluate pre-concentration and pre-purification can be used (Figure 6A, Table 4). Metal cation and ^{68}Ge content can be reduced by regular elution and elution prior to the synthesis as well as eluate and product purification (Figure 6B,C).

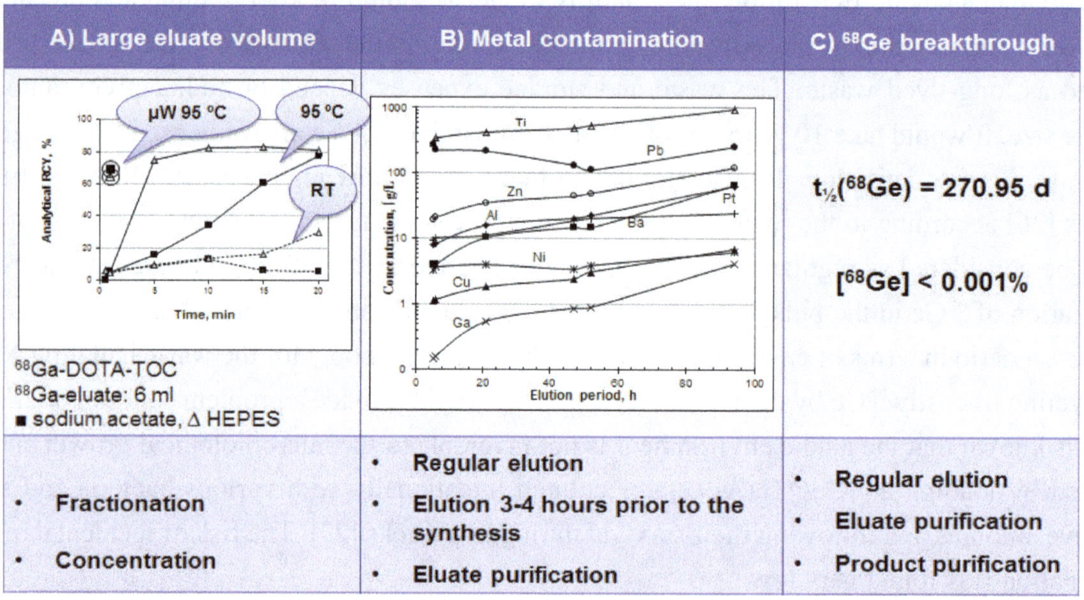

Figure 6. (**A**) Time course of ^{68}Ga complexation reaction conducted using the full original ^{68}Ga eluate (6 mL) at room temperature (**dashed line**), conventional heating in a heating block at 95 °C (**solid line**) and with microwave heating for 1 min at 90 ± 5 °C (**circled**) for two different buffer systems: ■ sodium acetate buffer, pH = 4.6, 20 nanomoles of DOTA-TOC; Δ HEPES buffer, pH = 4.2, 20 nanomoles of DOTA-TOC; (**B**) Metal ion content in 6 mL of the generator eluate as a function of the elution time period; (**C**) ^{68}Ge breakthrough with respective limit defined in European Pharmacopoeia (Ph. Eur.) monograph and methods for the reduction of the content level in the eluate and final product.

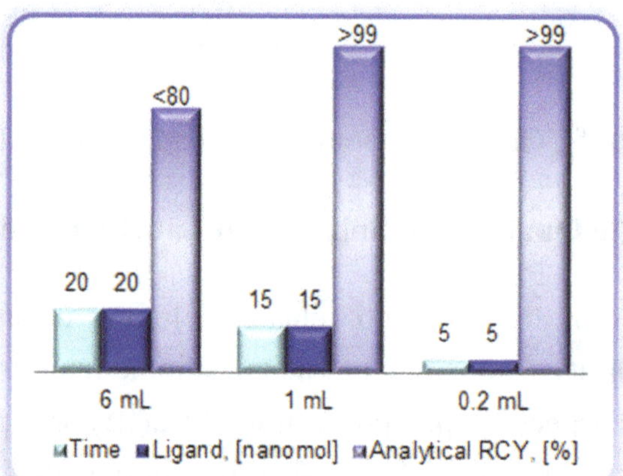

Figure 7. Reaction heating time (min), ligand amount (DOTA-TOC, (nanomole)), and analytical radiochemical yield (%) of the [^{68}Ga]Ga-DOTA-TOC synthesis using full volume of the generator eluate (6 mL), peak fraction of the generator eluate (1 mL), and pre-concentrated/pre-purified generator eluate (0.2 mL, anion exchange method).

The collection of the top fraction decreases the eluate volume and increases ^{68}Ga concentration (Figure 8A) [18,28]. Consequently, it improves the radioactivity incorporation, decreases the reaction time and required ligand amount (Figure 8B). However, it cannot remove metal cation impurities and parent ^{68}Ge.

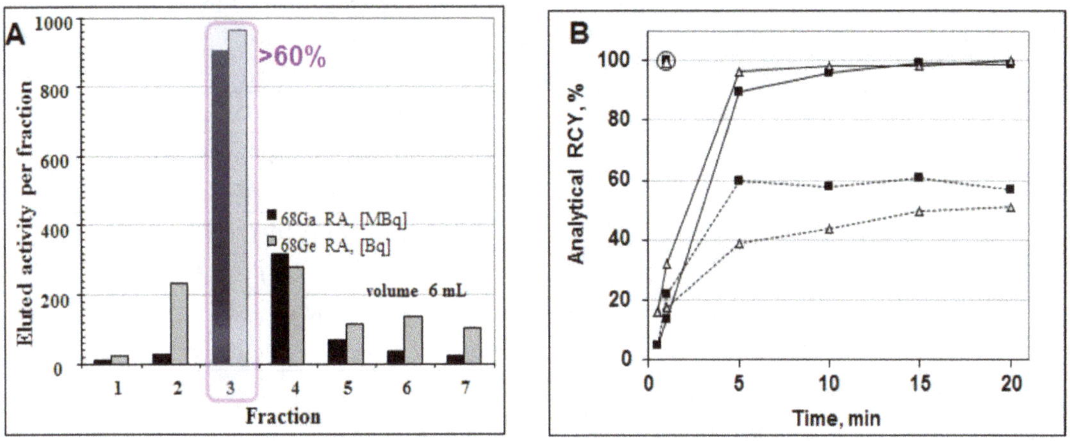

Figure 8. (**A**) Elution profile of the $^{68}Ge/^{68}Ga$ generator where one fraction was 1 mL (except for fraction 1 (0.3 mL) and fraction 7 (0.7 mL)), giving a total eluted volume of 6 mL. The profiles for the ^{68}Ga elution and the ^{68}Ge breakthrough are similar; the ^{68}Ge breakthrough is ~10^{-3}%. Fraction 3 (1 mL) contains over 60% of the available ^{68}Ga radioactivity; (**B**) Time course of ^{68}Ga complexation reaction conducted using 1 mL peak fraction of the generator eluate at room temperature (**dashed line**), conventional heating at 95 °C in a heating block (**solid line**), and with microwave heating at 90 ± 5 °C for 1 min (**circled**) for two different buffer systems: ■ sodium acetate buffer, pH = 4.6, 20 nmol of DOTA-TOC; Δ HEPES buffer, pH = 4.2, 5 nmol of DOTA-TOC.

The methods for the eluate pre-concentration and pre-purification prior to the labeling synthesis are based on anion exchange chromatography, cation exchange chromatography or their combination (Table 4) [18,29–36]. Anion exchange method uses water for ^{68}Ga recovery in 200 μL [18]. Cation exchange uses acetone/HCl mixture eluent resulting in 400 μL [34]. This method was modified in order to avoid the use of acetone that might cause formation of organic impurities [37] and appearance of acetone in the formulated product. Instead of acetone, sodium chloride [29,31] and ethanol [36] eluents were introduced as well as combined method with cation exchange for the eluate purification followed by anion exchange to eliminate the acetone [32]. However, it should be mentioned that the organic impurity formation can be avoided by storing the acetone/HCl eluent without light access and in the freezer (e.g., −20 °C). Common advantage of the pre-concentration methods is the possibility to use several tandem generators or eluates collected from several generators with the same final volume and enhanced ^{68}Ga amount/concentration and generator shelf-life. Anion exchange method utilizes $[^{68}GaCl_4]^-$ complex formation from ~4 M HCl medium and its absorption to the anion exchange resin (Figure 9A, Table 4). While Ge(IV) forms the anionic complex at the molarity above 5 and thus does not retain on the resin and passes through. The method allows 30–90 fold eluate volume reduction to 200 μL and is independent on the generator eluate molarity. It purifies the eluate from Ge, Al, In and Ti cations, can be accomplished within 4–6 min, and is amenable to automation. The small volume and higher concentration of ^{68}Ga

allows for reduced amount of the ligand and faster reaction with quantitative radioactivity incorporation and high specific radioactivity (SRA) of the tracer (Figures 7 and 9B).

Table 4. Basic methods of ^{68}Ge/^{68}Ga generator eluate utilization.

Method	Eluent	Volume	Cation Impurity Reduction	^{68}Ge Elimination
Full volume, 5–8 mL	H_2O/HCl	>5000 µL	Not purified	none
Fractionation, 1 mL	H_2O/HCl	1000 µL	Not purified	none
Eluate Concentration and Purification				
Anion exchange	H_2O	200 µL	One step: Al (>99%), In (>99%), Ti (90%)	Complete
Cation exchange	Acetone/HCl	400 µL	Two steps: Zn (×10^5), Ti (×10^2), Fe (×10)	10^4 fold
	NaCl/HCl	500 µL	NA	NA
	EtOH/HCl	1000 µL	Two steps: Ti (11%), Fe (×7)	400 fold
Combined cation/anion exchange	•Acetone/HCl •H_2O/HCl	1000 µL	NA	10^5 fold

Both fractionation and pre-concentration methods use hydrochloric acid in the eluent and thus require buffers for the correct pH adjustment necessary for the complexation. Moreover, weak buffer complexation capability is also essential in order to act as a stabilizing agent and prevent ^{68}Ga(III) precipitation and colloid formation (Figure 10A). A number of buffering systems such as HEPES, acetate, succinate, formate, tris, and glutamate were studied with HEPES, acetate and succinate buffers demonstrating better characteristics [18,38]. In particular, HEPES and acetate buffers are both biocompatible, with no toxicity issue, providing relevant pH, and functioning as stabilizing agents. However, at lower ligand concentration, HEPES is more preferable (Figure 10B). Nevertheless from the regulatory point of view acetate has an advantage since HEPES is not approved for the human use and thus purification and additional quality control (QC) analyses are required resulting in further time and resource consumption (Figure 10C).

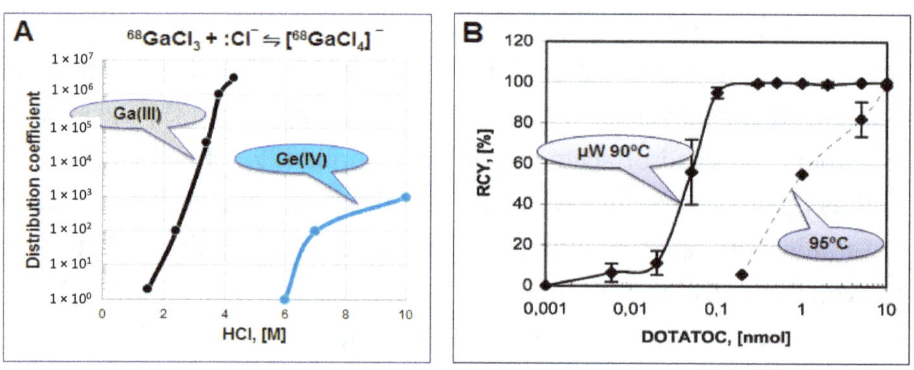

Figure 9. (**A**) Distribution coefficient D for the adsorption of Ga(III) and Ge(IV) chloride anions on an anion-exchange resin; (**B**) Influence of the DOTA-TOC amount on the decay-corrected radiochemical yield of the ^{68}Ga complexation reaction in HEPES buffer system using the full available ^{68}Ga radioactivity in 200 µL volume obtained after the pre-concentration and purification step. **Solid line**: 1 min microwave heating at 90 ± 5 °C, **dashed line**: 5 min conventional heating at 95 °C.

A

pH	Species	Solubility
0-3	Ga^{3+}; $[Ga(H_2O)_6]^{3+}$	soluble
3-7	$Ga(OH)_3$	insoluble
>7	$[Ga(OH)_4]^-$	soluble

B

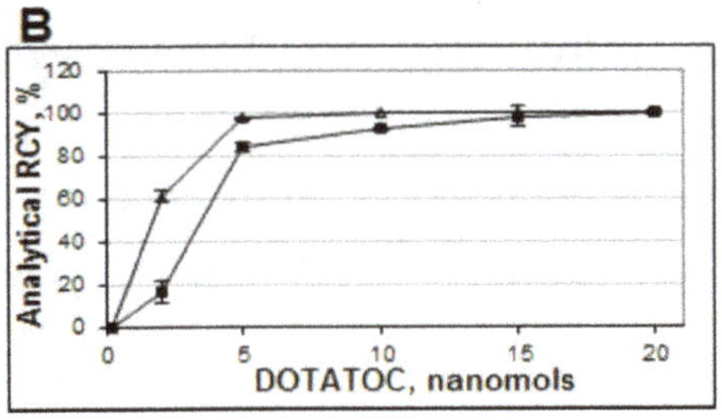

C

	HEPES buffer	Acetate buffer
Biocompatible	+	+
Toxicology (LD_{50})	Quail: 316 mg/kg)	Rat: 90 mL/kg
Stabilizing agent	+	+
Transchelation	+	+
pH	+	+
Human use	–	+
Purification	Required	Not required
QC	Required	Not required

Figure 10. (**A**) Table showing formation of various species dependent on pH; (**B**) Influence of the buffering system (■ sodium acetate, Δ HEPES) on the ^{68}Ga radioactivity incorporation for different DOTA-TOC quantities (1 min microwave heating at 90 ± 5 °C). The reaction was conducted using the 1 mL peak fraction of the original generator eluate; (**C**) Table comparing characteristics of acetate and HEPES buffers.

The use of pre-concentration methods, especially from several generator eluates, increases ^{68}Ga concentration and thus the risk of radiolysis caused by the formation of free radicals such as hydroxyl and superoxide radicals in aqueous solutions. Thus the labeling of radiosensitive compounds, e.g., peptides and proteins comprising methionine, tryptophan and cysteine amino acid residues (Figure 11A) may require presence of radical scavengers such as ascorbic acid, gentisic acid, thiols, human serum albumin, or ethanol. For example, 10%–20% of ethanol may improve the synthesis outcome considerably (Figure 11B). Moreover, ethanol is biocompatible without toxicity or immunoreactivity issues, GMP compatible, most often does not interfere with labeling reaction, and has no biological target binding capability. In addition, it can also aid the solubility of lipophilic precursors. The radical scavengers, e.g., sodium ascorbate, can also be added post synthesis to the formulated tracer.

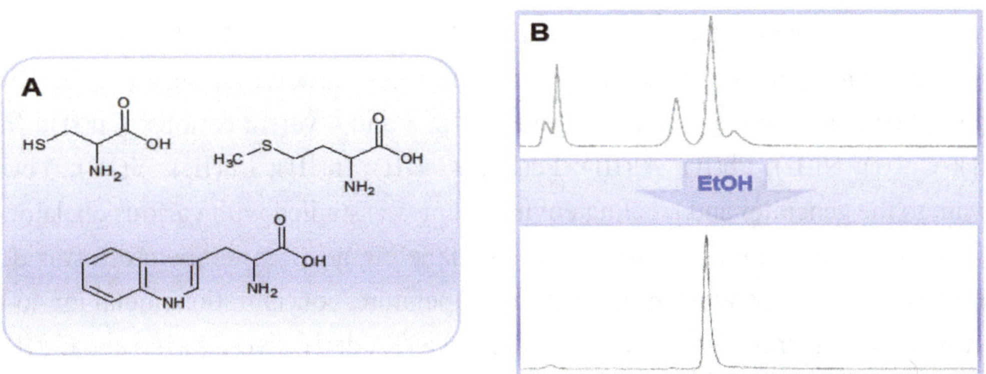

Figure 11. (**A**) Chemical structures of methionine, tryptophan and cysteine amino acid residues; (**B**) Radio-HPLC chromatograms of a crude ^{68}Ga-labeled protein comprising ~60 amino acid residues including several tryptophan and methionine amino acid residues without (**upper panel**) and with (**lower panel**) ethanol.

The generator eluate inevitably contains a number of metal cations that may interfere with the ^{68}Ga-labeling reaction (Figure 6B). Stable Zn(II) which is the product of ^{68}Ga decay (Equation (2)) is rather strong competitor in complexation with DOTA-comprising agents (Figure 12A). In generator column the accumulation of Zn(II) increases continuously (Figure 12B). At the time of secular equilibrium when the maximum amount of ^{68}Ga is accumulated, the amount of Zn(II) exceeds 10 times that of ^{68}Ga. When generator is eluted this excess is discarded and after ~2 half-lives the ratio of ^{68}Ga to Zn(II) is still over one (Figure 11B). So, regular elution and elution prior to the synthesis may allow 5.5-fold reduction of Zn(II) concentration (Figure 6B). Other solutions to overcome the reaction interference from Zn(II) could be the purification of the eluate prior to the labeling synthesis, enhanced amount of the ligand, or the use of chelators with high selectivity for Ga(III).

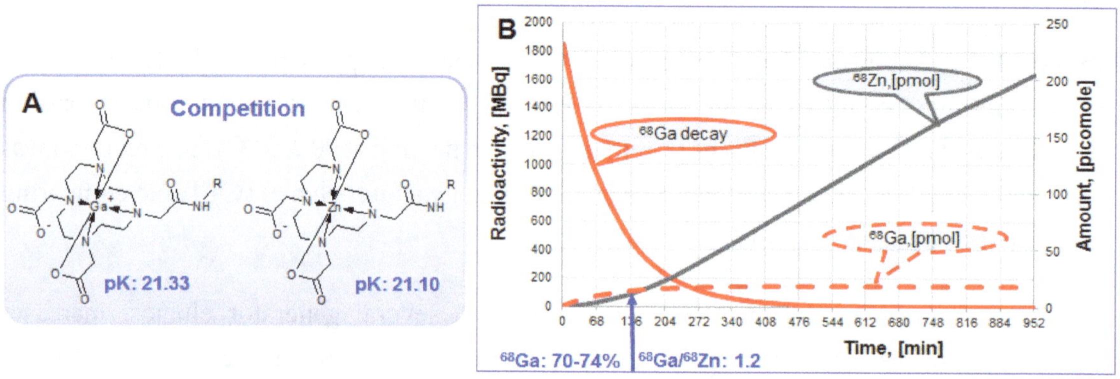

Figure 12. (**A**) Zn(II) forms thermodynamically stable complex with DOTA derivatives and interferes ^{68}Ga-labeling reaction, especially in the excessively high concentration; (**B**) Theoretical graphs (50 mCi generator) showing ^{68}Ga decay (MBq) and accumulation of radioactive ^{68}Ga and stable Zn(II) in picomoles within the time frame of secular equilibrium.

The eluate and reaction solutions contain other metal cations apart from Zn(II) that can compete with ^{68}Ga(III), requiring higher amount of the ligand and consequently decreasing specific radioactivity. The metal cations compete with Ga(III) in different manner dependent on their chemical and physical properties such as size, charge, and surface charge density. They might form faster and more stable complexes with the same chelator or like Ti(IV) and Zr(IV) form colloids and absorb ^{68}Ga(III) preventing it from the complexation. The reaction of a number of 2, 3 and 4 valent cations (Cu(II); Zn(II); Fe(II); Sn(II); Ca(II); Co(II); Ni(II); Pb(II); Al(III); Fe(III); Ga(III); In(III); Lu(III); Y(III); Yb(III); Ti(IV); Zr(IV)) relevant to the generator and labeling environment was studied with various chelators [1,39–44], especially with NOTA derivatives for which the fast labeling at room temperature was demonstrated earlier (Figure 13) [40]. Such parameters as reaction temperature, concentration, metal ion-to-ligand ratio, pH, and microwave heating mode were investigated. For DOTA derivatives, Al(III) and Ca(II) were found less critical and could be tolerated up to a concentration equal to that of the peptide bioconjugate [39,42]. The effect of the cations weakened in the following order Cu(II) > In(III) > Fe(III) > Fe(II). The radioactivity incorporation of 24% even in the presence of >1000 fold excess of Fe(III) indicated some selectivity of DOTA for Ga(III) [39]. NOTA derivatives could be radiolabeled at room temperature with over 98% yield, even in the presence of up to 10 ppm of other metal ion impurities such as Zn(II), Cu(II), Fe(III), Al(III), Sn(IV) and Ti(IV) [40,44]. Phosphinate chelators, TRAP-H, NOPO, and TRAP-Pr demonstrated efficient ^{68}Ga-labeling at a wide range of pH and as acidic as pH 1 using very low amount of the ligand and thus resulting in high SRA [41,43]. In contrast to carboxylate-based chelators (NOTA and DOTA) incorporation of ^{68}Ga(III) by the phosphinate chelators (TRAP-H, NOPO, and TRAP-Pr) was never entirely inhibited by the presence of Zn(II), not even at concentrations of 30 mM. Moreover, TRAP and NOPO were able to rapidly exchange coordinated Zn(II) with ^{68}Ga(III), indicating high selectivity of these chelators for Ga(III). Fusarinine C, a siderophore-based chelator, also demonstrated high selectivity for ^{68}Ga(III) resulting in SRA of up to 1.8 GBq/nmol [45]. Thus, the ^{68}Ga-labeling efficiency in the presence of metal cation impurities can be improved by: eluting generator regularly and prior to the synthesis; pre-purification of the generator eluate by anion or cation exchange chromatography; increasing the concentration of the ligand in order to compensate for the total metal cation concentration; and employing chelators with high selectivity for Ga(III).

^{68}Ga has been used to label small biologically active organic molecules, biological macromolecules, complexes of variable charge and lipophilicity as well as particles [1,4–6]. The majority of the imaging agents are synthesized using tagging techniques wherein a vector molecule is first conjugated to a chelator moiety for the subsequent complexation with ^{68}Ga (e.g., Figure 14A) [1]. The most frequently used chelators are derivatives of DOTA and NOTA that can stably complex ^{68}Ga(III), respectively, at elevated and room temperature (Figure 14B,C). The latter is very important in case of temperature sensitive fragile macromolecules and also it is amenable to cold type kit production in radiopharmacy practice. The advantage of DOTA is that the same vector molecule can potentially be used both for diagnosis and radiotherapy labeling it with various radionuclides such as ^{68}Ga, ^{90}Y or ^{177}Lu (Figure 1, lower panel).

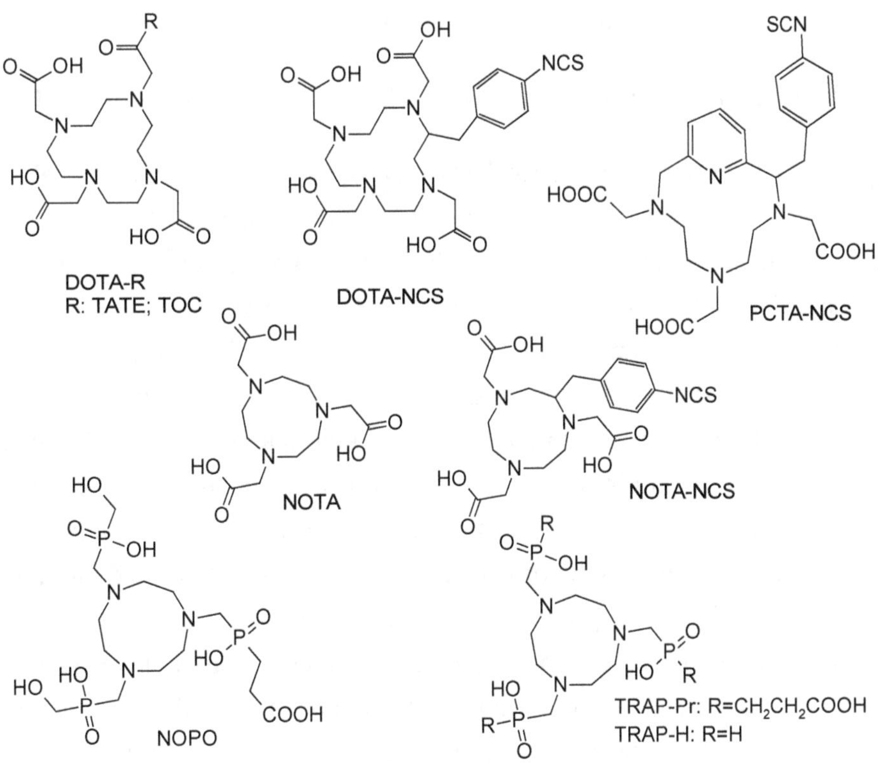

Figure 13. Chemical structures of example macrocyclic chelators and their derivatives that were studied in the competitive complexation reaction with various metal cations.

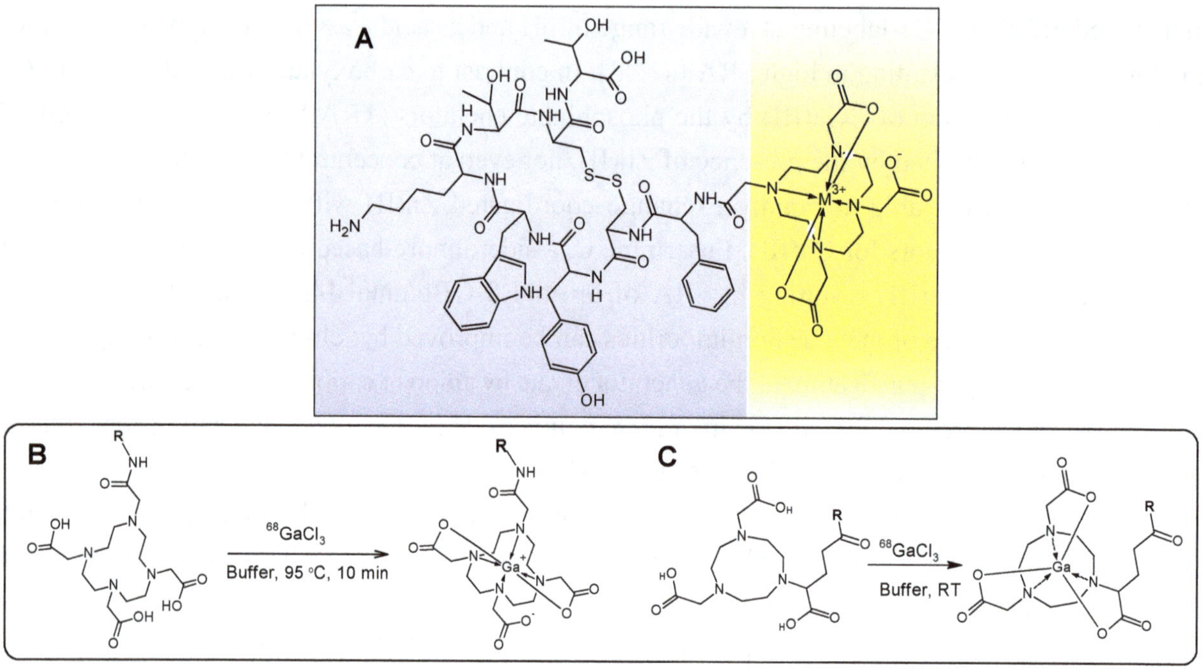

Figure 14. (**A**) Chemical structure of DOTA-TATE where the biologically active vector peptide (TATE, **purple background**) is conjugated to DOTA chelate moiety (**yellow background**) encaging the metal cation; (**B**,**C**) schematic presentation of ^{68}Ga-labeling , respectively, with DOTA- and NOTA-based ligands, where R stands for a macromolecule such as peptide, protein, oligonucleotide, glycoprotein, antibody or low molecular weight vector that can deliver the radionuclide to the binding site.

4. Influence of Biological and Clinical Endpoint Applications on the Chemistry Choice

Table 4 and Figure 7 summarize the three basic approaches of the generator eluate use with the respective key characteristics. Taking into consideration the poor labeling efficiency (Figures 6A and 7), the method using full generator eluate volume directly for the labeling is basically excluded. The choice between fractionation and pre-concentration methods depends on the requirements to specific radioactivity of the imaging agent that in turn is defined by target binding site limit, pharmacological side effects or ligand cost; demand on the small solution volume and high ^{68}Ga concentration; selectivity of the chelators towards ^{68}Ga(III); tracer production method, e.g., automated synthesis; or kit type preparation. If high specific radioactivity is required, then the pre-purified and pre-concentrated eluate might be preferred. While fractionation method which is simpler can be used if the amount of the ligand is not limited or the chelators have high selectivity for Ga(III). If the smallest volume and highest concentration of ^{68}Ga is required as, for example for the production of ^{68}Ga-carbon nanoparticles [46] the anion exchange concentration might be the first choice. Kit type preparation would most probably exclude pre-concentration and pre-purification methods due to the potentially high hand dose as well as multistep protocol.

SRA might be critical for endpoint biological and medical applications thus putting demand on the chemistry and such parameters as metal cation contamination, volume, and amount of the ligand. Figure 15 demonstrates an *in vitro* example where the synthesis method using anion exchange pre-concentration and pre-purification of the eluate assuring high SRA was necessary in order to obtain the saturation pattern (Figure 15B,C) and image contrast reproducibility, which could be achieved in the plateau range above SRA of 100 MBq/nmol (Figure 15D) [39]. Thus the synthesis with high SRA allowed the investigation of the influence of specific radioactivity on the binding of the tracer in frozen sections of rhesus monkey brain expressing SSTR (Figure 15A). Clear saturation allowing determination of dissociation constant, K_d and B_{max} could be observed (Figure 15B,C). The ratio of the amount of the receptor bound tracer to free tracer (Bound/Free (B/F)), which is also a signal to background ratio reflects contrast of an image. When presented as a function of SRA (Figure 15D) it provides important information with regard to the detection limit and reproducibility of a biological assay. In particular, the reduction of SRA corresponds to the decrease of B/F ratio and results in declined image contrast and poor detection. The most critical range of SRA values is around the inflection point where slight change of SRA may result in poor reproducibility of the image quantification. B/F becomes independent on SRA variation after it reaches the plateau. *In vivo* and *in vitro* experiments using tracers with optimized SRA would demonstrate high reproducibility and robustness.

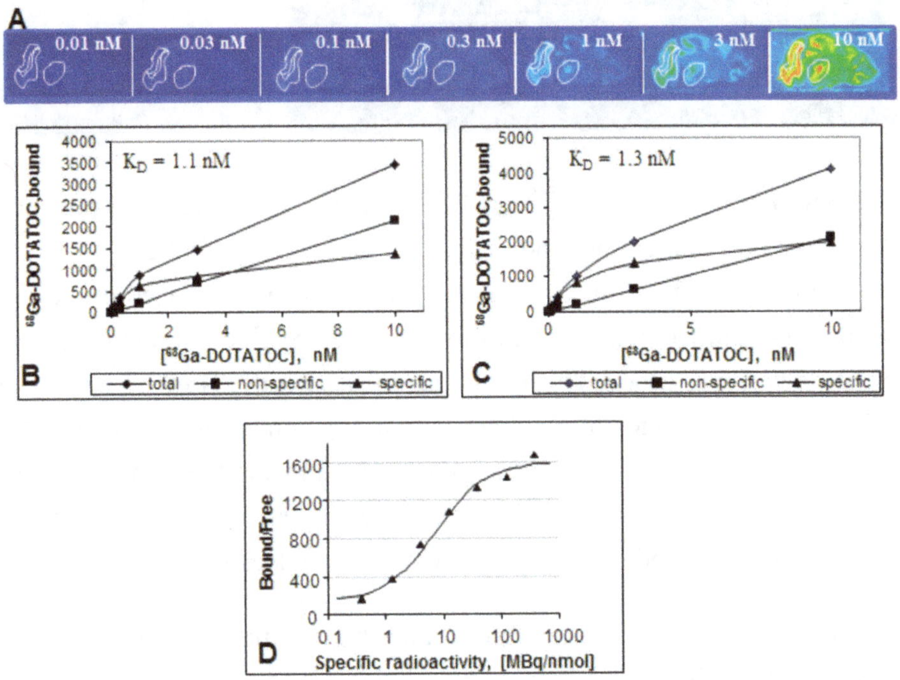

Figure 15. (**A**) Frozen section autoradiography showing [^{68}Ga]Ga-DOTA-TOC binding to SSTR of rhesus monkey thalamus and cortex. The brain sections were incubated with different concentrations of [^{68}Ga]Ga-DOTA-TOC (0.01–10 nM) for 30 min at room temperature; (**B,C**) Saturation of [^{68}Ga]Ga-DOTA-TOC binding to SSTR of Rhesus monkey thalamus (**B**) and cortex (**C**); (**D**) The ratio of the ligand bound to the receptor and the free ligand as a function of the SRA. The data were fitted to a sigmoid two-parametric model.

The choice of the synthesis method and SRA optimization are also driven by the *in vivo* agent performance in terms of the target and background uptake. It can be illustrated by a study wherein three sequential examinations with gradually increasing total amount of injected peptide were performed in the same patient on the same day (Figure 16) [10]. The anion exchange pre-concentration method was necessary to employ in order to provide a wide range of SRA values. The correlation between the lesion image contrast and SRA was not linear but followed Gaussian distribution pattern. As the peptide amount increased to 50 µg the uptake in the metastases improved, while it was decreased in liver and spleen (Figure 16, upper panel). This example also stresses the importance of individualized patient management. Thus, for all but one patient the tumor and normal tissue uptake decreased after i.v. injection of 500 µg peptide (Figure 16, upper panel). For the one patient tumor uptake increased continuously (Figure 16, lower panel). Such uptake pattern variability is most probably related to the receptor density variation and would presumably indicate different therapeutic protocols.

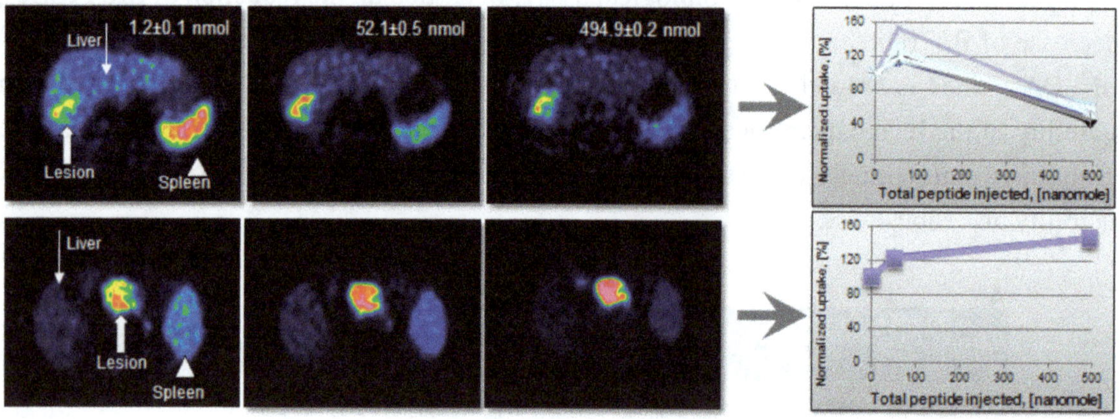

Figure 16. (Upper panel) Transaxial [^{68}Ga]-DOTA-TOC-PET images of a patient with liver metastases from a colonic carcinoid who underwent three sequential PET-CT examinations. The tracer accumulation pattern in tumor tissue **(thick arrow)** increased in the second PET examination by pre-treatment with 50 µg of unlabeled octreotide but decreased again in the third examination that was proceeded by 500 µg of octreotide. **(Lower panel)** Transaxial [^{68}Ga]-DOTA-TOC-PET images of a patient with a large endocrine pancreatic tumor who underwent three sequential PET-CT examinations. In contrast to the tumor uptake pattern in the other patients, as illustrated in the upper panel, the tumor accumulation **(thick arrow)** in this particular patient increased gradually over the three PET examinations.

The high ligand amount allowed lower SRA [10] and thus the use of simpler fractionation method that was employed in another clinical study wherein the optimized amount of the injected peptide [10] allowed high contrast and accurate comparison of two somatostatin ligand analogues ([^{68}Ga]-DOTA-TOC and [^{68}Ga]-DOTA-TATE, Figure 17) [47]. The identical imaging protocols and amount of administered peptide provided reliable comparison conditions. No statistically significant difference could be found in the tumor uptake of [^{68}Ga]Ga-DOTA-TOC and [^{68}Ga]Ga-DOTA-TATE in terms of both SUV and net uptake rate, K_i (Figure 17A, B). Thus, both tracers were found equally useful for staging and patient selection for peptide receptor radionuclide therapy (PRRT) in neuroendocrine tumors (NETs) with [^{177}Lu]Lu-DOTA-TATE. However, the marginal difference in the healthy organ distribution and excretion may render [^{68}Ga]Ga-DOTA-TATE preferable for the planning of PRRT where DOTA-TATE is used as vector. SUV did not correlate linearly with K_i and as such did not seem to reflect somatostatin receptor density accurately at higher SUV values, suggesting that K_i was the outcome measure of choice for quantification of somatostatin receptor density and assessment of treatment outcome (Figure 17B). No statistically significant difference could be observed in dosimetry estimations either (Figure 17C) [48].

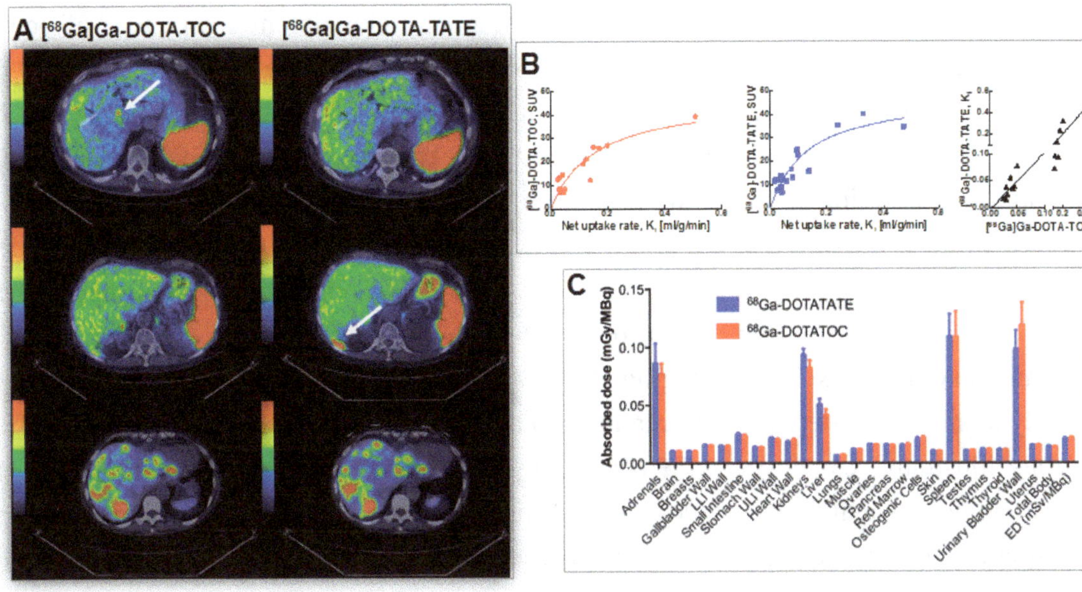

Figure 17. (**A**) Transaxial PET/CT fusion images of liver demonstrating cases of higher detection rate for: [^{68}Ga]Ga-DOTA-TOC (**A, upper panel**); [^{68}Ga]Ga-DOTA-TATE (**A, middle panel**); as well as equal detection rate (A, lower panel). Whole-body scans were conducted at 1 h p.i.. Arrows point at hepatic metastases; (**B**) SUV is presented as a function of net uptake rate K_i in tumors for [^{68}Ga]Ga-DOTA-TOC (**red**) and [^{68}Ga]-DOTA-TATE (**blue**). The solid lines are hyperbolic fits and are for visualization purposes only. Correlation between net uptake rate K_i at 1 h p.i. for [^{68}Ga]Ga-DOTA-TOC and [^{68}Ga]Ga-DOTA-TATE (**black**). The solid line is Deming regression with slope 1.06 and intercept 0.0. The axes are split in order to clarify the relationship at low uptake rates; (**C**) Absorbed doses in all organs included in OLINDA/EXM 1.1. LLI: lower large intestine; ULI: upper large intestine; ED: effective dose. Error bars indicate standard error of the mean.

Analogous results were found in another clinical study of patients affected by breast cancer using an Affibody® molecule, [^{68}Ga]Ga-ABY025 [11,12]. The detection rate and the image contrast were higher in the case of higher peptide amount. Again high ligand amounts allowed lower SRA and thus the use of simpler fractionation method. The patients received bolus intravenous administration of the low (LD) and high (HD) peptide content radiopharmaceuticals on two occasions one week apart. In some cases the lesion was not localized during the LD examination and the liver physiological uptake was rather high, while at HD the lesion was evident already at 1 h post injection and the image contrast increased with the time.

Common perception is that high affinity ligands may require tracers of high SRA. However, in the translation from cells to *in vitro* tissue and further to *in vivo* distribution, the influence of the affinity on the tracer performance may not be straightforward. The binding affinity is a parameter most often determined *in vitro* in cell cultures thus excluding *in vivo* physiological parameters. Binding affinity using frozen brain sections and biodistribution in rat were investigated for two somatostatin analogues presenting minor structural difference in C-terminal where the carboxyl group in threonine amino acid residue is exchanged to hydroxyl group (Figure 18A,D). This structural difference resulted in IC_{50} value over 10-fold difference as determined in transfected cells expressing SSTR subtype 2 [49]. However, the difference could not be observed in frozen tissue section autoradiography experiment where IC_{50} of octreotide against the two agents did not demonstrate a statistically significant difference (Figure 18B,E) [30]. There was no difference in *in vivo* and *ex vivo* biodistribution in rats in organs physiologically expressing SSTRs such as adrenals, pituitary gland and pancreas (Figure 18G). The pattern of peptide mass influence on the biodistribution was also similar for the two analogues (Figure 18C,F). As mentioned above, the clinical study also revealed no statistically significant differences in the uptake and detection rate dependent on the affinity difference [47]. In some cases [^{68}Ga]Ga-DOTA-TOC detected more lesions than [^{68}Ga]Ga-DOTA-TATE and vice versa (Figure 17) or the detection rate was the same. The dosimetry investigation, which is essential in order to exclude damaging effect of the radiation to the vital organs, did not reveal any statistically significant difference between the two analogues either, resulting in identical effective dose. These are illustrative examples of the complexity of the translation from the *in vitro* to *in vivo* applications. It indicated that lower values of SRA might be acceptable and thus simpler labeling techniques using fractionation method would be sufficient.

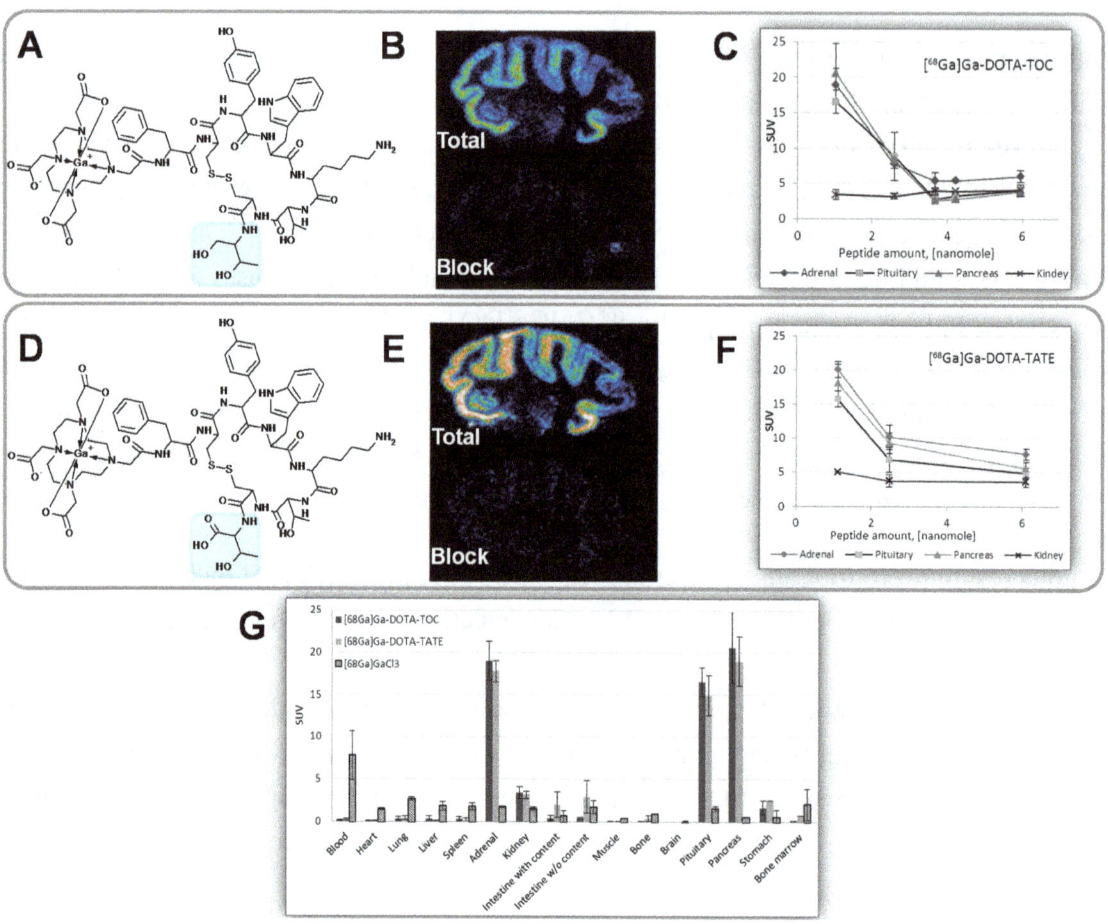

Figure 18. (**A**) Chemical structure of [^{68}Ga]Ga-DOTA-TOC ($IC_{50} = 2.5 \pm 0.5$; cell culture); (**B**) Rhesus monkey brain frozen section autoradiography ($IC_{50} = 23.9 \pm 7.9$); (**C**) *In vivo* rat organ distribution for variable injected peptide amount; (**D**) Chemical structure of [^{68}Ga]Ga-DOTA-TATE ($IC_{50} = 0.2 \pm 0.004$; cell culture); (**E**) Rhesus monkey brain frozen section autoradiography ($IC_{50} = 19.4 \pm 8.3$); (**F**) *In vivo* rat organ distribution for variable injected peptide amount; (**G**) Rat organ distribution of [^{68}Ga]Ga-DOTA-TOC and [^{68}Ga]Ga-DOTA-TATE 1 h post injection of 1 nmol of the peptide.

However, in the case of potent ligands such as Exendin-4, the amount that can be administered without induction of pharmacological effect can be very limited. Thus in the clinical examination of a patient affected by insulinoma using [^{68}Ga]Ga-DO3A-Exendin-4, the maximum amount of the administered peptide was limited to 0.5 μg/kg consequently requiring higher SRA values and respective tracer production methods involving pre-concentration and pre-purification of the generator eluate. [^{68}Ga]Ga-DO3A-Exendin-4/PET-CT demonstrated its uniqueness for the management of this disease group of patients. In particular, [^{68}Ga]Ga-DO3A-Exendin-4/PET-CT clearly localized the lesions while conventional morphological and established physiological diagnostic techniques failed to do so (Figure 19) [50]. Thus it is important to invest resources into the tracer production development.

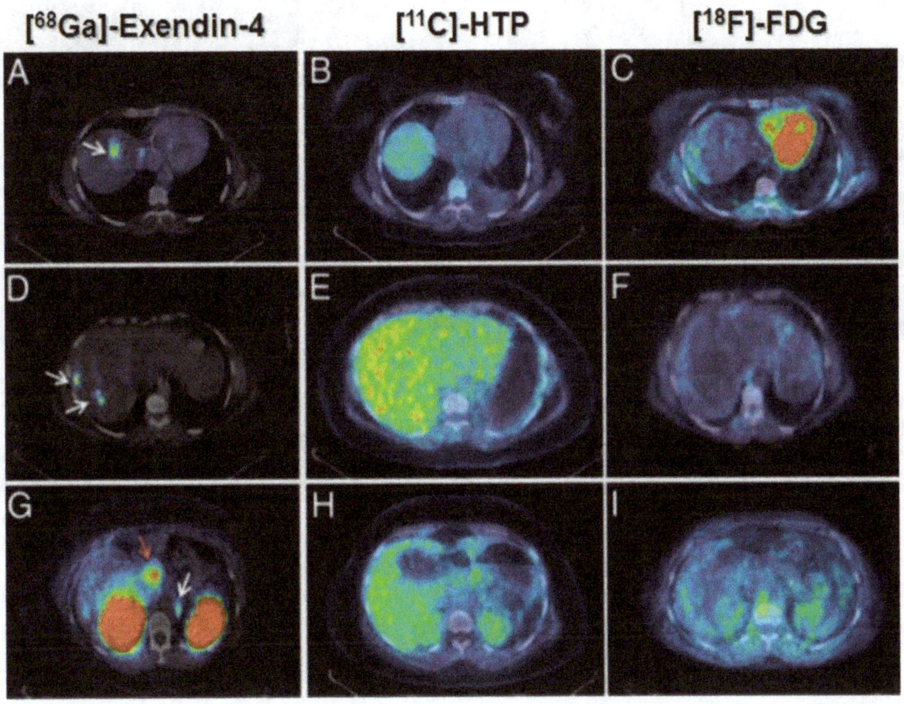

Figure 19. [^{68}Ga]Ga-DO3A-Exendin-4/PET-CT revealed several GLP-1R positive lesions (white arrows) in the liver (**A,D**) and a paraortallymph node (**G**). Beta cells in normal pancreas (red arrow) have significant expression of GLP-1R and can also be visualized by this technique (**G**). No pancreatic or hepatic lesions could be detected by PET/CT using established tumor markers such as [^{11}C]HTP (**B,E,H**) and [^{18}F]FDG (**C,F,I**).

One more aspect that influences the choice of the imaging radionuclide labeling chemistry is the possibility of subsequent radiotherapy in the light of internal radiotheranostics. In particular the choice of the chelator is essential since any structural modification of the ligand molecule may influence its biological function and it is of outmost importance to keep the *in vivo* performance and targeting properties of the imaging and radiotherapeutic analogues as similar as possible (Figure 1). It is particularly important for targeted imaging in oncology wherein the tumor-type specific precise localization of tumors and metastases becomes possible allowing for pre-therapeutic quantification of receptor status, uptake kinetics and dosimetry and thus enabling accurate therapy selection and planning as well as monitoring response to the therapy resulting in personalized medicine (Figure 1). For example, the use of DOTA derivatives for both imaging radionuclide such as ^{68}Ga(III) and therapeutic radionuclide such as ^{177}Lu(III) results in relatively minor alteration in the ligand and thus might be more preferable. These radionuclides have the same charge and fit the cavity of DOTA macrocycle forming stable complexes. However, having different coordination sphere, they form complexes of different geometry, *cis*-pseudooctahedral and monocapped square antiprismatic geometry, respectively, for Ga(III) and Lu(III) [51,52]. Even minor changes in the structure of a ligand may alter its binding parameters and biodistribution pattern and thus characterization of biological activity of each specific agent must be conducted. With regard to ^{68}Ga- and ^{177}Lu-labeled Exendin-4 analogues the biodistribution pattern and dosimetry estimations correlated despite the differences in the radionuclide-chelator complex moiety [53,54].

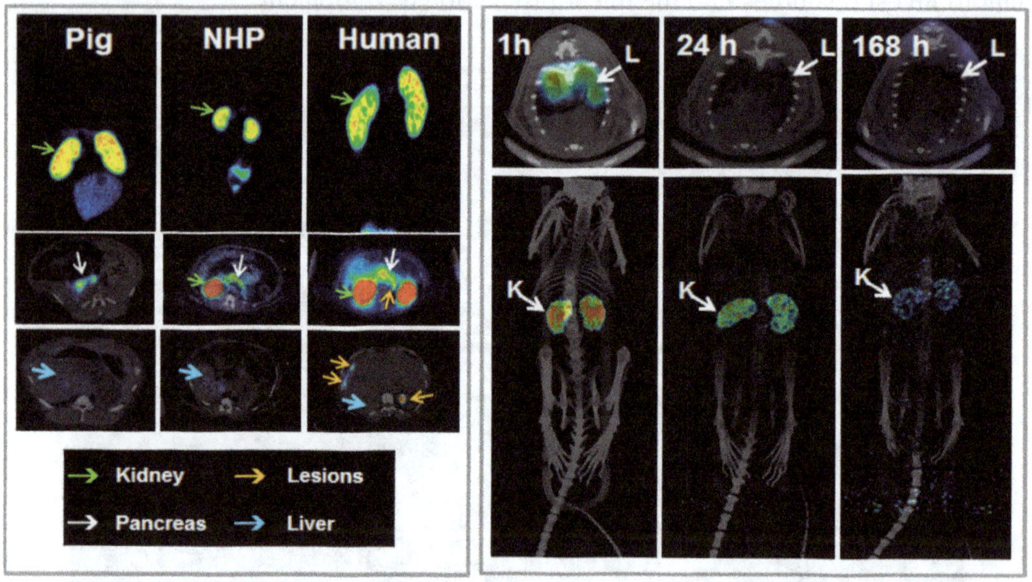

Figure 20. (Left panel) *In vivo* biodistribution of [^{68}Ga]Ga-DO3A-VS-Cys^{4o}-Exendin-4 as analyzed by PET-CT imaging in the pig (0.025 µg/kg; 60 min), non-human primate (NHP) (0.01 µg/kg; 90 min), and human (0.17 µg/kg; 40 min, 100 min and 120 min). The pancreas (**white arrow**) was delineated within 10 min post injection in all species. The low hepatic uptake (**blue arrow**) shows the potential for outlining insulinoma tumor metastasis (**orange arrow**, human images). The MIP coronal images demonstrate the highest uptake of the tracer in the kidneys (green arrow) in all species. (**Right panel**) Representative fused SPECT-CT images of [^{177}Lu]-DO3A-VS-Cys^{40}-Exendin-4 in rats at different time points. Lungs could be outlined at 1 h p.i. and showed faster clearance in later time points (**upper panel**). MIP images of whole body scan showing dominance of kidneys as excretory organ of tracer (**lower panel**).

Dosimetry investigation plays a crucial role in the radiopharmaceutical development especially in the context of internal radiotheranostics. The dosimetry estimations conducted with ^{68}Ga-conterparts can presumably predict the applicability of the corresponding radiotherapeutic counterpart and thus save resources and expenses otherwise spent of the futile development of a radiotherapeutic pharmaceutical. The influence of the SRA on the biodistribution discussed in this section also applies here. However, SRA is a function of the half-life and thus direct comparison between the short-lived and long-lived radionuclides can be misleading. Therefore, it is the amount of the injected ligand that should be kept similar in the experiments. As mentioned above, [^{68}Ga]Ga-DO3A-Exendin-4/PET-CT demonstrated very promising results [50] indicating that internal radiotherapy using ^{177}Lu-labeled analogue might be a valuable therapeutic tool in the management of patients affected by insulinomas. However, estimation of [^{68}Ga]Ga-DO3A-Exendin-4 dosimetry (Figure 20, left panel) [54] demonstrated high kidney absorbed dose that could preclude the use of [^{177}Lu]Lu-DO3A-Exendin-4. This finding motivated the investigation of [^{177}Lu]Lu-DO3A-Exendin-4 dosimetry using rat biodistribution for the extrapolation and estimation of human dosimetry parameters (Figure 20, right panel) [53]. The amount of the injected peptide was kept similar to that of [^{68}Ga]Ga-DO3A-Exendin-4 and biodistribution pattern was comparable. The results confirmed that given the high kidney absorbed dose the amount of the acceptable administered radiation dose might be insufficient for the tumor control and thus render the treatment futile. Therefore the kidney protection and peptidase inhibition that may allow reduction of kidney absorbed dose and amplification of the tumor absorbed doses are required in order to develop [^{177}Lu]Lu-DO3A-Exendin-4 for the radiotherapy.

The *in vivo* pre-clinical and clinical examples demonstrate necessity for the optimization of the SRA of the imaging/therapeutic agents in each particular case. The optimization requires wide range of SRA values and in order to provide it the highest possible SRA must be achieved using respective labeling techniques.

5. Regulatory Aspects

Generator is involved in the GMP production process and should comply with the requirements that would assure: product quality; patient safety; traceability of the process; reliability and robustness of the performance. Quality assurance system is necessary to ensure that quality and safety of ^{68}Ga-based radiopharmaceuticals is adequate for the intended use. The qualification and validation of the performance of a chromatographic generator includes the investigation of its elution profile, elution efficiency, the extent of radionuclidic contamination of the eluate, contamination of the eluate with other metal cations and column material. To be suitable for the use in nuclear medicine, a generator must have favorable properties when these vital parameters are examined. The primary document to adhere is the European Pharmacopoeia monograph on Gallium (^{68}Ga) chloride solution and Gallium (^{68}Ga) edotreotide injection [16,17]. Other helpful documents are the EudraLex (Volume 4, GMP) annexes (Annex 1, Manufacture of sterile med products; Annex 3, Manufacture of radiopharmaceuticals; Annex 13, Investigational medicinal products); European Pharmacopoeia monographs (Radiopharmaceutical Preparations (0125) Ph. Eur.; Parenteral preparations (0520) Ph. Eur.; Bacterial endotoxins (20614) Ph. Eur.); Medical internal radiation dose format (MIRD); and International commission on radiological protection (ICRP). European Pharmacopoeia monographs on the compounding of radiopharmaceuticals and extemporaneous preparation of radiopharmaceuticals is in progress. The contribution of EANM, SNM and researchers around the world to the current advances in the regulatory aspects of PET radiopharmaceutical is considerable. Such issues as: regulatory documentation regarding small scale preparation of radiopharmaceuticals and the impact of the obligation to apply for manufacturing authorization or clinical trial; compliance with regulatory requirements for radiopharmaceutical production in clinical trials; quality of starting materials and final drug products/radiopharmaceuticals were thoroughly analyzed [55–60]. Guidelines on Good Radiopharmacy Practice (GRPP) [61]; patient examination protocols, interpretation and reporting of the patient examination results [62,63]; Investigational Medicinal Product Dossier; and Exploratory

Investigational New Drug that reduce the demand on toxicity studies and respective cost burden as well as allow easier understanding of the regulatory requirements [64–66] improve professional communication and standardization. Recognition of the microdosing concept (≤100 µg or ≤30 nanomoles for peptides/proteins) [67–70] by EMEA and FDA allows validation requirements relevant to PET radiopharmaceuticals. The GMP validation expenses could further be decreased by the reduction of toxicology studies to biodistribution and dosimetry investigation specially that the latter provides more accurate and sensitive detection of distribution throughout the organs at the same time allowing monitoring adverse effects, clinical signs, clinical chemistries, hematology, histopathology, *etc.* This approach would also reduce the number of sacrificed animals adhering to the ethical norms. The work on global standardization, growth, and dissemination conducted by International Atomic Energy Agency also play essential role in the facilitation of PET introduction into clinical routine. The advent of regulatory documentation specific to PET radiopharmaceuticals introduces more clarity and improves communication between the PET community and regulatory authorities, nevertheless it should be mentioned that currently the facilitation of the entry of novel pharmaceuticals still relies mostly on magisterial and officinal preparation in combination with compassionate use under responsibility of the prescribing physician.

The parameters of a $^{68}Ge/^{68}Ga$ generator that should be validated according to the specifications given in the Ph. Eur. monograph on the gallium chloride solution [16,17] are summarized in Figure 21. In addition, ^{68}Ga accumulation kinetics allows choice of the generator elution and tracer production frequency. Daily elution or elution 3–4 h prior to synthesis is recommended in order to keep the metal cation impurities at lower level. In the case of a pharmaceutical grade generator the validation might be reduced to the qualification and determination of the ^{68}Ge breakthrough and elution efficiency as well as a test synthesis with a validated tracer, if supported by the local quality assurance and regulation.

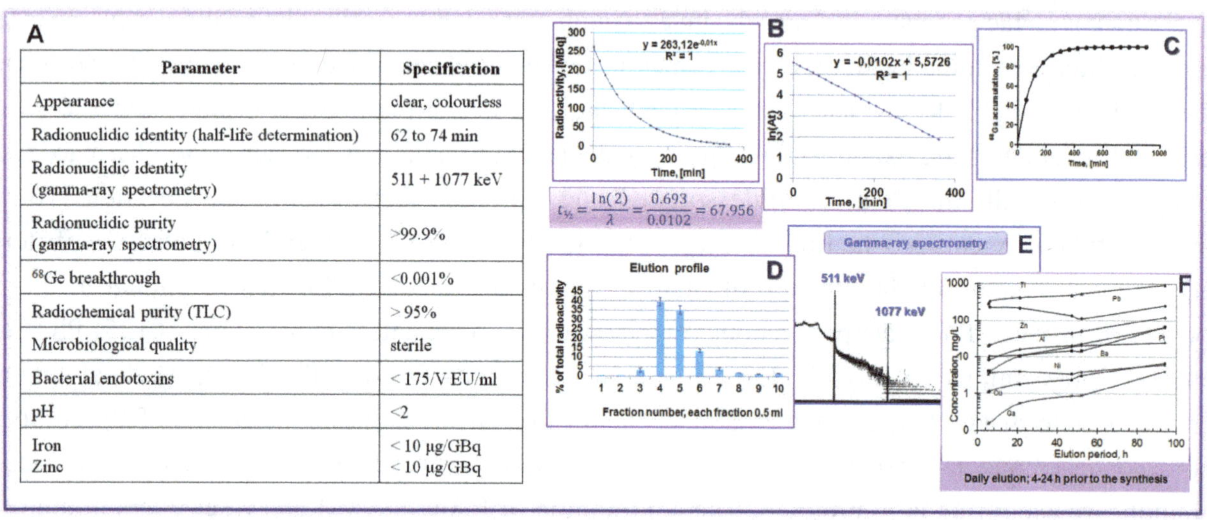

Parameter	Specification
Appearance	clear, colourless
Radionuclidic identity (half-life determination)	62 to 74 min
Radionuclidic identity (gamma-ray spectrometry)	511 + 1077 keV
Radionuclidic purity (gamma-ray spectrometry)	>99.9%
^{68}Ge breakthrough	<0.001%
Radiochemical purity (TLC)	>95%
Microbiological quality	sterile
Bacterial endotoxins	< 175/V EU/ml
pH	<2
Iron Zinc	< 10 µg/GBq < 10 µg/GBq

Figure 21. $^{68}Ge/^{68}Ga$ generator validation: (**A**) Table summarizing the validation parameters and the respective specifications; (**B**) $t_{½}$ determination; (**C**) ^{68}Ga accumulation; (**D**) elution profile; (**E**) radionuclide purity; and (**F**) recommendation to elute generator prior to the synthesis.

The content of the long-lived parent ^{68}Ge in the eluate is addressed in order to assure radiation safety of the patient. The limit of 0.001% defined in the Ph. Eur. monographs was estimated assuming high and infinite accumulation of the radionuclide in sensitive organs, in particular bone marrow [71].

However, experimental evidence was necessary for the justification of the assumption. Thus, the organ distribution of ^{68}Ge(IV) in rat was conducted for the extrapolation and estimation of human dosimetry parameters in order to provide experimental evidence for the determination of ^{68}Ge(IV) limit [72]. While the dosimetry investigation of ^{68}Ge had not been performed, the metabolism, toxicity, carcinogenicity, mutagenicity, teratogenicity as well as myopathy and nephropathy of germanium in its various chemical forms had been studied previously for various administration routs [72]. In summary, germanium as a chemical element is of low risk to man without biological function or pharmacological activity, and with fast elimination without organ accumulation. Thus with regard to radioactive ^{68}Ge(IV) where the amount of the element is negligible, the safety issue is reduced to ionizing radiation and, in particular the buildup of ^{68}Ga(III) (as *in vivo* generator) at the sites of deposition of ^{68}Ge(IV). The dosimetry study showed that the maximum allowed administered radioactivity amount could be 645 MBq for female and 935 MBq for male, which was 35,000–50,000 higher than the level defined in the Ph. Eur. monograph. To put this in perspective, a fresh 50 mCi ^{68}Ge/^{68}Ga generator would allow for a breakthrough of ^{68}Ge(IV) of 35 to 50% before reaching the limit doses.

In addition, the preparation and administration of ^{68}Ge(IV) was conducted in the presence and absence of [^{68}Ga]Ga-DOTA-TOC simultaneous labeling synthesis. The presence of the tracer did not influence the distribution of the ^{68}Ge. It was also shown that ^{68}Ge(IV) was not chelated by DOTA-TOC and thus deposition of ^{68}Ge in the sites of DOTA-based imaging agents accumulation is also excluded. The content of ^{68}Ge and [^{68}Ga]Ga-DOTA-TOC was monitored by HPLC with tandem UV and radio detectors where the signal from [^{68}Ga]Ga-DOTA-TOC disappeared within 24 h while the signal from ^{68}Ge remained unchanged. The respective fractions were collected and periodically measured resulting in half-life values, respectively, for ^{68}Ga and ^{68}Ge (Figure 22).

These results imply that the ^{68}Ge(IV) limit currently recommended by monographs could be increased at least 100 times without compromising patient safety. This finding together with the availability of pharmaceutical grade generator, absence of the complexation with DOTA derivatives and knowledge that Ge(IV) does not bind to plasma proteins may facilitate the clinical introduction of kit type preparation of ^{68}Ga-based imaging agents. Kit type formulation development is ongoing at both academic and industrial establishments. Several countries are working within the frame of IAEA coordinated research project (F22050) [73].

In general terms, a radionuclide generator is defined as a medicinal product according to the current legislation [74]. However, dissimilarities between: different radionuclide generators; the use of the generator eluate; and tracer production processes are not taken into account. For example, the eluate from ^{82}Sr/^{82}Rb and ^{99}Mo/^{99m}Tc generators enters the blood stream either directly from the generator or after the labeling reaction in the product vial (kit formulation), and thus it must be assured to be sterile, isotonic and pyrogen free (medicinal product) especially considering that sodium chloride eluent is a favorable media for microbial growth. The principle difference with regard to ^{68}Ge/^{68}Ga generator used in a GMP manufacturing process is that the eluate solution is removed after the labeling reaction by product purification and the final product is sterile filtered. This can be illustrated by comparison of a typical ^{99m}Tc-based registered radiopharmaceutical preparation process with ^{68}Ga-based imaging agent manufacturing process. The preparation under pharmaceutical practice using kit formulation technique considers direct mixing of the generator eluate with the reagents in the product vial with subsequent formulation in the same vial and release without product purification, sterile filtration and quality control

(Figure 23, left column). This process results in a final radiopharmaceutical containing generator eluate components for the direct patient injection and thus the eluate quality must be assured by marketing authorization. While ^{68}Ga-radiopharmaceuticals are usually manufactured under GMP environment where generator eluate either directly or after pre-purification is added to a reaction vessel, followed by the product purification, formulation, sterile filtration and release after the quality control (Figure 23, right column). Thus the final radiopharmaceutical does not contain original generator eluate solution and is sterile filtered. Essentially the manufacturing process is similar to that of cyclotron produced radionuclide-based tracers. This implies that generators with and without marketing authorization could potentially be used in such production process. The efficiency of the worldwide dissemination of ^{68}Ga-radiopharmaceuticals with the patient benefit as priority would increase considerably if the essence of the manufacturing process would navigate the regulatory definition of generator produced ^{68}Ga. It should be specified in each particular case dependent on the production process (kit formulation or GMP manufacturing) if it is a starting material, radionuclide precursor, active pharmaceutical ingredient or active pharmaceutical ingredient starting material. The definition would influence the choice of the generator type, namely with or without marketing authorization, potentially reducing the cost and increasing accessibility.

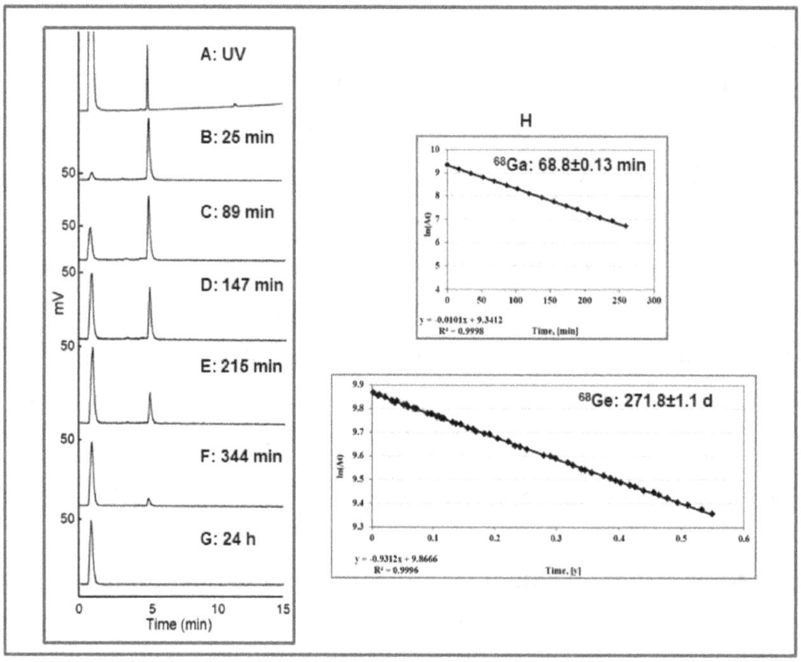

Figure 22. (**A**) UV-HPLC chromatogram of the authentic reference, [^{Nat}Ga]-DOTA-TOC (the void signal corresponds to the buffer); (**B–F**) Radio-HPLC chromatograms of [^{68}Ga]Ga-DOTA-TOC produced in the presence of [^{68}Ge]$GeCl_4$. The analysis was conducted, respectively, at 25, 89, 147, 215, and 344 min post synthesis. The signals with R_t of 1.0 ± 0.02 min and 4.90 ± 0.02 min correspond, respectively, to the ionic ^{68}Ge(IV) and [^{68}Ga]Ga-DOTA-TOC; (**G**) Radio-HPLC chromatogram taken 24 h after the production of [^{68}Ga]Ga-DOTA-TOC in the presence of [^{68}Ge]$GeCl_4$. The signal with R_t of 1.0 ± 0.02 min corresponds to the ionic ^{68}Ge(IV) and the signal at 4.90 ± 0.02 min corresponding to [^{68}Ga]Ga-DOTA-TOC was not detected; (**H**) Determination of the $t_{½}$ for ^{68}Ga and ^{68}Ge measuring respective collected chromatography fractions.

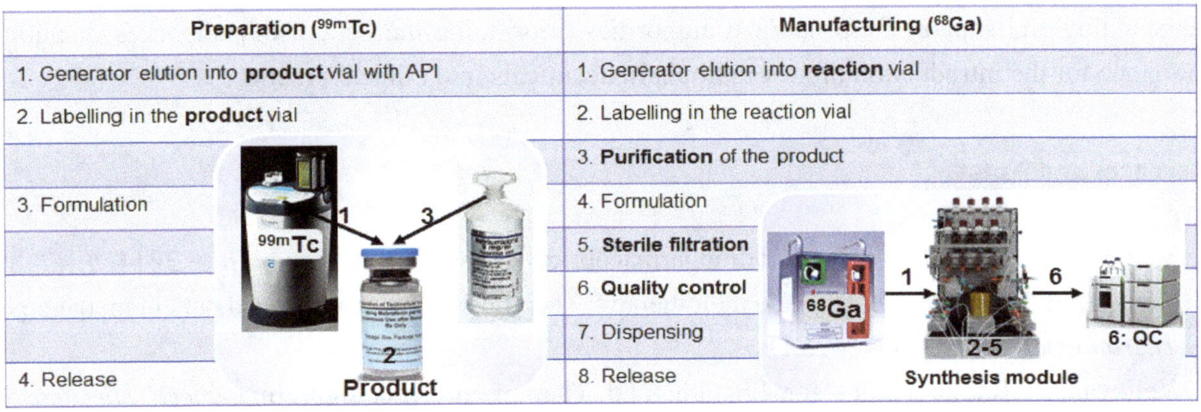

Figure 23. (**Left column**) Typical preparation steps of a ^{99m}Tc-based registered radiopharmaceutical; (**Right column**) Basic steps of an automated manufacturing of a ^{68}Ga-based radiopharmaceutical.

Radiopharmaceutical manufacturing automation provides possibility for the harmonized and standardized multicenter clinical studies that in turn may accelerate the introduction of new radiopharmaceuticals as well as their regulatory approval. Automation is important for the radioprotection, high reliability, reproducibility and robustness of the production as well as in-line traceability of the process for GMP compliance [75–77]. The increasing clinical demand of ^{68}Ga-based tracers prompted the need for the automation. There are a number of automated synthesizers either in-house built apparatus or available on the market as standard or custom made products. Stationary tubing systems require regular cleaning and cross contamination may occur in such systems. Disposable cassette systems offer improved microbiological safety with respect to sterility and endotoxin content as well as exclude chemical cross contamination. Better cGMP compliance and simplification of the process is possible since cleaning and sanitation of the tubings, containers, and purification cartridges is avoided. The stationary tubing system on the other hand provides more flexibility and lower radiopharmaceutical production price. Fractionation, anion and cation pre-concentration methods have been automated. A number of disposable cassettes for the production of tracers for the targeted imaging of SSTR, chemokine, integrin receptors, prostate specific membrane antigene as well as inflammation visualization agent, citrate, has entered the market.

6. Conclusions

Methods for the manual and automated GMP compliant production of ^{68}Ga-based agents have been developed. They are based on eluate fractionation or eluate concentration and purification approaches. The choice of the labeling method depends on the endpoint pre-clinical and clinical application with respective requirements to the imaging agent characteristics. The market of generators and automated synthesis systems is expanding. The automated production improves the practicality of harmonized and standardized multicenter clinical studies facilitating the introduction of new radiopharmaceuticals. The development of kit type preparation is also feasible, although there are yet no registered ^{68}Ga-radiopharmaceuticals on the market at present. Considerable advances have been made in PET radiopharmaceutical regulation and legislation still there is a number of particular questions and aspects to be addressed. Currently, understanding and support from national authorities prioritizing the benefit of patients is of outmost importance for the introduction of new radiopharmaceuticals into clinical practice.

References and Notes

1. Velikyan, I. Prospective of ^{68}Ga-radiopharmaceutical development. *Theranostics* **2014**, *4*, 47–80.
2. Velikyan, I. Molecular imaging and radiotherapy: Theranostics for personalized patient management. *Theranostics* **2012**, *2*, 424–426.
3. Velikyan, I. Radionuclides for Imaging and Therapy in Oncology; In *Cancer Theranostics*; Chen, X., Wong, S., Eds.; Elsevier: Amsterdam, The Netherlands, 2014; pp. 285–325.
4. Velikyan, I. Positron emitting [^{68}Ga]Ga-based imaging agents: Chemistry and diversity. *Med. Chem.* **2011**, *7*, 338–372.
5. Velikyan, I. The diversity of ^{68}Ga-based imaging agents. *Recent Results Cancer Res.* **2013**, *194*, 101–131.
6. Velikyan, I. Continued rapid growth in Ga applications: Update 2013 to june 2014. *J. Label. Compd. Radiopharm.* **2015**, 99–121.
7. Blom, E.; Langstrom, B.; Velikyan, I. ^{68}Ga-labeling of biotin analogues and their characterization. *Bioconjugate Chem.* **2009**, *20*, 1146–1151.
8. Eriksson, O.; Carlsson, F.; Blom, E.; Sundin, A.; Langstrom, B.; Korsgren, O.; Velikyan, I. Preclinical evaluation of a ^{68}Ga-labeled biotin analogue for applications in islet transplantation. *Nucl. Med. Biol.* **2012**, *39*, 415–421.
9. Selvaraju, R.K.; Velikyan, I.; Johansson, L.; Wu, Z.; Todorov, I.; Shively, J.; Kandeel, F.; Korsgren, O.; Eriksson, O. *In vivo* imaging of the glucagonlike peptide 1 receptor in the pancreas with ^{68}Ga-labeled do3a-exendin-4. *J. Nucl. Med.* **2013**, *54*, 1458–1463.
10. Velikyan, I.; Sundin, A.; Eriksson, B.; Lundqvist, H.; Sorensen, J.; Bergstrom, M.; Langstrom, B. *In vivo* binding of [^{68}Ga]-dotatoc to somatostatin receptors in neuroendocrine tumours—Impact of peptide mass. *Nucl. Med. Biol.* **2010**, *37*, 265–275.
11. Sorensen, J.; Velikyan, I.; Wennborg, A.; Feldwisch, J.; Tolmachev, V.; Sandberg, D.; Nilsson, G.; Olofsson, H.; Sandstrom, M.; Lubberink, M.; *et al.* Measuring her2-expression in metastatic breast cancer using ^{68}Ga-aby025 pet/ct. *Eur. J. Nucl. Med. Mol. Imaging* **2014**, *41*, S226.
12. Velikyan, I.; Wennborg, A.; Feldwisch, J.; Orlova, A.; Tolmachev, V.; Lubberink, M.; Sandstrom, M.; Lindman, H.; Carlsson, J.; Sorensen, J. Gmp compliant preparation of a ^{68}Gallium-labeled affibody analogue for breast cancer patient examination: First-in-man. *Eur. J. Nucl. Med. Mol. Imaging* **2014**, *41*, S228–S229.
13. Bé, M.M.; Schönfeld, E. Table de Radionucléide. 2012. Available online: http://www.nucleide.org/DDEP_WG/DDEPdata.htm (accessed on 25 June 2015).
14. McCutchan, E.A. Nuclear Data Sheets for A = 68. *Nucl. Data Sheets* **2012**, *113*, 1735–1870.
15. García-Toraño, E.; Peyrés Medina, V.; Romero, E.; Roteta, M. Measurement of the half-life of ^{68}Ga. *Appl. Radiat. Isot.* **2014**, *87*, 122–125.
16. European Pharmacopeia 7.7 (01/2013:2482 Gallium (68Ga) Edotreotide injection). *Eur Pharm.* **2011**, *23*, 310–313.

17. European Pharmacopeia. Gallium (68 Ga) chloride solution for radiolabelling. European Directorate for the Quality of Medicines. *Eur Pharm.* **2013**, *2464*, 1060–1061.
18. Velikyan, I.; Beyer, G.J.; Langstrom, B. Microwave-supported preparation of ^{68}Ga-bioconjugates with high specific radioactivity. *Bioconjugate Chem.* **2004**, *15*, 554–560.
19. Rosch, F. Past, present and future of ^{68}Ge/^{68}Ga generators. *Appl. Radiat. Isot.* **2013**, *76*, 24–30.
20. Nakayama, M.; Haratake, M.; Koiso, T.; Ishibashi, O.; Harada, K.; Nakayama, H.; Sugii, A.; Yahara, S.; Arano, Y. Separation of Ga-68 from Ge-68 using a macroporous organic polymer containing n-methylglucamine groups. *Anal. Chim. Acta* **2002**, *453*, 135–141.
21. Le, V.S. ^{68}Ga generator integrated system: Elution-purification-concentration integration. *Recent Results Cancer Res.* **2013**, *194*, 43–75.
22. Saha Das, S.; Chattopadhyay, S.; Alam, M.; Madhusmita; Barua, L.; Das, M.K. Preparation and evaluation of sno2-based ^{68}Ge/^{68}Ga generator made from ^{68}Ge produced through natzn(α,xn) reaction. *Appl. Radiat. Isot.* **2013**, *79*, 42–47.
23. Chakravarty, R.; Chakraborty, S.; Ram, R.; Dash, A.; Pillai, M.R.A. Long-term evaluation of "barc ^{68}Ge/^{68}Ga generator" based on the nanoceria-polyacrylonitrile composite sorbent. *Cancer Biother. Radiopharm.* **2013**, *28*, 631–637.
24. Gleason, G.I. A positron cow. *Int. J. Appl. Radiat. Isot.* **1960**, *8*, 90–94.
25. Yano, Y. Radiopharmaceuticals from Generator-Produced Radionuclides; In *Preparation and Control of ^{68}Ga Radiopharmaceuticals*; International Atomic Energy Agency: Vienna, Austria, 1971; pp. 117–125.
26. De Blois, E.; Chan, H.S.; Roy, K.; Krenning, E.P.; Breeman, W.A.P. Reduction of ^{68}Ge activity containing liquid waste from ^{68}Ga pet chemistry in nuclear medicine and radiopharmacy by solidification. *J. Radioanal. Nucl. Chem.* **2011**, *288*, 303–306.
27. Petrik, M.; Schuessele, A.; Perkhofer, S.; Lass-Florl, C.; Becker, D.; Decristoforo, C. Microbial challenge tests on nonradioactive tio2-based ^{68}Ge/^{68}Ga generator columns. *Nucl. Med. Commun.* **2012**, *33*, 819–823.
28. Breeman, W.A.; de Jong, M.; de Blois, E.; Bernard, B.F.; Konijnenberg, M.; Krenning, E.P. Radiolabelling dota-peptides with ^{68}Ga. *Eur. J. Nucl. Med. Mol. Imaging* **2005**, *32*, 478–485.
29. Schultz, M.K.; Mueller, D.; Baum, R.P.; Leonard Watkins, G.; Breeman, W.A. A new automated nacl based robust method for routine production of gallium-68 labeled peptides. *Appl. Radiat. Isot.* **2013**, *76*, 46–54.
30. Velikyan, I.; Xu, H.; Nair, M.; Hall, H. Robust labeling and comparative preclinical characterization of dota-toc and dota-tate. *Nucl. Med. Biol.* **2012**, *39*, 628–659.
31. Mueller, D.; Klette, I.; Baum, R.P.; Gottschaldt, M.; Schultz, M.K.; Breeman, W.A.P. Simplified nacl based ^{68}Ga concentration and labeling procedure for rapid synthesis of ^{68}Ga radiopharmaceuticals in high radiochemical purity. *Bioconjugate Chem.* **2012**, *23*, 1712–1717.
32. Loktionova, N.S.; Belozub, A.N.; Filosofov, D.V.; Zhernosekov, K.P.; Wagner, T.; Turler, A.; Rosch, F. Improved column-based radiochemical processing of the generator produced ^{68}Ga. *Appl. Radiat. Isot.* **2011**, *69*, 942–946.
33. Gebhardt, P.; Opfermann, T.; Saluz, H.P. Computer controlled Ga-68 milking and concentration system. *Appl. Radiat. Isot.* **2010**, *68*, 1057–1059.

34. Zhernosekov, K.P.; Filosofov, D.V.; Baum, R.P.; Aschoff, P.; Bihl, H.; Razbash, A.A.; Jahn, M.; Jennewein, M.; Rosch, F. Processing of generator-produced ^{68}Ga for medical application. *J. Nucl. Med.* **2007**, *48*, 1741–1748.

35. Meyer, G.J.; Macke, H.; Schuhmacher, J.; Knapp, W.H.; Hofmann, M. ^{68}Ga-labelled dota-derivatised peptide ligands. *Eur. J. Nucl. Med. Mol. Imaging* **2004**, *31*, 1097–1104.

36. Eppard, E.; Wuttke, M.; Nicodemus, P.L.; Rosch, F. Ethanol-based post-processing of generator-derived ^{68}Ga toward kit-type preparation of ^{68}Ga-radiopharmaceuticals. *J. Nucl. Med.* **2014**, *55*, 1023–1028.

37. Petrik, M.; Ocak, M.; Rupprich, M.; Decristoforo, C. Impurity in ^{68}Ga-peptide preparation using processed generator eluate. *J. Nucl. Med.* **2010**, *51*, 495.

38. Bauwens, M.; Chekol, R.; Vanbilloen, H.; Bormans, G.; Verbruggen, A. Optimal buffer choice of the radiosynthesis of Ga-68-dotatoc for clinical application. *Nucl. Med. Commun.* **2010**, *31*, 753–758.

39. Velikyan, I.; Beyer, G.J.; Bergstrom-Pettermann, E.; Johansen, P.; Bergstrom, M.; Langstrom, B. The importance of high specific radioactivity in the performance of ^{68}Ga-labeled peptide. *Nucl. Med. Biol.* **2008**, *35*, 529–536.

40. Velikyan, I.; Maecke, H.; Langstrom, B. Convenient preparation of ^{68}Ga-based pet-radiopharmaceuticals at room temperature. *Bioconjugate Chem.* **2008**, *19*, 569–573.

41. Notni, J.; Simecek, J.; Hermann, P.; Wester, H.J. Trap, a powerful and versatile framework for Gallium-68 radiopharmaceuticals. *Chem. Eur. J.* **2011**, *17*, 14718–14722.

42. Oehlke, E.; Le, V.S.; Lengkeek, N.; Pellegrini, P.; Jackson, T.; Greguric, I.; Weiner, R. Influence of metal ions on the ^{68}Ga-labeling of dotatate. *Appl. Radiat. Isot.* **2013**, *82*, 232–238.

43. Simecek, J.; Hermann, P.; Wester, H.J.; Notni, J. How is ^{68}Ga labeling of macrocyclic chelators influenced by metal ion contaminants in ^{68}Ge/^{68}Ga generator eluates? *ChemMedChem* **2013**, *8*, 95–103.

44. Chakravarty, R.; Chakraborty, S.; Dash, A.; Pillai, M.R.A. Detailed evaluation on the effect of metal ion impurities on complexation of generator eluted ^{68}Ga with different bifunctional chelators. *Nucl. Med. Biol.* **2013**, *40*, 197–205.

45. Zhai, C.; Summer, D.; Rangger, C.; Haas, H.; Haubner, R.; Decristoforo, C. Fusarinine c, a novel siderophore-based bifunctional chelator for radiolabeling with Gallium-68. *J. Label. Compd. Radiopharm.* **2015**, *58*, 209–214.

46. Borges, J.B.; Velikyan, I.; Långström, B.; Sörensen, J.; Ulin, J.; Maripuu, E.; Sandström, M.; Widström, C.; Hedenstierna, G. Ventilation distribution studies comparing technegas and gallgas using $^{68}GaCl_3$ as the label. *J. Nucl. Med.* **2011**, *52*, 206–209.

47. Velikyan, I.; Sundin, A.; Sörensen, J.; Lubberink, M.; Sandström, M.; Garske-Román, U.; Lundqvist, H.; Granberg, D.; Eriksson, B. Quantitative and qualitative intrapatient comparison of ^{68}Ga-dotatoc and ^{68}Ga-dotatate: Net uptake rate for accurate quantification. *J. Nucl. Med.* **2014**, *55*, 204–210.

48. Sandström, M.; Velikyan, I.; Garske-Román, U.; Sörensen, J.; Eriksson, B.; Granberg, D.; Lundqvist, H.; Sundin, A.; Lubberink, M. Comparative biodistribution and radiation dosimetry of ^{68}Ga- dotatoc and ^{68}Ga-dotatate in patients with neuroendocrine tumors. *J. Nucl. Med.* **2013**, *54*, 1755–1759.

49. Reubi, J.C.; Schär, J.C.; Waser, B.; Wenger, S.; Heppeler, A.; Schmitt, J.S.; Mäcke, H.R. Affinity profiles for human somatostatin receptor subtypes sst1-sst5 of somatostatin radiotracers selected for scintigraphic and radiotherapeutic use. *Eur. J. Nucl. Med. Mol. Imaging* **2000**, *27*, 273–282.
50. Eriksson, O.; Velikyan, I.; Selvaraju, R.K.; Kandeel, F.; Johansson, L.; Antoni, G.; Eriksson, B.; Sörensen, J.; Korsgren, O. Detection of metastatic insulinoma by positron emission tomography with [^{68}Ga]exendin-4-a case report. *J. Clin. Endocrinol. Metab.* **2014**, *99*, 1519–1524.
51. Aime, S.; Barge, A.; Botta, M.; Fasano, M.; Danilo Ayala, J.; Bombieri, G. Crystal structure and solution dynamics of the lutetium(iii) chelate of dota. *Inorg. Chim. Acta* **1996**, *246*, 423–429.
52. Heppeler, A.; Froidevaux, S.; Macke, H.R.; Jermann, E.; Behe, M.; Powell, P.; Hennig, M. Radiometal-labelled macrocyclic chelator-derivatised somatostatin analogue with superb tumour-targeting properties and potential for receptor-mediated internal radiotherapy. *Chem. Eur. J.* **1999**, *5*, 1974–1981.
53. Velikyan, I.; Bulenga, T.N.; Selvaraju, K.R.; Lubberink, M.; Espes, D.; Rosenstrom, U.; Eriksson, O. Dosimetry of [177Lu]-DO3A-VS-Cys40-Exendin-4—impact on the feasibility of insulinoma internal radiotherapy. *Am. J. Nucl. Med. Mol. Imaging* **2015**, *5*, 109–126.
54. Selvaraju, R.; Bulenga, T.N.; Espes, D.; Lubberink, M.; Sörensen, J.; Eriksson, B.; Estrada, S.; Velikyan, I.; Eriksson, O. Dosimetry of [^{68}Ga]Ga-DO3A-VS-Cys40-Exendin-4 in rodents, pigs, non-human primates and human-repeated scanning in human is possible. *Am. J. Nucl. Med. Mol. Imaging* **2015**, *5*, 259–269.
55. Decristoforo, C.; Penuelas, I.; Elsinga, P.; Ballinger, J.; Winhorst, A.D.; Verbruggen, A.; Verzijlbergen, F.; Chiti, A. Radiopharmaceuticals are special, but is this recognized? The possible impact of the new clinical trials regulation on the preparation of radiopharmaceuticals. *Eur. J. Nucl. Med. Mol. Imaging* **2014**, *41*, 2005–2007.
56. Decristoforo, C.; Peñuelas, I. Towards a harmonized radiopharmaceutical regulatory framework in europe? *Q. J. Nucl. Med. Mol. Imaging* **2009**, *53*, 394–401.
57. Verbruggen, A.; Coenen, H.H.; Deverre, J.R.; Guilloteau, D.; Langstrom, B.; Salvadori, P.A.; Halldin, C. Guideline to regulations for radiopharmaceuticals in early phase clinical trials in the EU. *Eur. J. Nucl. Med. Mol. Imaging* **2008**, *35*, 2144–2151.
58. Norenberg, J.P.; Petry, N.A.; Schwarz, S. Operation of a radiopharmacy for a clinical trial. *Semin. Nucl. Med.* **2010**, *40*, 347–356.
59. Lange, R.; Ter Heine, R.; Decristoforo, C.; Peñuelas, I.; Elsinga, P.H.; van Der Westerlaken, M.M.L.; Hendrikse, N.H. Untangling the web of european regulations for the preparation of unlicensed radiopharmaceuticals: A concise overview and practical guidance for a risk-based approach. *Nucl. Med. Commun.* **2015**, *36*, 414–422.
60. Aerts, J.; Ballinger, J.R.; Behe, M.; Decristoforo, C.; Elsinga, P.H.; Faivre-Chauvet, A.; Mindt, T.L.; Peitl, P.K.; Todde, S.C.; Koziorowski, J. Guidance on current good radiopharmacy practice for the small-scale preparation of radiopharmaceuticals using automated modules: A european perspective. *J. Label. Compd. Radiopharm.* **2014**, *57*, 615–620.
61. Elsinga, P.; Todde, S.; Penuelas, I.; Meyer, G.; Farstad, B.; Faivre-Chauvet, A.; Mikolajczak, R.; Westera, G.; Gmeiner-Stopar, T.; Decristoforo, C. Guidance on current good radiopharmacy practice (cgrpp) for the small-scale preparation of radiopharmaceuticals. *Eur. J. Nucl. Med. Mol. Imaging* **2010**, *37*, 1049–1062.

62. Virgolini, I.; Ambrosini, V.; Bomanji, J.B.; Baum, R.P.; Fanti, S.; Gabriel, M.; Papathanasiou, N.D.; Pepe, G.; Oyen, W.; de Cristoforo, C.; *et al.* Procedure guidelines for pet/ct tumour imaging with ^{68}Ga-dota-conjugated peptides: ^{68}Ga-dota-toc, ^{68}Ga-dota-noc, ^{68}Ga-dota-tate. *Eur. J. Nucl. Med. Mol. Imaging* **2010**, *37*, 2004–2010.

63. Janson, E.T.; Sorbye, H.; Welin, S.; Federspiel, B.; Gronbaek, H.; Hellman, P.; Ladekarl, M.; Langer, S.W.; Mortensen, J.; Schalin-Jantti, C.; *et al.* Nordic guidelines 2014 for diagnosis and treatment of gastroenteropancreatic neuroendocrine neoplasms. *Acta Oncol.* **2014**, *53*, 1284–1297.

64. Marchetti, S.; Schellens, J.H.M. The impact of fda and emea guidelines on drug development in relation to phase 0 trials. *Br. J. Cancer* **2007**, *97*, 577–581.

65. Mills, G. The exploratory ind. *J. Nucl. Med.* **2008**, *49*, 45N–47N.

66. Todde, S.; Windhorst, A.D.; Behe, M.; Bormans, G.; Decristoforo, C.; Faivre-Chauvet, A.; Ferrari, V.; Gee, A.D.; Gulyas, B.; Halldin, C.; *et al.* Eanm guideline for the preparation of an investigational medicinal product dossier (impd). *Eur. J. Nucl. Med. Mol. Imaging* **2014**, *41*, 2175–2185.

67. Lappin, G.; Kuhnz, W.; Jochemsen, R.; Kneer, J.; Chaudhary, A.; Oosterhuis, B.; Drijfhout, W.J.; Rowland, M.; Garner, R.C. Use of microdosing to predict pharmacokinetics at the therapeutic dose: Experience with 5 drugs. *Clin. Pharmacol. Ther.* **2006**, *80*, 203–215.

68. Garner, R.C.; Lappin, G. The phase 0 microdosing concept. *Br. J. Clin. Pharmacol.* **2006**, *61*, 367–370.

69. Bergstrom, M.; Grahnen, A.; Langstrom, B. Positron emission tomography microdosing: A new concept with application in tracer and early clinical drug development. *Eur. J. Clin. Pharmacol.* **2003**, *59*, 357–366.

70. *Guidance for Industry, Investigators, and Reviewers*; Exploratory ind Studies. U.S. Department of Health and Human Services: Washington, DC, USA, 2006.

71. Decristoforo, C.; Pickett, R.D.; Verbruggen, A. Feasibility and availability of ^{68}Ga-labelled peptides. *Eur. J. Nucl. Med. Mol. Imaging* **2012**, *39*, S31–S40.

72. Velikyan, I.; Antoni, G.; Sorensen, J.; Estrada, S. Organ biodistribution of germanium-68 in rat in the presence and absence of [^{68}Ga]ga-dota-toc for the extrapolation to the human organ and whole-body radiation dosimetry. *Am. J. Nucl. Med. Mol. Imaging* **2013**, *3*, 154–165.

73. International Atomic Energy Agency. Development of Ga-68 Based Pet-Radiopharmaceuticals for Management of Cancer and Other Chronic Diseases. Available online: http://cra.iaea.org/cra/explore-crps/all-active-by-programme.html (accessed on 25 June 2015).

74. Directive 2001/83/ec of the European Parliament and of the Council of 6 November 2001 on the Community Code Relating to Medicinal Products for Human Use. Available online: http://ec.europa.eu/health/files/eudralex/vol-1/dir_2001_83_consol_2012/dir_2001_83_cons_2012_en.pdf (Updated 2012) (accessed on 25 June 2015).

75. Decristoforo, C. Gallium-68—A new opportunity for pet available from a long shelflife generator—automation and applications. *Curr. Radiopharm.* **2012**, *5*, 212–220.

76. Boschi, S.; Lodi, F.; Malizia, C.; Cicoria, G.; Marengo, M. Automation synthesis modules review. *Appl. Radiat. Isot.* **2013**, *76*, 38–45.

2

Synthesis, Radiolabelling and *In Vitro* Characterization of the Gallium-68-, Yttrium-90- and Lutetium-177-Labelled PSMA Ligand, CHX-A''-DTPA-DUPA-Pep

Benjamin Baur [1,†,*], Christoph Solbach [1,†], Elena Andreolli [1,2], Gordon Winter [1], Hans-Jürgen Machulla [1] and Sven N. Reske [1]

[1] Clinic for Nuclear Medicine, University of Ulm, Albert-Einstein-Allee, 89081 Ulm, Germany; E-Mails: christoph.solbach@uniklinik-ulm.de (C.S.); elena.andreolli@gmail.com (E.A.); gordon.winter@uniklinik-ulm.de (G.W.); hans.machulla@uniklinik-ulm.de (H.-J.M.); sven.reske@uniklinik-ulm.de (S.N.R.)

[2] Department of Health Sciences, University of Milano-Bicocca, Milan 20900, Italy

[†] These authors contributed equally to this work.

* Author to whom correspondence should be addressed; E-Mail: benjamin.baur@uniklinik-ulm.de

---

Abstract: Since prostate-specific membrane antigen (PSMA) has been identified as a diagnostic target for prostate cancer, many urea-based small PSMA-targeting molecules were developed. First, the clinical application of these Ga-68 labelled compounds in positron emission tomography (PET) showed their diagnostic potential. Besides, the therapy of prostate cancer is a demanding field, and the use of radiometals with PSMA bearing ligands is a valid approach. In this work, we describe the synthesis of a new PSMA ligand, CHX-A''-DTPA-DUPA-Pep, the subsequent labelling with Ga-68, Lu-177 and Y-90 and the first *in vitro* characterization. In cell investigations with PSMA-positive LNCaP C4-2 cells, K_D values of $\leq 14.67 \pm 1.95$ nM were determined, indicating high biological activities towards PSMA. Radiosyntheses with Ga-68, Lu-177 and Y-90 were developed under mild reaction conditions (room temperature, moderate pH of 5.5 and 7.4, respectively) and resulted in nearly quantitative radiochemical yields within 5 min.

Keywords: PSMA; prostate-specific membrane antigen; PET; positron emission tomography; prostate cancer; DUPA; Ga-68; Y-90; Lu-177; radionuclide therapy

---

1. Introduction

Prostate cancer (PCa) is still one of the leading causes of cancer deaths among men. Despite using novel therapeutic approaches, mortality from metastasizing prostate cancer is still high [1]. Therefore, the early diagnosis of prostate cancer to prevent tumor dissemination is highly desirable. Furthermore, effective treatment strategies for disseminated prostate cancer are urgently needed. Comprehensibly, targeting of PCa or its metastases is a demanding task in the field of molecular imaging with positron emission tomography (PET) and for targeted internal radiation therapy.

Prostate-specific membrane antigen (PSMA) is a peptidase that catalyzes the hydrolysis of *N*-acetyl-L-aspartyl-L-glutamate (NAAG) into the corresponding *N*-acetyl-L-aspartate (NAA) and L-glutamate [2]. The use of PSMA as a target for diagnostic and therapeutic agents is a highly valid approach. Compared to healthy human prostate tissue, in almost all PCa tumors, the expression of PSMA is 10–80 fold higher.

Besides, the PSMA levels are increased in the neovasculature of other solid tumors, as well [3–6]. Therefore, selective addressing of PSMA with small molecules labelled with a positron emitting radionuclide is a considerable approach for the diagnosis of prostate cancer with PET.

Based on the chemical structure of NAAG, several glutamate-urea-glutamate-based peptides bearing a 2-[3-(1,3-dicarboxypropyl)-ureido]pentanedioic acid (DUPA) moiety were developed in the last few years [7]. These molecules showed high affinity and specific binding to PSMA, as demonstrated in binding studies using PSMA expressing LNCaP cell lines. Beside the slightly modified chemical structure, these molecules differ mainly in the selection of the chelator for the complexation of the desired radionuclide [7–9].

Due to their proven excellent affinity to PSMA, it is desirable to develop radionuclide-based therapeutic strategies using adapted PSMA targeting. In radiometal therapy approaches, the application of Y-90 and Lu-177 is favored. The use of Y-90 ($E_{\beta max}$: 2.3 MeV, $t_{½}$: 64 h) is more appropriate in the treatment of larger tumor lesions, while Lu-177 ($E_{\beta max}$: 0.5 MeV, $t_{½}$: 6.7 d) is more suitable for the treatment of smaller lesions and metastases, accompanied by a minimization of kidney dose in comparison to the application of Y-90 labelled peptides [10]. Moreover, due to the contemporary beta- and gamma-emission, Lu-177 is a useful diagnostic tool for scintigraphy of tumoral uptake [11].

For both diagnostic and therapeutic application, 1,4,7,10-tetraazacyclododecane-*N*,*N*',*N*'',*N*'''-tetraacetic acid (DOTA) is the mostly used chelator for the complexation of radiometals, like Ga-68, Lu-177 and Y-90, to small molecules [12,13]. However, DOTA can show some undesirable characteristics for therapy. Possible immunogenicity in humans has been published, as well as unfavorable kinetics in the complexation of radiometals [14,15]. Furthermore, labelling reactions using DOTA as the chelating agent are usually carried out at high temperatures under acidic conditions and long reaction times [16]. The preferred labelling procedure for peptides should consist of a simple, fast and quantitative labelling step at room temperature and neutral pH to avoid decomposition. Therefore, the use of alternative chelators is a demanding approach. In addition, the chelator must provide sufficient stability *in vivo*.

The preceding developments based on the chelator, diethylenetriaminepentaacetic acid (DTPA), lead to the promising cyclohexyl substituted analogue, cyclohexyl-diethylene triamine pentaacetic acid (CHX-A''-DTPA) [17]. It showed high stability *in vivo*, and radiolabelling with Y-90 was achieved under mild conditions (pH = 6 at room temperature) [17]. Thus, CHX-A''-DTPA is a highly promising alternative to the mostly used DOTA. Previous work using the PSMA ligand (5S,8S,22S,26S)-1-amino-5,8-dibenzyl-4,7,10,19,24-pentaoxo-3,6,9,18,23,25-hexaazaoctacosane-22,26,28-tricarboxylic acid (DUPA-Pep), conjugated with DOTA, revealed a high PSMA-affinity with a K_D of 21.6 ± 0.4 nM measured in a PSMA-positive LNCaP C4-2 cell assay [18]. Furthermore, the first clinical application of [^{68}Ga]Ga-DOTA-DUPA-Pep showed the feasibility of *in vivo* targeting. [^{68}Ga]Ga-HBED-PSMA showed promising clinical results for prostate cancer patients so far [19,20].

Thus, in the present study, we describe the synthesis of CHX-A"-DTPA-DUPA-Pep (scheme 1), subsequent labelling with Ga-68, Y-90 and Lu-177, and the investigation of its biological activity as a new potential PSMA ligand for the diagnosis and therapy of prostate cancer.

Scheme 1. Synthesis of cyclohexyldiethylenetriamine pentaacetic acid (5*S*,8*S*,22*S*,26*S*)-1-amino-5,8-dibenzyl-4,7,10,19,24-pentaoxo-3,6,9,18,23,25-hexaazaoctacosane-22,26,28-tri-carboxylic acid trifluoroacetate (CHX-A"-DTPA-DUPA-Pep).

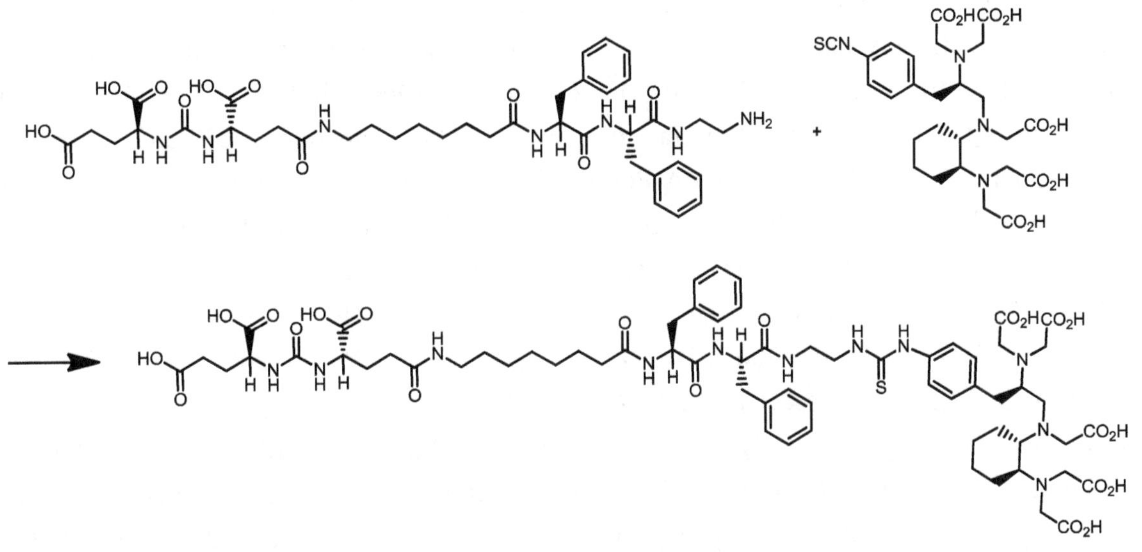

2. Experimental

[^{90}Y]YCl_3 and [^{177}Lu]$LuCl_4$, in 0.04 M HCl were purchased from Eckert and Ziegler and Isotope Technologies, respectively. The ^{68}Ge/^{68}Ga generator was obtained from IDB Holland BV. All chemicals and solvents were purchased from Aldrich, Fluka, Applichem, Waters and Merck and used without further purification. (5*S*,8*S*,22*S*,26*S*)-1-Amino-5,8-dibenzyl-4,7,10,19,24-pentaoxo-3,6,9,18,23,25-hexaazaoctacosane-22,26,28-tricarboxylic acid trifluoroacetate ("DUPA-Pep" trifluoroacetate) was obtained from ABX (Germany). *N*-[(*R*)-2-Amino-3-(*p*-isothiocyanato-phenyl) propyl]-trans-(*S*,*S*)-cyclohexane-1,2-diamine-*N*,*N*,*N'*-,*N''*,*N''*-pentaacetic acid (*p*-SCN-Bn-CHX-A"-DTPA) was achieved from Macrocyclics (Dallas, TX, USA). Diethylenetriaminepentaacetic acid (≥99%) was obtained from Fluka (Buchs, Switzerland). Solvents for analytics were of HPLC-grade purity. Chemicals for organic synthesis were of >98% purity. Chemicals for radiolabelling were of trace metal® grade. An analytical assay was carried out by thin-layer chromatography (TLC) with Silica gel 60 RP-18 F_{254}S (on alumina sheets of 5 × 7.5 cm, Merck) as the stationary phase, visualized by UV-detection for preparative synthesis and by phosphorimager analysis (FLA3000. Raytest, Straubenhardt, Germany) for radiosynthesis. In addition, a radio high-pressure liquid chromatography system (radio-HPLC, P680 Dionex, Idstein, Germany), equipped with NaI(TI)-scintillation detector (GABI, Raytest) and a UV-Vis detector (UVD 170U, Dionex), was used for the identification of the labelled peptide. For the control of radiochemical yields (RCYs), a γ-counter (Cobra™ II, Packard Instrument, Canberra, Australia) was applied. ^{1}H- and ^{13}C- nuclear magnetic resonance spectra were recorded by a 400 MHz Bruker Avance spectrometer (Bruker, Karlsruhe, Germany) at ambient temperature. MS spectra were measured using a Triple Stage Quadrupole TSQ 70 Finnigan-MAT-mass spectrometer (Finnigan-MAT, Bremen, Germany).

2.1. Organic Synthesis of CHX-A"-DTPA-DUPA-Pep

DUPA-Pep trifluoroacetate (10 mg, 12.5 μmol) was dissolved in DMSO (1 mL), and DIPEA (15 μL, 90 μmol) and *p*-SCN-Bn-CHX-A"-DTPA·3HCl (Macrocyclics, Dallas, TX., USA) (7 mg, 11 nmol) were added. The reaction was carried out for 16 h. The product was purified by preparative HPLC consisting of a C18 column (Gemini 5μ C18, 250 × 21 mm, Phenomenex, Aschaffenburg, Germany) as the stationary phase and by use of gradient elution technique (gradient profile: 0–3 min 20% MeCN in H_2O (0.1% TFA), 3–15 min from 20% to 40% MeCN in H_2O (0.1% TFA), 15–30 min 40% MeCN in H_2O (0.1% TFA); a flow rate of 7 mL/min, UV detection at 220 and 254 nm) as the mobile phase gave CHX-A"-DTPA-DUPA-Pep (12.5 mg, 8.6 μmol, 72%) as a colorless solid after lyophilization with a purity of >98% (HPLC). ^{1}H NMR (400 MHz, DMSO-d_6) δ = 1.2 (m, 14H); 1.7 (m, 4H); 2,0 (m, 8 H); 2.2 (m, 2H); 2.7 (m, 1H); 2.8 (m, 1H); 3.0 (m, 6H); 3.2 (m, 4H); 3.4 (m, 4H); 3.6 (m, 7H); 4.1 (m, 5H); 4.5 (m, 3H); 6.4 (m, 2H); 7.3 (m, 14H); 7.8 (m, 2H); 8.0 (m, 3H); 9.6 (s, 1H); 12.6 (s, 5H). ^{13}C NMR (300 MHz, DMSO-d_6) δ = 25.1 ($2CH_2$); 26.3 (CH_2); 27.5 (2*CH_2); 28.3 (2*CH_2); 28.3 (2*CH_2); 28.4 (CH_2); 28.5 (CH_2); 29.1 (CH_2); 29.8 (CH_2); 31.6 (CH_2); 35.1 (CH_2); 37,0 (CH_2); 37.2 (2*CH_2); 37.7 (CH_2); 37.9 (2*CH_2); 38.5 (3*CH_2); 48.3 (2*CH_2); 51.6 (2*CH); 52.1 (CH); 53.6 (2*CH); 53.9 (2*CH); 126.1 (CH (phenylalanine)); 126.3 (CH (phenylalanine)); 127.9 (2*C2 phenyl(desferal)); 128.0 (2*C3 phenyl(desferal)); 129.1 (4*CH (phenylalanine)); 129.2 (4*CH (phenylalanine)); 137.5 (C1, C6 phenyl(desferal)); 137.9 (2*C (phenylalanine)); 155.3 (2*C = O); 157.2 (HN-(C = O)-NH); 158.2 (2*C = O); 171.0 (2*COOH); 171.1 (COOH); 172.1 (2*COOH); 173.7 (COOH); 174.1 (2*COOH); 174.2 (C = S). ESI-HRMS (*m/z*): MALDI calcd. for $C_{65}H_{89}N_{11}O_{21}S$, 1391,60; found, $[M + H]^+$1392.60177.

2.2. Radionuclide Production and Radiochemistry

2.2.1. Production of [^{68}Ga]Ga-Chloride

Ga-68 ($t_{½}$ = 67.7 min, $β^+$: 89%, $E_{β^+ max}$, 1.9 MeV; EC: 11%, $E_{γ\ max}$: 4.0 MeV) was prepared as described by Meyer *et al.* [21]. Briefly, Ga-68 was eluted from a TiO_2-based ^{68}Ge/^{68}Ga generator with *ca.* 2 mL of 1 M HCl and collected into a vial containing 1 mL of 9.5 M HCl. The resulting solution was loaded onto a strong anion exchange resin (100 mg Dowex 1 × 8), and the activity was retained as the $[GaCl_4]^-$ complex. After elution with 200 μL of water, the pH of the solution was neutralized by adding the appropriate volume of 2 M Na_2CO_3.

2.2.2. Radiosynthesis of [^{68}Ga]Ga-CHX-A''-DTPA-DUPA-Pep

The Ga-68 activity in neutral aqueous solution (13 µL; 9.3–9.6 MBq) was added to a freshly prepared solution of CHX-A''-DTPA-DUPA-Pep, dissolved in DMSO (2 mg/mL) and 0.25 M HEPES buffer (pH 7.4, 500 µL), resulting in a total volume of 514–563 µL and a final pH of 7.4. Different amounts of peptide (1, 10, 25, 50 and 100 µg; 0.7, 7.2, 18, 36 and 72 nM) were used to study the dependence of RCY on peptide concentration and reaction time. The reaction was carried out at room temperature for 60 min. At different reaction times (1, 5, 10, 30 and 60 min), 1-µL aliquots were withdrawn and analyzed by radio-TLC on RP-18 thin layer plates as the stationary phase and 0.1% TFA/MeOH 30/70 *v*/*v* as the mobile phase.

2.2.3. Radiosynthesis of [^{90}Y]Y-CHX-A''-DTPA-DUPA-Pep

Y-90 activity in 0.04 M HCl solution (20 µL; 3.7–3.8 MBq) was added to a freshly prepared solution of CHX-A''-DTPA-DUPA-Pep, dissolved in DMSO (2 mg/mL) and 0.5 M NH_4OAc buffer (pH 5.5, 500 µL), resulting in a total volume of 533–570 µL and a final pH of 5.5. Different amounts of peptide (25, 50 and 100 µg; 18, 36 and 72 nM) were used to study the dependence of RCY on peptide concentration and reaction time. The reaction was carried out at room temperature for 60 min. At different reaction times (5, 10, 30 and 60 min), 1-µL aliquots were withdrawn and analyzed by radio-TLC on RP-18 thin layer plates as the stationary phase and 0.1% TFA/MeOH 30/70 *v*/*v* as the mobile phase.

2.2.4. Radiosynthesis of [^{177}Lu]Lu-CHX-A''-DTPA-DUPA-Pep

Lu-177 activity in 0.04 M HCl solution (5 µL; 6.3–6.7 MBq) was added to a freshly prepared solution of CHX-A''-DTPA-DUPA-Pep, dissolved in DMSO (2 mg/mL) and 0.5 M NH_4OAc buffer (pH 5.5, 500 µL), resulting in to total volume of 510–555 µL and a final pH of 5.5. Different amounts of peptide (10, 25, 50 and 100 µg; 7.2, 18, 36 and 72 nM) were used to study the dependence of RCY on peptide concentration and reaction time. The reaction was carried out at room temperature for 60 min. At different reaction times (5, 10, 30 and 60 min), 1-µL aliquots were withdrawn and analyzed by radio-TLC on RP-18 thin layer plates as the stationary phase and 0.1% TFA/MeOH 30/70 *v*/*v* as the mobile phase.

2.2.5. Radio-TLC Analysis

RCYs of the labelling reactions described above were determined in dependency on reaction time and peptide concentration. One microliter was withdrawn from every reaction mixture at different definite time points for radio-TLC analysis. RP-18 Silica gel plates were used as the stationary phase and 0.1% TFA/MeOH 30/70 *v*/*v* as the mobile phase, in which the free radiometal remains at the baseline (R_f: 0.01). The R_f value of CHX-A''-DTPA-DUPA-Pep was found to be 0.73 (λ: 254 nm), while the R_f value of radio labelled compound was found to be *ca.* 0.78 (phosphorimager). Quantitative assays of radioactive spots were carried out by phosphorimager to determine the amount of radio labelled chelate and free radiometal.

2.2.6. Radio-HPLC Analysis

Radiochemical purity was determined by gradient radio-HPLC analysis. A C18 column (Phenomenex Gemini, 5 µm, C18, 250 × 4.6 mm) was used as stationary phase. Gradient elution technique was performed by the use of Solvent A (H_2O, 0.1% TFA) and Solvent B (MeCN, 0.1% TFA) as the mobile phase (gradient profile: 85% A at 5 min; 85%–30% A from 5 to 14 min, 30%–85% A from 14 to 16 min; flow rate: 2 mL/min). The retention time of [^{68}Ga]Ga-CHX-A''-DTPA-DUPA-Pep was 9.4 min (Figure 1).

Figure 1. Exemplary chromatograms of [^{68}Ga]Ga-CHX-A''-DTPA-DUPA-Pep in the radioactivity channel (upper signal; the first peak shows the total activity injected detector bypass for recovery rate calculation) and CHX-A''-DTPA-DUPA-Pep in the UV-channel (bottom signal; λ: 254 nm).

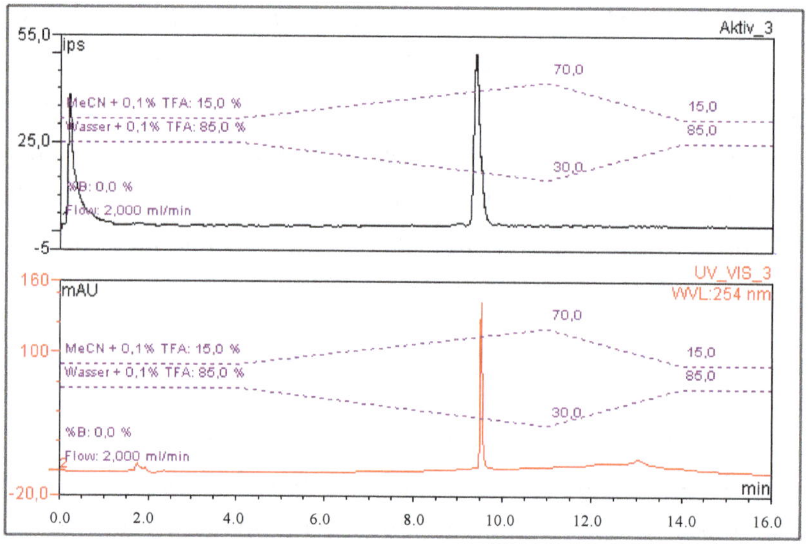

2.3. *Stability of Labelled CHX-A''-DTPA-DUPA-Pep*

The stability of the labelled peptide in human serum and phosphate buffered saline (PBS) was verified via radio-HPLC after 30 min, 2, 4 and 8 h for [^{68}Ga]Ga-CHX-A''-DTPA-DUPA-Pep and by radio-TLC on RP-18 thin layer plates as the stationary phase and 0.1% TFA/MeOH 30/70 *v*/*v* as the mobile phase after 1 h, 3 h, 6 h, 24 h, 48 h and 72 h for [^{177}Lu]Lu-CHX-A''-DTPA-DUPA-Pep and [^{90}Y]Y-CHX-A''-DTPA-DUPA-Pep. The radiochemical stability of the labelled compounds was determined in serum and PBS buffer at 37 °C. The total volume was 1.2 mL (980 µL of serum or buffer and 220 µL of product solution). In stability tests, 12 MBq of Ga-68 and 4.5 MBq of each radionuclide, Lu-177 and Y-90, were applied. Two hundred microliters of the mixture were withdrawn at each time point, and the samples were analyzed by radio-HPLC. Radio-TLC analyses were performed without further reprocessing.

The PBS samples were injected into a radio-HPLC system without further work-up. Serum samples of the Y-90 and Lu-177 labelled compound were tested without further work-up by radio-TLC. Serum samples for radio-HPLC-investigations underwent a serum protein precipitation work-up procedure before injection. Briefly: an equal volume of EtOH (200 µL) was added to the samples. Subsequently, the samples were centrifuged for 10 min at 10,000 rpm. Ultrafiltration of the supernatant was performed using an Amicon ultra centrifugal filter (3 KDa NMWL, Millipore, Darmstadt, Germany) for 10 min at 10,000 rpm. The filtrate was analyzed by radio-HPLC.

Exchange experiments with 500-fold excess of DTPA and additionally with hydrolysed *p*-SCN-Bn-CHX-A"-DTPA were performed for each of the three radiolabeled CHX-A"-DTPA-DUPA-Pep compounds. Briefly, after radiolabelling with Ga-68, Y-90 and Lu-177, a 500-fold excess of DTPA or hydrolysed *p*-SCN-Bn-CHX-A"-DTPA (in 500 µL of 0.5 M NH_4OAc buffer (pH 5.5)) was added to the sealed reaction mixture stored at RT. Aliquots were withdrawn at two time points (30 min and 240 min) and analyzed by radio-TLC procedure (RP-18 Silica gel plates as the stationary phase and 0.1% TFA/MeOH 30/70 *v*/*v* as the mobile phase).

2.4. Cell Culture and Analysis of Binding Specificity of CHX-A"-DTPA-DUPA-Pep

The PSMA-positive cell line, LNCaP C4-2, was obtained from ViroMed Laboratories (Minnetonka, MN, USA) and grown in T-media (Dulbecco's Modified Eagle's Medium (DMEM), high glucose, Gibco) and 20% Ham's F-12 (Biochrom, Berlin, Germany) supplemented with 5% fetal bovine serum, 5 µg/mL insulin (Sigma, St. Louis, MO., USA), 13.65 pg/mL triiodothyronine (Sigma), 5 µg/mL apo-transferrin (Sigma), 0.244 µg/mL D-biotin (Sigma) and 25 µg/mL adenine (Sigma). As a negative control, PC-3 cells (DSMZ, ACC 465) were maintained in DMEM and 10% Ham's F12 with 10% FBS, 1% penicillin/streptomycin and 2 mM glutamine. All cell lines were incubated at 37 °C under constant humidity and an atmosphere of 5% CO_2.

To determine the binding coefficient (K_D) of the radio-labelled peptide, 5×10^5 cells/well were grown in coated 12-well plates in 1 mL of medium for 48 h. The cells were washed twice with PBS, and 900 µL fresh media were added. Radiolabelled peptide was added, resulting in final concentrations of 480, 240, 120, 60, 30, 15 and 7.5 nM. In parallel, the PSMA-inhibitor (2-PMPA) was applied in a final concentration of 30 µM to determine unspecific binding. All samples were prepared in triplicate. Following 60 min of incubation at 37 °C, cells were washed twice to remove unbound activity and afterwards lysed in 1 mL of 0.5 M NaOH. Activity was measured in a gamma counter (COBRA™ II, Packard Instrument). Aliquots of the solution added to the cells were also measured for the calculation of the cellular uptake as %ID. Data were analyzed using GraphPad Prism 5.02 (one site, total and non-specific binding evaluation).

2.5. Statistical Aspects

All experiments were conducted with $n \geq 3$. Data are expressed as the mean ± SD.

3. Results and Discussion

3.1. Organic Synthesis of CHX-A"-DTPA-DUPA-Pep

CHX-A"-DTPA-DUPA-Pep synthesis was successfully achieved by coupling DUPA-Pep and p-SCN-Bn-CHX-A"-DTPA in the presence of DIPEA as the base. After preparative HPLC purification and lyophilization of the purified fraction, the peptide was obtained as a white powder in yields of 72% and a purity of ≥98% (HPLC).

3.2. Radiochemistry

Radiolabelling with Ga-68 was performed in HEPES buffer (pH = 7.4) at room temperature by adding the prepared solution of $[^{68}Ga]GaCl_3$ to the peptide reaction mixture. The radiochemical yields were evaluated in dependence on the reaction time and the amount of peptide via radio-TLC (Table 1, Figure 2). Starting from 18 nM (25 µg) of CHX-A"-DTPA-DUPA-Pep, the RCY lay over 95% after 30 min of reaction time. Increasing the amount of peptide, to 72 nM (100 µg), a RCY >95% was obtained after 1 min of reaction time. Due to nearly quantitative labelling, the product solution was applied without further purification.

Table 1. Dependence of the radiochemical yield (RCY) of $[^{68}Ga]$Ga-CHX-A"-DTPA-DUPA-Pep on the peptide amount (concentration) and the reaction time at room temperature.

Amount (µg)	RCY % (1 min)	RCY % (5 min)	RCY % (10 min)	RCY % (30 min)	RCY % (60 min)
1	0.2 ± 0 .1	0.2 ± 0.0	0.3 ± 0.1	0.5 ± 0.1	0.6 ± 0.1
10	3.7 ± 0.3	14.0 ± 0.3	21.9 ± 0.8	41.3 ± 4.0	56.5 ± 5.8
25	29.0 ± 1.5	70.0 ± 1.3	85.6 ± 0.8	96.6 ± 0.3	97.1 ± 0.6
50	69.4 ± 0.9	95.4 ± 0.4	96.6 ± 0.6	96.6 ± 0.2	97.2 ± 0.7
100	95.1 ± 0.3	95.8 ± 0.1	96.1 ± 0.1	97.3 ± 0.1	97.7 ± 0.6

Figure 2. Dependence of the RCY of $[^{68}Ga]$Ga-CHX-A"-DTPA-DUPA-Pep on the peptide amount (concentration) and reaction time at room temperature.

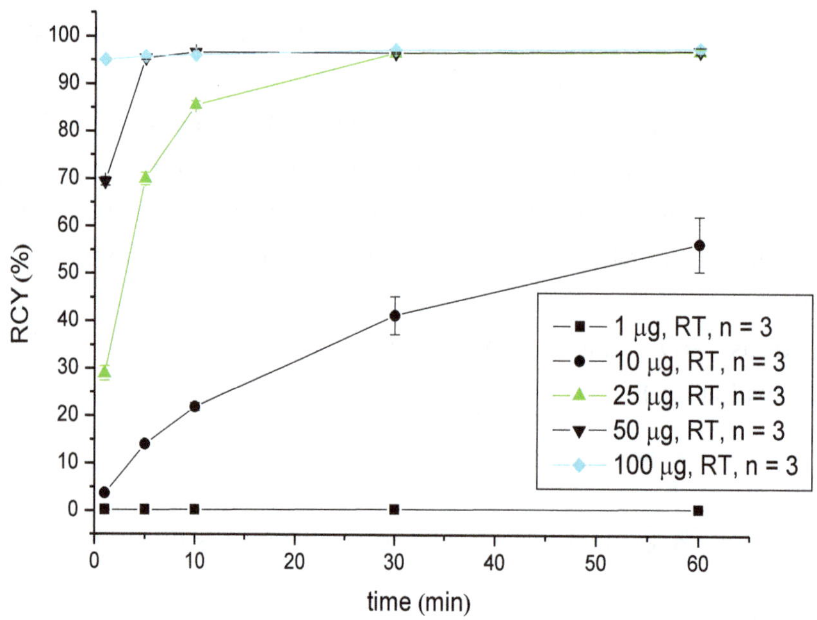

Regarding radiometals for radiotherapy (Lu-177 and Y-90), the radiolabelling was performed at pH 5.5 in 0.5 M NH_4OAc buffer and showed RCYs >95% for low amounts of peptide (25 µg (18 nM) in the case of ^{90}Y-labelling and 10 µg (7.2 nM) in the case of ^{177}Lu-labelling) after 5 min of reaction time. A practically quantitative RCY of >99% was obtained in both radiosyntheses after 30 min of reaction time when the highest amount of peptide (100 µg; 72 nM) was used (Tables 2 and 3, Figures 3 and 4).

Table 2. Dependence of the RCY of [^{90}Y]Y-CHX-A"-DTPA-DUPA-Pep on peptide amount (concentration) and reaction time at room temperature.

Amount (µg)	RCY % (5 min)	RCY % (10 min)	RCY % (30 min)	RCY % (60 min)
25	98.2 ± 0.2	97.3 ± 1.0	98.7 ± 0.2	97.9 ± 0.1
50	98.6 ± 0.1	98.2 ± 0.2	98.5 ± 0.3	99.0 ± 0.1
100	98.4 ± 0.4	98.2 ± 0.2	99.3 ± 0.2	99.0 ± 0.1

Table 3. Dependence of the RCY of [^{177}Lu]Lu-CHX-A"-DTPA-DUPA-Pep on peptide amount (concentration) and reaction time at room temperature.

Amount (µg)	RCY % (5 min)	RCY % (10 min)	RCY % (30 min)	RCY % (60 min)
10	96.2 ± 1.0	95.2 ± 0.8	98.6 ± 0.4	96.7 ± 0.3
25	95.7 ± 0.5	97.2 ± 0.7	93.4 ± 0.4	96.1 ± 1.1
50	95.4 ± 0.1	96.7 ± 0.2	98.5 ± 0.4	98.4 ± 0.7
100	98.4 ± 0.1	98.6 ± 0.3	99.3 ± 0.2	99.6 ± 0.2

Figure 3. Dependence of the RCY of [^{90}Y]Y-CHX-A"-DTPA-DUPA-Pep on peptide amount (concentration) and reaction time at room temperature.

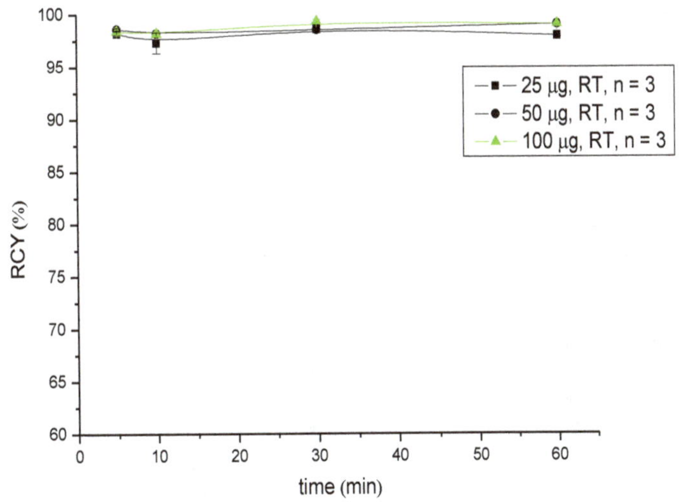

Figure 4. Dependence of the RCY of [^{177}Lu]Lu-CHX-A"-DTPA-DUPA-Pep on peptide amount (concentration) and reaction time at room temperature.

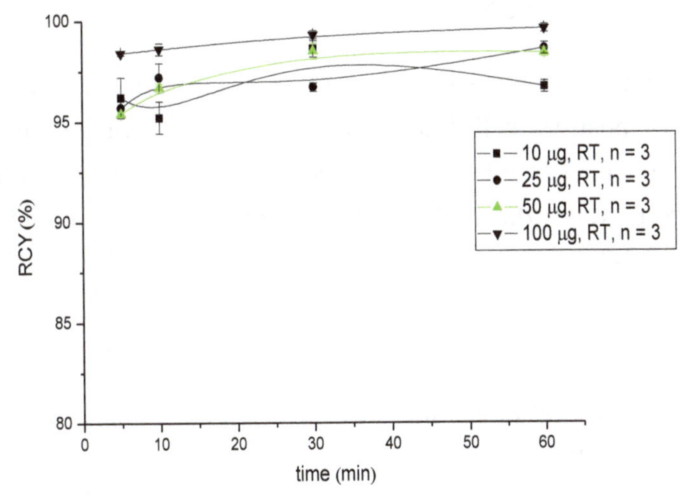

3.3. Stability Investigations

A high incorporation level and high complex stability is strongly desired in therapeutic applications, due to the severe myelotoxicity associated with Y-90 and the long half-life of Lu-177 (6.74 d). Thus, in order to verify the stability of the Y-90 and Lu-177 complexes, stability studies were performed in human serum and PBS at 37 °C. Additionally, the stability of the Ga-68 labelled compound was investigated. Radio-TLC analysis of [^{177}Lu]Lu- and [^{90}Y]Y-CHX-A"-DTPA-DUPA-Pep after 1 h, 3 h, 6 h, 24 h, 48 h and 72 h confirmed the stability of the radiolabelled product. Moreover, the incubation of the [^{68}Ga]Ga-CHX-A"-DTPA-DUPA-Pep for 30 min, 1 h, 2 h, 4 h and 8 h at 37 °C resulted in no detectable changes, as shown by radio-HPLC (Figure 5). Exchange experiments with a 500-fold excess of DTPA and with a 500-fold excess of hydrolysed *p*-SCN-Bn-CHX-A"-DTPA confirmed the stability of the investigated radiolabelled complexes. No radiometal labelled chelator (DTPA or hydrolysed *p*-SCN-Bn-CHX-A"-DTPA) was observed.

Figure 5. Stability study of [^{68}Ga]Ga-CHX-A"-DTPA-DUPA-Pep in human serum: overlaid radio-HPLC chromatograms after 8 h (1), 4 h (2), 2 h (3) and 30 min (4). The first peak shows the total activity injected (the detector bypass for the recovery rate calculation).

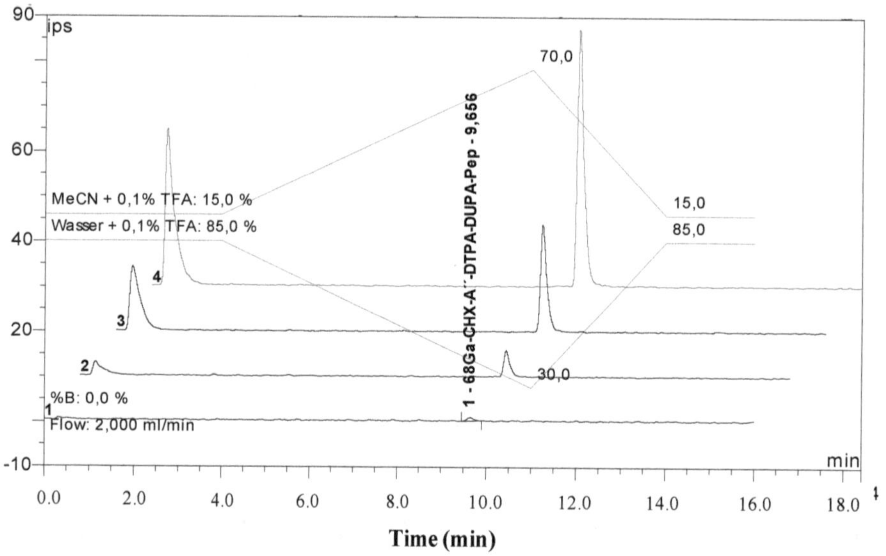

3.4. Determination of In Vitro Binding Specificity

The binding coefficient was investigated for all radiolabelled CHX-A"-DTPA-DUPA-Pep derivatives. In the PSMA-positive cell line, LNCaP C4-2, K_D values of 14.67 ± 1.95 nM for ^{177}Lu-labelled peptide, 8.0 ± 1.1 nM for Y-90 labelled peptide and 12.09 ± 0.66 nM for ^{68}Ga-labelled CHX-A"-DTPA-DUPA-Pep were determined. No specific binding could be observed for the PSMA-negative cell line, PC-3.

4. Conclusions

The synthesis of the DTPA-derivative bearing the PSMA targeting ligand, CHX-A"-DTPA-DUPA-Pep, was straightforward and efficient.

The radiolabelling of the new PSMA ligand with diverse radiometals, for both diagnosis and therapy, was investigated, and optimized conditions were developed.

Labelling with Ga-68 was performed at room temperature under neutral conditions. Significant differences in RCY were observed. Radio labelling with Ga-68 succeeds in a short reaction time with high radiochemical yields; ≥95% when 50 µg (36 nM) of the peptide was used. Additionally, the labelling of CHX-A"-DTPA-DUPA-Pep with Y-90 and Lu-177 was successfully developed. In both cases, the RCY was >95% after 5 min at room temperature using 25 µg (18 nM) peptide Y-90 and 10 µg (7.2 nM) Lu-177, respectively. In conclusion, RCYs over 95% up to quantitative yields were obtained for each radionuclide at room temperature at a moderate pH value.

In cell uptake experiments with the PSMA-positive cell line, LNCaP C4-2, the biological activity of CHX-A"-DTPA-DUPA-Pep was tested exemplarily for the Ga-68- and Lu-177- radiolabelled peptide. The obtained K_D values of 14.67 ± 1.95 nM for the Ga-68 labelled peptide, 8.0 ± 1.1 nM for the Y-90 labelled peptide and 12.09 ± 0.66 nM for the Lu-177 labelled peptide demonstrate high biological activity towards PSMA. The stability of the labelled peptide was confirmed in both human serum and PBS buffer. Additionally performed exchange experiments by use of DTPA and hydrolysed *p*-SCN-Bn-CHX-A"-DTPA confirmed the complex stability. The application of CHX-A"-DTPA as a chelator allows the choice of the suited radionuclide with respect to the selected (clinical) application. In the next step, it has to be elucidated if Ga-68, Y-90 and Lu-177 labelled CHX-A"-DTPA-DUPA-Pep may be useful ligands for the diagnosis and therapy of prostate cancer.

Acknowledgments

We gratefully acknowledge the funding of the University of Milano-Bicocca (Milan, Italy) through a PhD fellowship in Biomedical Technology.

Author Contributions

B.B. and C.S. coordinated the study, supervised the experiments and wrote the manuscript. B.B. and E.A. performed the chemical, the radiochemical syntheses and the stability experiments. G.W. performed the *in vitro* measurements. H.-J.M. and S.R. gave advice in the interpretation of the data and reviewed the manuscript. All authors approved the final manuscript.

References

1. Siegel, R.; Ward, E.; Brawley, O.; Jemal, A. Cancer statistics, 2011: The impact of eliminating socioeconomic and racial disparities on premature cancer deaths. *CA Cancer J. Clin.* **2011**, *61*, 212–236.
2. Robinson, M.B.; Blakely, R.D.; Couto, R.; Coyle, J.T. Hydrolysis of the brain dipeptide n-acetyl-l-aspartyl-l-glutamate. Identification and characterization of a novel n-acetylated alpha-linked acidic dipeptidase activity from rat brain. *J. Biol. Chem.* **1987**, *262*, 14498–14506.

3. Olson, W.C.; Heston, W.D.; Rajasekaran, A.K. Clinical trials of cancer therapies targeting prostate-specific membrane antigen. *Rev. Recent Clin. Trials* **2007**, *2*, 182–190.
4. Hao, G.; Zhou, J.; Guo, Y.; Long, M.A.; Anthony, T.; Stanfield, J.; Hsieh, J.T.; Sun, X. A cell permeable peptide analog as a potential-specific pet imaging probe for prostate cancer detection. *Amino Acids* **2011**, *41*, 1093–1101.
5. Su, S.L.; Huang, I.P.; Fair, W.R.; Powell, C.T.; Heston, W.D. Alternatively spliced variants of prostate-specific membrane antigen rna: Ratio of expression as a potential measurement of progression. *Cancer Res.* **1995**, *55*, 1441–1443.
6. Wernicke, A.G.; Varma, S.; Greenwood, E.A.; Christos, P.J.; Chao, K.S.C.; Liu, H.; Bander, N.H.; Shin, S.J. Prostate-specific membrane antigen expression in tumor-associated vasculature of breast cancers. *APMIS* **2013**, doi:10.1111/apm.12195.
7. Kularatne, S.A.; Venkatesh, C.; Santhapuram, H.K.; Wang, K.; Vaitilingam, B.; Henne, W.A.; Low, P.S. Synthesis and biological analysis of prostate-specific membrane antigen-targeted anticancer prodrugs. *J. Med. Chem.* **2010**, *53*, 7767–7777.
8. Malik, N.; Machulla, H.J.; Solbach, C.; Winter, G.; Reske, S.N.; Zlatopolskiy, B. Radiosynthesis of a new psma targeting ligand ([18f]fpy-dupa-pep). *Appl. Radiat. Isot.* **2011**, *69*, 1014–1018.
9. Eder, M.; Schafer, M.; Bauder-Wust, U.; Hull, W.E.; Wangler, C.; Mier, W.; Haberkorn, U.; Eisenhut, M. 68ga-complex lipophilicity and the targeting property of a urea-based psma inhibitor for pet imaging. *Bioconjug. Chem.* **2012**, *23*, 688–697.
10. Stabin, M.G.; Siegel, J.A. Physical models and dose factors for use in internal dose assessment. *Health Phys.* **2003**, *85*, 294–310.
11. Van Essen, M.; Krenning, E.P.; de Jong, M.; Valkema, R.; Kwekkeboom, D.J. Peptide receptor radionuclide therapy with radiolabelled somatostatin analogues in patients with somatostatin receptor positive tumours. *Acta Oncol.* **2007**, *46*, 723–734.
12. Kwekkeboom, D.J.; Teunissen, J.J.; Bakker, W.H.; Kooij, P.P.; de Herder, W.W.; Feelders, R.A.; van Eijck, C.H.; Esser, J.P.; Kam, B.L.; Krenning, E.P. Radiolabeled somatostatin analog [177lu-dota0,tyr3]octreotate in patients with endocrine gastroenteropancreatic tumors. *J. Clin. Oncol.* **2005**, *23*, 2754–2762.
13. Otte, A.; Herrmann, R.; Heppeler, A.; Behe, M.; Jermann, E.; Powell, P.; Maecke, H.R.; Muller, J. Yttrium-90 dotatoc: First clinical results. *Eur. J. Nucl. Med.* **1999**, *26*, 1439–1447.
14. Kosmas, C.; Snook, D.; Gooden, C.S.; Courtenayluck, N.S.; Mccall, M.J.; Meares, C.F.; Epenetos, A.A. Development of humoral immune-responses against a macrocyclic chelating agent (dota) in cancer-patients receiving radioimmunoconjugates for imaging and therapy. *Cancer Res.* **1992**, *52*, 904–911.
15. Kodama, M.; Koike, T.; Mahatma, A.B.; Kimura, E. Thermodynamic and kinetic studies of lanthanide complexes of 1,4,7,10,13-pentaazacyclopentadecane-n,n',n'',n''',n''''-pentaacetic acid and 1,4,7,10,13,16-hexaazacyclooctadecane-n,n',n'',n''',n'''',n'''''-hexaacetic acid. *Inorg. Chem.* **1991**, *30*, 1270–1273.
16. Wadas, T.J.; Wong, E.H.; Weisman, G.R.; Anderson, C.J. Coordinating radiometals of copper, gallium, indium, yttrium, and zirconium for pet and spect imaging of disease. *Chem. Rev.* **2010**, *110*, 2858–2902.

17. Kobayashi, H.; Wu, C.; Yoo, T.M.; Sun, B.F.; Drumm, D.; Pastan, I.; Paik, C.H.; Gansow, O.A.; Carrasquillo, J.A.; Brechbiel, M.W. Evaluation of the *in vivo* biodistribution of yttrium-labeled isomers of chx-dtpa-conjugated monoclonal antibodies. *J. Nucl. Med.* **1998**, *39*, 829–836.
18. Winter, G.; Zlatopolskiy, B.; Kull, T.; Bertram, J.; Genze, F.; Cudek, G.; Machulla, H.-J.; Reske, S. 68ga-dota-dupa-pep as a new peptide conjugate for molecular imaging of prostate carcinoma. *J. Nucl. Med. Meet. Abstr.* **2011**, *52*, 1597.
19. Reske, S.N.; Winter, G.; Baur, B.; Machulla, H.J.; Kull, T. Comment on afshar-oromieh *et al.*: Pet imaging with a [68ga]gallium-labelled psma ligand for the diagnosis of prostate cancer: Biodistribution in humans and first evaluation of tumour lesions. *Eur. J. Nucl. Med. Mol. Imaging.* **2013**, *40*, 969–970.
20. Afshar-Oromieh, A.; Malcher, A.; Eder, M.; Eisenhut, M.; Linhart, H.G.; Hadaschik, B.A.; Holland-Letz, T.; Giesel, F.L.; Kratochwil, C.; Haufe, S.; *et al.* Pet imaging with a [68ga] gallium-labelled psma ligand for the diagnosis of prostate cancer: Biodistribution in humans and first evaluation of tumour lesions. *Eur. J. Nucl. Med .Mol. Imaging* **2013**, *40*, 486–495.
21. Meyer, G.J.; Macke, H.; Schuhmacher, J.; Knapp, W.H.; Hofmann, M. 68a-labelled dota-derivatised peptide ligands. *Eur. J. Nucl. Med. Mol. Imaging* **2004**, *31*, 1097–1104.

3

Folate Receptor Targeted Alpha-Therapy Using Terbium-149

Cristina Müller [1,*], Josefine Reber [1], Stephanie Haller [1], Holger Dorrer [2,3], Ulli Köster [4], Karl Johnston [5], Konstantin Zhernosekov [2], Andreas Türler [2,3] and Roger Schibli [1,6]

[1] Center for Radiopharmaceutical Sciences ETH-PSI-USZ, Paul Scherrer Institute, 5232 Villigen-PSI, Switzerland; E-Mails: josefine.reber@gmail.com (J.R.); stephanie.haller@psi.ch (S.H.); roger.schibli@psi.ch (R.S.)

[2] Laboratory of Radiochemistry and Environmental Chemistry, Paul Scherrer Institute, 5232 Villigen-PSI, Switzerland; E-Mails: holger.dorrer@psi.ch (H.D.); konstantin.zhernosekov@gmail.com (K.Z.); andreas.tuerler@psi.ch (A.T.)

[3] Laboratory of Radiochemistry and Environmental Chemistry, Department of Chemistry and Biochemistry University of Bern, 3012 Berne, Switzerland

[4] Institut Laue-Langevin, 38000 Grenoble, France; E-Mail: koester@ill.fr

[5] Physics Department, ISOLDE/CERN, 1211 Geneva, Switzerland; E-Mail: karl.johnston@cern.ch

[6] Department of Chemistry and Applied Biosciences, ETH Zurich, 8093 Zurich, Switzerland

* Author to whom correspondence should be addressed; E-Mail: cristina.mueller@psi.ch

---

Abstract: Terbium-149 is among the most interesting therapeutic nuclides for medical applications. It decays by emission of short-range α-particles (E_α = 3.967 MeV) with a half-life of 4.12 h. The goal of this study was to investigate the anticancer efficacy of a ^{149}Tb-labeled DOTA-folate conjugate (cm09) using folate receptor (FR)-positive cancer cells *in vitro* and in tumor-bearing mice. ^{149}Tb was produced at the ISOLDE facility at CERN. Radiolabeling of cm09 with purified ^{149}Tb resulted in a specific activity of ~1.2 MBq/nmol. *In vitro* assays performed with ^{149}Tb-cm09 revealed a reduced KB cell viability in a FR-specific and activity concentration-dependent manner. Tumor-bearing mice were injected with saline only (group A) or with ^{149}Tb-cm09 (group B: 2.2 MBq; group C: 3.0 MBq). A significant tumor growth delay was found in treated animals resulting in an increased average survival time of mice which received ^{149}Tb-cm09 (B: 30.5 d; C: 43 d) compared to untreated controls (A: 21 d). Analysis of blood parameters revealed no signs of acute toxicity to the kidneys or liver in treated mice over the time of investigation.

These results demonstrated the potential of folate-based α-radionuclide therapy in tumor-bearing mice.

Keywords: terbium-149; alpha-therapy; folate receptor; DOTA-folate; KB tumors; ^{149}Tb-cm09; albumin binder, radionuclide therapy

---

1. Introduction

Targeted radionuclide therapy using β^--particle-emitting radionuclides (e.g., ^{131}I, ^{90}Y, ^{177}Lu) of variable energies is employed in clinical routine. For this purpose a variety of tumor-targeted biomolecules have been used, ranging from small-molecular weight compounds (e.g., ^{131}I-MIBG), to peptides (e.g., ^{177}Lu-DOTATATE) and monoclonal antibodies (^{90}Y-Ibritumomab, Zevalin®) [1,2]. A promising option for a potential improvement of the therapeutic efficacy of radioendotherapy may be the selection of appropriate radionuclides. α-Particles of medically interesting radionuclides provide a 200- to 1,000-fold higher linear energy transfer (LET) than β^--particles [3,4]. Therefore, and because of the much shorter path-length (25–100 μm) of α-particles compared to β^--particles (0.05–12 mm), α-particle-emitting nuclides may be interesting for targeted radionuclide therapy of micrometastases or even single cancer cells.

Allen *et al.* suggested the radiolanthanide ^{149}Tb as the preferred radionuclide for α-radionuclide therapy [3]. A decay scheme with a list of significant emitted radiation of ^{149}Tb and its daughter nuclides has been previously published by Beyer *et al.* [5]. ^{149}Tb decays with a half-life of 4.12 h by emission of short-range α-particles (E_α = 3.967 MeV, I = 16.7%) [4,5]. In addition, it emits γ-rays of an energy (E_γ = 165 keV, 26.4%) potentially suitable for single photon emission computed tomography (SPECT) and positrons ($E_{\beta+\ average}$ = 638 keV, 3.8%) which may be detected via positron emission tomography (PET) (Figure 1A) [4,6]. However, there also exists suitable diagnostic matched nuclides such as ^{155}Tb ($T_{1/2}$ = 5.32 d, E_γ= 87 keV, I = 32% and 105 keV, I = 25%) and ^{152}Tb ($T_{1/2}$ = 17.5 h, $E_{\beta+\ average}$ = 1.08 MeV, I = 17%) for imaging purposes via SPECT and PET, respectively [7]. Tb can be stably coordinated by macrocyclic chelators (e.g., DOTA) as it has been recently demonstrated using the β^--emitting nuclide ^{161}Tb [7–9]. ^{149}Tb is among the most attractive candidates of α-emitting radiometals for targeted radionuclide therapy. Other α-emitters have either a very short half-life (^{213}Bi: $T_{1/2}$ = 46 min, ^{212}Bi: $T_{1/2}$ = 61 min) or a complicated decay cascade of 4 to 5 α-emissions (^{225}Ac: $T_{1/2}$ = 10.0 d, ^{227}Th: $T_{1/2}$ = 18.7 d) [4,10,11]. The longer-lived *in vivo* generator ^{212}Pb/^{212}Bi ($T_{1/2}$ = 10.64 h) might be a more favorable solution but could suffer from release of the ^{212}Bi from the DOTA complex [12]. In such cases the decay of the daughter nuclides may occur in non-targeted organs which could cause undesired toxicity to healthy tissue [13]. In spite of the fact that the α-emitting ^{211}At ($T_{1/2}$ = 7.21 h) is considered appropriate for medical use with regard to the physical properties, a major impediment to practical applications is the low *in vivo* stability of astatine bonds with aromatic carbon bonds [14]. However, current availability of ^{149}Tb is poor due to production routes which are not easily accessible [6]. Potential production routes include irradiation of rare ^{152}Gd targets with high energy protons (>50 MeV) or the use of light ions as projectiles of >500 MeV protons for spallation reactions. However, in both cases mass separation is required to avoid radioisotopic impurities.

Figure 1. (**A**) The α-particle-emitting [149]Tb as one of four medically interesting terbium-nuclides which belong to the series of chemical elements called lanthanides (15 elements from La to Lu); (**B**) Chemical structure of the radiolabeled DOTA-folate conjugate (cm09) with an albumin binding entity (speculative coordination sphere of the Tb-DOTA-complex).

A

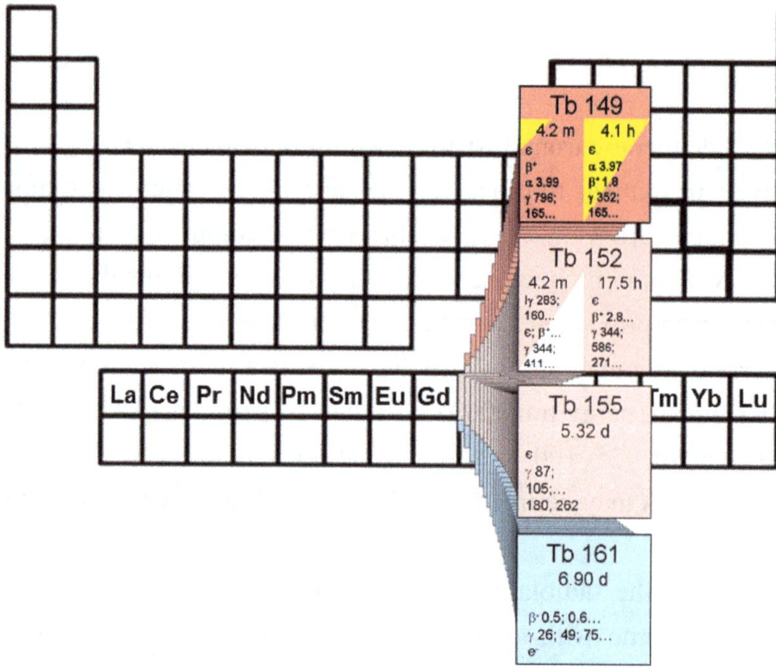

B

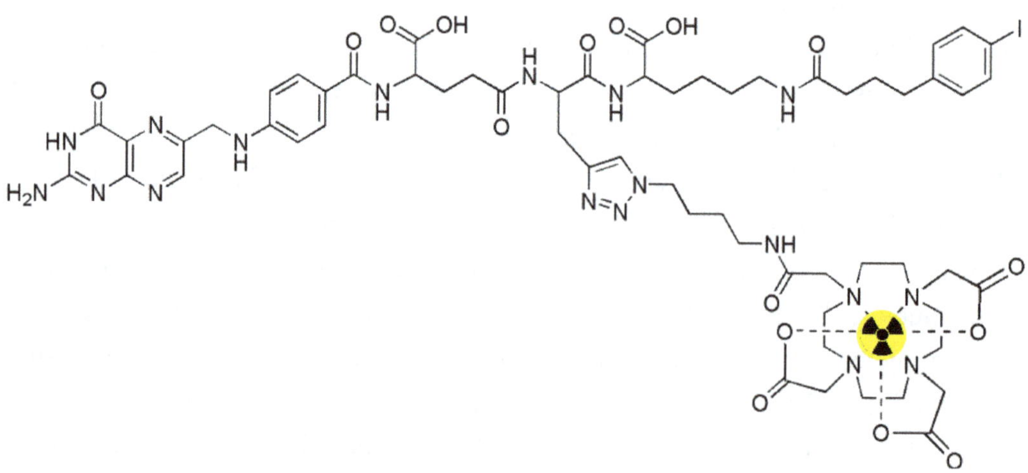

The aim of the present study was to complement our preliminary *in vivo* results [7] by a further study using [149]Tb for *in vitro* cell viability assays and *in vivo* using a well-established tumor mouse model. We employed the recently developed DOTA-folate conjugate (herein referred to as cm09, Figure 1B) and human KB cancer cells which express the folate receptor (FR) at high levels. From our previous *in vivo* studies performed with ^{177}Lu-cm09, it is known that the novel folate radioconjugate is applicable for preclinical therapy studies in the KB tumor mouse model where it provides an excellent tumor accumulation of radioactivity and as a consequence high antitumor efficacy [15].

2. Experimental

2.1. Chemicals and Reagents for Production and Purification of ^{149}Tb

Gold foils (thickness: 0.1 mm, purity: 99.95%, Goodfellow Cambridge Ltd. Huntingdon, UK) were electrolytically coated with a thin layer of zinc (purity ≥99.9%). The acids in this work (HNO_3 suprapur and HCl suprapur) were obtained from VWR International GmbH (Dietikon, Switzerland) and diluted with MilliQ water (18.2 MΩ·cm; Millipore AG, Zug, Switzerland). A solution of NH_3 (25%, suprapur) was obtained from VWR International GmbH. α-Hydroxyisobutyric acid (α-HIBA, purity: 99%), L-lactic acid ($C_3H_6O_3$, purity ≥99%) and NaOH monohydrate (Traceselect, purity ≥99.9995%) were obtained from Sigma-Aldrich International GmbH (St. Gallen, Switzerland).

2.2. Production of ^{149}Tb

^{149}Tb was produced at the isotope separation online facility ISOLDE (CERN, Geneva, Switzerland) as previously reported [7,16,17]. In brief, a tantalum target (50 g/cm^2) was irradiated with high-energy (~1.4 GeV) protons. After effusion of the spallation products from the heated target (~2,000 °C) they were ionized by surface ionization and resonant laser ionization. The monocations were extracted from the ion source, accelerated to 50 keV and separated in a magnetic field according to their mass [16,17]. Products of mass number 149 were implanted into a zinc-coated gold foil (70 mm^2) and shipped to PSI for the purification procedure.

2.3. Purification of ^{149}Tb

The zinc layer was dissolved in a solution mixture of HNO_3/NH_4NO_3 (0.2 M NO_3^-, pH 1, 500 μL) at 50 °C. Isolation of ^{149}Tb from isobar and pseudo-isobar impurities and stable Zn was accomplished by cation exchange chromatography. For this purpose a column (5 mm × 35 mm) filled with a strongly acidic macroporous cation exchange resin was employed as recently reported [7,18]. ^{149}Tb and ^{149}Gd were eluted with α-HIBA (0.13 M) at a flow rate of 0.33 mL/min allowing their separation [7]. Further radioactive impurities and stable Zn remained on the column. Regeneration of the column was carried out using higher concentrated α-HIBA (1.0 M). The collected fractions (330 μL each) which contained ^{149}Tb-α-HIBA were acidified by addition of HCl (4 M, 17 μL). The acidic solution was loaded on a second cation exchange chromatography column (4 mm × 4 mm). α-HIBA, NH_4^+ and HCl were removed by a washing step using MilliQ water. The elution of ^{149}Tb was performed by a solution of L-lactate (0.4 M) previously adjusted to a pH value of 4.7 with sodium hydroxide. The eluted ^{149}Tb-fraction was diluted with the 1.7-fold volume of MilliQ water to adjust the osmolarity to a physiological value (~300 mOsm).

2.4. Preparation of ^{149}Tb-cm09 and Stability in Blood Plasma

Radiolabeling was performed by addition of 18 μL of the DOTA-folate (cm09) stock solution (10 mM, corresp. to 18 nmol of cm09) to the obtained solution of ^{149}Tb (25 MBq) in L-lactate (pH 4.7). The reaction mixture was incubated for 10 min at 95 °C. Quality control was performed by HPLC using a C-18 reversed phase column (Xterra MS C-18, 5 μm, 15 cm × 4.6 cm, Waters, Milford,

MA, USA). The mobile phase consisted of MilliQ water with 0.1% trifluoroacetic acid (A) and methanol (B) with a linear gradient from 5% to 80% B over 25 min at a flow rate of 1 mL/min. The product (R_t = 19.5 min) was obtained with a radiochemical purity of >96%. After addition of Na-DTPA (10 μL, 5 mM, pH 5) the labeling solution (1.0–1.2 MBq/nmol) was directly used for *in vitro* and *in vivo* application. The stability of ^{149}Tb-cm09 was investigated by incubation of the radioconjugate (50 μL, ~1 MBq) in human plasma (250 μL) at 37 °C. Aliquots (50 μL) were taken for analysis after 30 min, 1 h and 4 h. The proteins were precipitated by addition of methanol (200 μL) and the supernatants were analyzed using HPLC.

2.5. Cell Culture

KB cells (human cervical carcinoma cell line, HeLa subclone; ACC-136) were purchased from the German Collection of Microorganisms and Cell Cultures (DSMZ, Braunschweig, Germany). Cells were cultured as monolayers at 37 °C in a humidified atmosphere containing 5% CO_2. Importantly KB cells were cultured in a folate-free special cell culture medium, FFRPMI (modified RPMI, without folic acid, vitamin B_{12} and phenol red; Cell Culture Technologies GmbH, Gravesano/Lugano, Switzerland). FFRPMI media was supplemented with 10% heat-inactivated fetal calf serum (FCS), L-glutamine and antibiotics (penicillin/streptomycin/fungizone). Routine culture treatment was performed twice a week.

2.6. In Vitro Cell Viability Studies

Inhibition of KB cell viability was investigated using a 3-(4,5-dimethylthiazol-2-yl)-2,5-diphenyltetrazolium bromide (MTT) assay [19]. The cells were harvested and seeded in 96-well plates at 2.5 × 10^3 cells per well in a final volume of 200 μL FFRPMI medium with supplements. After 24 h incubation for cell adhesion, the medium was removed and the cells were incubated with ^{149}Tb-cm09 (0.05–500 kBq in 200 μL medium/well) alone or in combination with excess folic acid (200 nM) for 4 h at 37 °C. Cell incubation with FFRPMI medium only was performed as a control experiment. After incubation, the supernatants were removed and KB cells were washed with PBS (200 μL/well) before addition of supplemented FFRPMI medium (200 μL/well). Cells were then allowed to grow for 4 days before analysis as previously reported [20]. After addition of 30 μL of an MTT solution (5 mg/mL) to each well, the well-plates were incubated for an additional 4 h at 37 °C. The medium was removed and the dark-violet formazan crystals were dissolved in dimethyl sulfoxide. The absorbance was determined at 560 nm using a microplate reader (Victor X3, Perkin Elmer, Waltham, MA, USA). To quantify cell viability, the ratio of the absorbance of the test samples to the absorbance of control cell samples (=100% viability) was calculated using Microsoft Excel software (Microsoft Corp. Redmond, WA, USA).

2.7. In Vivo Therapy Studies

In vivo experiments were approved by the local veterinary department and conducted in accordance with the Swiss law of animal protection. Four to five-week-old female, athymic nude mice (CD-1 Foxn-1/nu) were purchased from Charles River Laboratories (Sulzfeld, Germany). They were fed with a folate-deficient rodent diet (ssniff Spezialdiäten GmbH, Soest, Germany) starting 5 days prior to tumor cell inoculation [21]. Endpoint criteria were defined as weight loss of >15% of the initial body weight (at day 0), tumor volume >1,000 mm^3, ulceration or bleeding of the tumor xenograft or abnormal behavior indicating pain or unease of the animal.

The therapy study was performed according to the injection protocol shown in Table 1. Twelve mice were subcutaneously inoculated with 5×10^6 KB tumor cells (suspended in 100 μL PBS) as previously reported 4 days before injection of the radioactive folate conjugate [15].

Table 1. Injection protocol of the *in vivo* therapy study.

	Number of mice [n]	Injection solution	Injected radioactivity [MBq]
Group A	4	L-lactate solution	-
Group B	4	^{149}Tb-cm09 in L-lactate solution	2.2
Group C	4	^{149}Tb-cm09 in L-lactate solution	3.0

At the time of treatment the tumors reached a volume 60–80 mm^3. Mice of group A were intravenously injected with only L-lactate solution whereas mice of group B and C received ^{149}Tb-cm09 (2.2 MBq and 3.0 MBq, respectively) in the same L-lactate solution. The amount of injected activity was the highest possible based on the availability of the nuclide sufficient to inject 4 mice. After start of the therapy mice were weighed three times a week over 35 days and tumor volumes were monitored by measuring two perpendicular diameters with a caliper and calculated according to the equation: $V = 0.5 \times L \times W^2$ (L is the length (large diameter) and W is the width (small diameter) of the tumor). Mice were removed from the study if one or several of the predefined endpoint criteria were reached which required euthanasia.

The therapeutic efficacy was expressed as the percentage of tumor growth inhibition (%TGI) calculated according to the formula: $\%TGI = 100 - (RTV_T/RTV_U \times 100)$, where RTV_T is the mean relative tumor volume of treated mice (groups B or C), and RTV_U is the mean relative tumor volume of untreated mice (group A) determined at day 21 when the first control mouse was euthanized. The tumor growth delay index (TGDI) was calculated according to the formula: $TGDI = TGD_T/TGD_U$. It was defined as the mean tumor growth delay ratio of treated (TGD_T) and untreated animals (TGD_U) which was required to increase the RTV 5-fold [22].

2.8. Determination of Plasma Parameters

Plasma parameters such as blood urea nitrogen (BUN), alkaline phosphatase (ALP), and total bilirubin (TBIL) were measured from all mice at day 14 after start of the therapy and before euthanasia of each mouse. BUN is a common parameter to determine potential damage to the kidneys whereas increased ALP and TBIL could be an indication for impaired liver function. Plasma samples were prepared by centrifugation of blood samples (150–200 μL per mouse) drawn from the sublingual vein of each mouse and collected in heparinized vials (Microvette, 200 mL Sarstedt, Nümbrecht, Germany). For each parameter a plasma volume of 10 μL was required for the analysis using a Fuji Dri-Chem 40000i analyzer (Polymed Medical Center AG, Glattbrugg, Switzerland).

2.9. Dosimetric Calculations

To estimate the equivalent absorbed dose for ^{149}Tb-cm09 in KB tumor xenografts, biodistribution data obtained with ^{161}Tb-cm09 were used. Based on these data the following calculations were made: (i) the cumulative radioactivity was calculated from integrated AUCs (MBq·s) of biodistribution data expressed in non decay-corrected percent injected activity [%IA] per tumor mass (assumed as 100 mg, due to an approximate calculated volume of the tumors at the start of the therapy); (ii) the adsorbed radiation dose in tumor xenografts was assessed for a sphere of 100 mg using the Unit Density Sphere Model from RADAR [23]; (iii) The absorbed dose (mGy/MBq) was calculated by multiplying the AUC (s; normalized to 1 MBq ID) with the S-value (mGy/MBq·s); and (iv) the dose (mGy) was calculated by multiplying the absorbed dose (mGy/MBq) with the amount of injected radioactivity.

2.10. Statistical Significance

Significance of the survival time and tumor growth delay was calculated by the performance of the *t*-test (Microsoft Excel). All analyses were two-tailed and considered as type 3 (two sample unequal variance). A p-value < 0.05 was considered statistically significant.

3. Results and Discussion

3.1. Production and Purification of ^{149}Tb

^{149}Tb was produced by proton-induced spallation of tantalum targets at ISOLDE/CERN on a zinc-covered gold foil containing isobar and pseudo-isobar nuclides of mass number 149. Upon arrival at PSI (~4 h after the end of collection) ~40 MBq ^{149}Tb, ~5 MBq ^{149}Gd, ~0.4 MBq ^{145}Eu (from α-decay of ^{149}Tb), ~70 MBq ^{133m}Ce, ~15 MBq ^{133}Ce and ~350 MBq ^{133}La were detected. The mass 133 pseudo-isobars appear at mass 149 as monoxide molecular ions. The radioactive solution which was obtained after dissolution of the zinc-layer was loaded on column I for chromatographic separation of ^{149}Tb. The elution was accomplished with a diluted solution of α-HIBA within only 25 min. The ^{149}Tb (~29 MBq, corresponding to 73% of total radioactivity) was isolated in a volume of 1.65 mL free of radioactive impurities. Under these isocratic elution conditions an excellent separation of ^{149}Tb and ^{149}Gd was achieved (Figure 2). Further radiolanthanide impurities such as ^{145}Eu, ^{133m}Ce, ^{133}Ce and ^{133}La as well as stable Zn were retained on the chromatographic column I and eluted afterwards using a higher concentrated α-HIBA solution for regeneration of the column.

After concentration of the ^{149}Tb-solution by adsorption at the cation exchanger of the second column, the product was obtained within 25 min as ^{149}Tb-L-lactate (0.4 M, pH 4.7) in a small volume of only 225 μL. Addition of 375 μL MilliQ water resulted in a solution of 0.15 M sodium L-lactate with a physiological osmolarity of ~300 mOsm. Determination of radioactivity revealed a total yield of ~25 MBq ^{149}Tb containing ~88 kBq ^{149}Gd—which decays via electron capture and γ-ray emission—as the only detectable radionuclide impurity generated by the decay of ^{149}Tb after separation on column I. The total yield of the separation process was ~63% (corresponding to a ~94% decay-corrected yield) and the whole isolation process including measurement of the single elution fractions was accomplished within 145 min. The L-lactate-based physiological formulation was suitable not only for the direct performance of radiolabeling of cm09 but allowed even *in vitro* and *in vivo* application without further purification steps.

Figure 2. Elution profile of chromatographic column I showing separation of ^{149}Tb (■, red) from ^{149}Gd (●, blue).

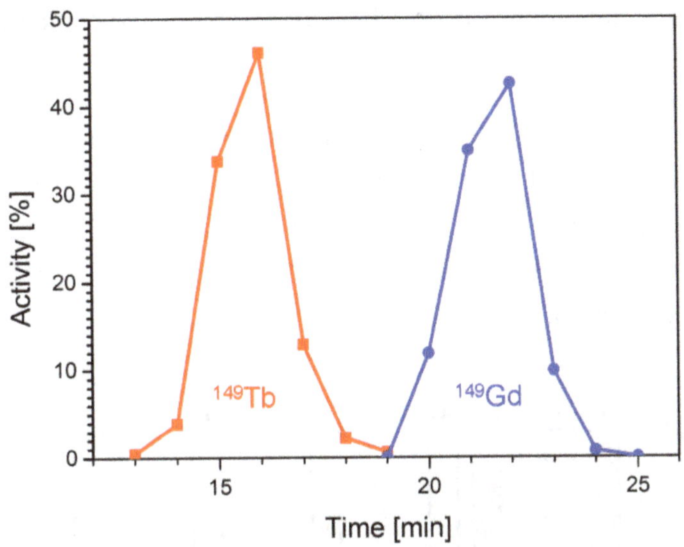

In comparison to our previous study [7] where we used ^{149}Tb for radiolabeling directly after elution from the first column in the α-HIBA solution (~0.15 M), the purification process was optimized in the present study. The advantages were two-fold: Firstly, using the second chromatographic column allowed concentration of the radioactivity in a smaller volume which was favorable for subsequent radiolabeling steps and *in vivo* application. Secondly, the elution was carried out with a solution of L-lactate providing ^{149}Tb in a more physiological solution compared to the α-HIBA solution which was employed in our previous studies.

3.2. Radiosynthesis of ^{149}Tb-cm09 and Stability in Blood Plasma

Radiolabeling of cm09 (18 nmol) with ^{149}Tb (25 MBq) resulted in a product peak of the radiolabeled product with a retention time (R_t) of 19.5 min. The chromatogram was equal to what was previously obtained with the ^{161}Tb-labeled match (^{161}Tb-cm09) [9]. On the other hand injection of free $^{149/161}$Tb(III) was eluted almost with the front (R_t = 3 min). These findings confirmed the identity of the product peak as ^{149}Tb-cm09 which was obtained with a radiochemical purity of >96% with only insignificant traces of free ^{149}Tb(III).

Incubation of ^{149}Tb-cm09 (1.0–1.2 MBq/nmol) in blood plasma at 37 °C revealed high stability (>98%) of the folate radioconjguate over at least 4 hours. These findings were expected as it was previously shown that ^{161}Tb-cm09 was completely stable in human blood plasma over several days [7,9].

3.3. In Vitro Application of ^{149}Tb-cm09

In vitro cell viability assays were performed to investigate the effect of ^{149}Tb-cm09. FR-positive KB tumor cells were incubated with increasing radioactivity concentrations of ^{149}Tb-cm09. It was found that the viability of the KB cells was inhibited in an activity-dependent manner (Figure 3). Application of a low radioactivity concentration of ^{149}Tb-cm09 (0.5 kBq/mL) resulted in an only 20%-reduction of the tumor cell viability. However, a 1,000-fold higher radioactivity concentration (500 kBq/mL) resulted in an almost complete loss of KB cell viability. Addition of excess folic acid to block cell surface exposed FRs abolished the effect of ^{149}Tb-cm09 completely even at high radioactivity concentrations. Under these conditions tumor cells grew normally and comparably to untreated control cells (Figure 3). These findings clearly indicated a FR-specific effect of ^{149}Tb-cm09.

Figure 3. *In vitro* viability of KB tumor cells is reduced upon exposure to increasing radioactivity concentrations of ^{149}Tb-cm09 (red bars). Incubation of cells with excess folic acid to block FRs protected KB cells from the ^{149}Tb-cm09-induced inhibitory effect (yellow bars). Exposure of cells to unlabeled cm09 (100 nM to 10 μM) had no effect on cell growth (data not shown).

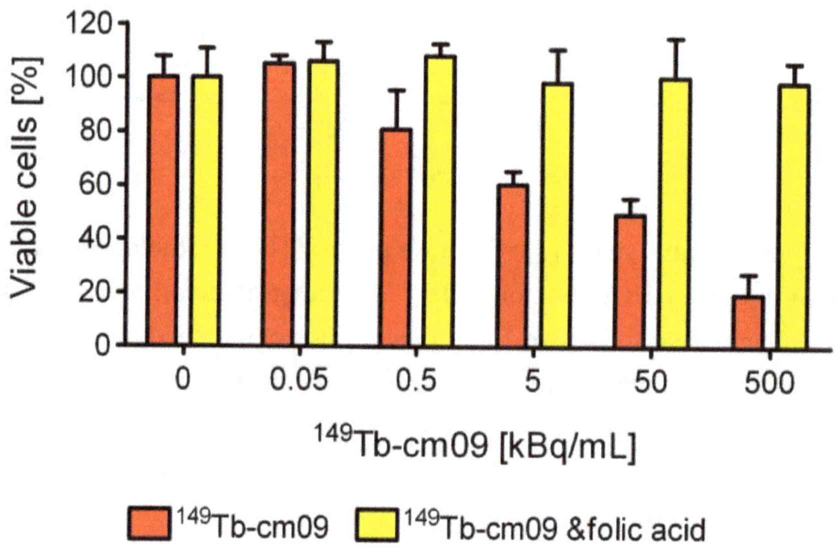

3.4. Therapy Study in Tumor-Bearing Mice Using ^{149}Tb-cm09

The therapy study in KB tumor-bearing nude mice showed significant tumor growth delay (TGD) in ^{149}Tb-cm09 treated mice compared to untreated control mice (Figure 4A). The tumor growth delay index for a 5-fold increased tumor volume compared to the tumor volume at the beginning of the study ($TGDI_5$) reached a value of 1.5 (p = 0.04) for mice of group B which were treated with 2.2 MBq ^{149}Tb-cm09. This means a 1.5-fold higher value than for untreated control mice ($TGDI_5$ = 1). In mice of group C, which received 3.0 MBq of ^{149}Tb-cm09, the $TGDI_5$ was even 2.0-fold (p = 0.01) increased compared to the $TGDI_5$ of untreated controls. At day 21 when the first control mouse had to be euthanized due to an oversized tumor the average relative tumor volume (RTV) was significantly smaller in treated mice of group B (p = 0.01) and group C (p = 0.001) compared to the tumor volume of untreated control mice (group A). At this time point of the study tumor growth was inhibited by 62% (group B) and 85% (group C), respectively, indicating a dose-dependent therapeutic efficacy of ^{149}Tb-cm09. The average survival time was increased by 45% (30.5 d, p = 0.01) in mice of group B and by 105% (43 d, p = 0.004) in mice of group C compared to control mice (group A, 21 d) (Figure 4B).

Figure 4. Results of FR-targeted radionuclide α-therapy using ^{149}Tb-cm09 in KB tumor-bearing mice. (**A**) Graph of the average relative tumor volume (RTV) of mice from each group ($n = 4$) during the time period when at least 3 mice were still alive; (**B**) Survival curves of mice from each group (group A: 21 d; group B: 30.5 d and group C: 43 d).

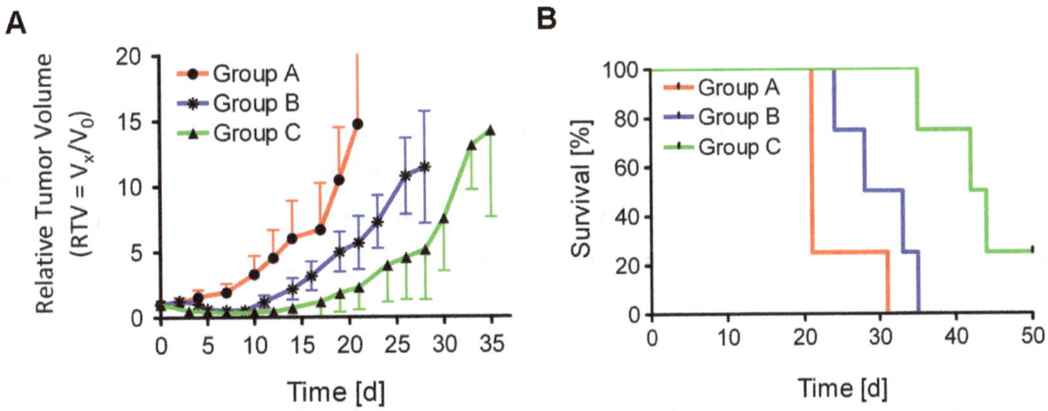

Analysis of blood plasma parameters (BUN, ALP and TBIL) did not reveal significant changes ($p > 0.05$) among control mice and mice treated with ^{149}Tb-cm09 (Table 2). This analysis indicated unimpaired renal and hepatobiliar function. Hence, it can be concluded that acute radiotoxic effects to the kidneys and the liver were not experienced by FR-targeted α-radionuclide therapy over the whole time of this study which lasted for 35 days. More detailed studies to investigate effects of ^{149}Tb-cm09 on kidney function will be necessary since undesired side-effects on the long-term cannot be excluded based on the examinations performed herein.

Table 2. Results of plasma analysis at day 14 and before terminal (in parentheses); (BUN = blood urea nitrogen, ALP = alkaline phosphatase, TBIL = total bilirubin).

	BUN [mmol/L]	ALP [U/L]	TBIL [μmol/L)
Group A	7.0 ± 1.8 (4.1 ± 0.5)	77 ± 10 (99 ± 16)	6.5 ± 2.5 (6.3 ± 1.0)
Group B	4.6 ± 0.6 (4.7 ± 0.4)	67 ± 5 (119 ± 7)	7.6 ± 4.7 (6.0 ± 1.0)
Group C	5.2 ± 1.3 (5.9 ± 1.4)	75 ± 14 (73 ± 21)	7.0 ± 0.8 (5.0 ± 1.0)

Overall the present results outperformed our previous data which were obtained upon administration of two injections of ^{149}Tb-cm09 at low quantities of radioactivity (1.1 MBq and 1.3 MBq, respectively) [7]. Compared to our previous therapy study, the present study design differed in that the mice received the whole amount of radioactivity in a single injection of either 2.2 MBq ^{149}Tb-cm09 (group B) or 3.0 MBq ^{149}Tb-cm09 (group C).

Beyer *et al.* conducted an experiment where ^{149}Tb-labeled rituximab (5.5 MBq per mouse) was investigated in a leukemia animal model using SCID mice with an intravenous graft of Daudi cells [5]. Their aim was to examine the efficacy of ^{149}Tb-rituximab to specifically kill circulating single cancer cells or small cell clusters *in vivo*. The therapy was started within 3 days upon intravenous xenografting of a lethal number of Daudi cells when most of the tumor cells were expected to be still in circulation [5]. Whereas untreated control mice had to be euthanized within the first 37 days a tumor-free survival was found for over 120 d in almost 90% of the ^{149}Tb-rituximab treated animals. Since application of the same amount of unlabeled rituximab did not show a therapeutic effect, the favorable outcome of this study could be ascribed to the α-radionuclide therapy [5]. In the present study injection of ^{149}Tb-cm09 reduced tumor growth of solid KB xenografts and increased the survival time significantly in mice of both treated groups (B and C) compared to untreated control mice (group A). These excellent results complement those of Beyer *et al.* by demonstrating the therapeutic potential of ^{149}Tb. However, our study design differed from that of Beyer *et al.* in three respects. (i) Instead of using an established antibody, we employed a small-molecular weight folate conjugate (cm09) as a targeting agent which previously proved the promising potential to be used for therapeutic purposes [15]; (ii) The amount of injected radioactivity was 2.2 MBq and 3.0 MBq, respectively, in our study compared to 5.5 MBq which were used in the study of Beyer *et al.* [5]; (iii) Finally the tumor mouse model which was used in our study was based on solid tumor xenografts of a human cervical cancer cell line while Beyer *et al.* used a tumor mouse model with circulating leukemia cells.

3.5. Dosimetric Calculations

In order to obtain an idea about the radioactive dose burden of ^{149}Tb-cm09 to KB tumor xenografts a dose estimation was made while taking only the self-radiation dose into account. According to the AUC obtained from tissue distribution data in mice injected with ^{161}Tb-cm09 [7] and the S-value of ^{149}Tb listed for a sphere of 100 mg an absorbed dose of 8.67 Gy/MBq was estimated for KB tumor xenografts. This resulted in an absorbed dose of ~19 Gy (group B) and ~26 Gy (group C) in tumors upon a single injection of 2.2 MBq and 3.0 MBq of ^{149}Tb-cm09, respectively.

Recently, we peformed a preclinical therapy study with 10 MBq of ^{161}Tb-cm09 using the same KB tumor mouse model [9]. In that case the dose to the tumor was calculated to a value of ~33 Gy and the corresponding $TGDI_5$ reached a value of ~2.2. In the present study the $TGDI_5$ for ^{149}Tb-cm09 was ~1.6 (2.2 MBq, ~19 Gy) and ~2.0 (3.0 MBq, ~26 Gy) indicating a slightly improved effect of the α-radionuclide therapy. However, for an exact comparison of α- and β^-/Auger-radionuclide therapy it would be necessary to perform a site-by-site study using ^{149}Tb-folate and ^{161}Tb-folate with an activity that results in the same calculated dose to the tumor.

4. Conclusions

In this study the potential of α-radionuclide therapy in general and of ^{149}Tb in particular was demonstrated using a folate-based biomolecule. Application of ^{149}Tb-cm09 was well-tolerated in mice and treated KB tumor xenografts efficiently. The experiments revealed significant tumor growth delay and an increased survival time of mice treated with ^{149}Tb-cm09 compared to untreated control mice. However, further studies will be required to investigate potential advantages of FR-targeted α-radionuclide therapy over β^--radionuclide therapy with regard to tumor response and potential damage to the kidneys.

Acknowledgments

We thank Nadja Romano, Maruta Bunka, the ISOLDE technical team and the ISOLDE RILIS team for technical assistance. This project was financially supported by the Swiss National Science Foundation (Ambizione Grant), COST (Action BM0607), the Swiss Cancer League (KLS-02762-02-2011), the Swiss South African Joint Research Programme (SSAJRP) and by the European Union via the ENSAR Project (contract 262010).

Author Contributions

C.M. coordinated the study, supervised the experiments and wrote the manuscript. J.R. and S.H. performed the *in vitro* and *in vivo* studies at PSI. H.D. performed the separation of ^{149}Tb at PSI. U.K. and K.J. coordinated and performed the production of ^{149}Tb at ISOLDE/CERN. K.Z. developed the separation procedure of ^{149}Tb and contributed to the study design. A.T. and R.S. gave advice in the interpretation of the data and critically reviewed the manuscript. All authors approved the final manuscript.

References

1. Oyen, W.J.; Bodei, L.; Giammarile, F.; Maecke, H.R.; Tennvall, J.; Luster, M.; Brans, B. Targeted therapy in nuclear medicine-current status and future prospects. *Ann. Oncol.* **2007**, *18*, 1782–1792.
2. Zoller, F.; Eisenhut, M.; Haberkorn, U.; Mier, W. Endoradiotherapy in cancer treatment—Basic concepts and future trends. *Eur. J. Pharmacol.* **2009**, *625*, 55–62.
3. Allen, B.J.; Blagojevic, N. Alpha- and beta-emitting radiolanthanides in targeted cancer therapy: The potential role of terbium-149. *Nucl. Med. Commun.* **1996**, *17*, 40–47.
4. Allen, B.J. Targeted alpha therapy: Evidence for potential efficacy of alpha-immunoconjugates in the management of micrometastatic cancer. *Australas. Radiol.* **1999**, *43*, 480–486.
5. Beyer, G.J.; Miederer, M.; Vranjes-Duric, S.; Comor, J.J.; Kunzi, G.; Hartley, O.; Senekowitsch-Schmidtke, R.; Soloviev, D.; Buchegger, F. Targeted alpha therapy *in vivo*: Direct evidence for single cancer cell kill using ^{149}Tb-rituximab. *Eur. J. Nucl. Med. Mol. Imaging* **2004**, *31*, 547–554.
6. Beyer, G.J.; Comor, J.J.; Dakovic, M.; Soloviev, D.; Tamburella, C.; Hagebo, E.; Allan, B.; Dmitriev, S.N.; Zaitseva, N.G.; Starodub, G.Y.; *et al.* Production routes of the alpha emitting ^{149}Tb for medical application. *Radiochim. Acta.* **2002**, *90*, 247–252.
7. Müller, C.; Zhernosekov, K.; Köster, U.; Johnston, K.; Dorrer, H.; Hohn, A.; van der Walt, N.T.; Türler, A.; Schibli, R. A unique matched quadruplet of terbium radioisotopes for PET and SPECT and for α- and β^--radionuclide therapy: An *in vivo* proof-of-concept study with a new receptor-targeted folate derivative. *J. Nucl. Med.* **2012**, *53*, 1951–1959.
8. Lehenberger, S.; Barkhausen, C.; Cohrs, S.; Fischer, E.; Grünberg, J.; Hohn, A.; Koster, U.; Schibli, R.; Türler, A.; Zhernosekov, K. The low-energy beta- and electron emitter ^{161}Tb as an alternative to ^{177}Lu for targeted radionuclide therapy. *Nucl. Med. Biol.* **2011**, *38*, 917–924.
9. Müller, C.; Reber, J.; Haller, S.; Dorrer, H.; Bernhardt, P.; Zhernosekov, K.; Türler, A.; Schibli, R. Direct *in vitro* and *in vivo* comparison of ^{161}Tb and ^{177}Lu using a tumour-targeting folate conjugate. *Eur. J. Nucl. Med. Mol. Imaging* **2014**, *41*, 476–485.

10. Imam, S.K. Advancements in cancer therapy with alpha-emitters: A review. *Int. J. Radiat. Oncol. Biol. Phys.* **2001**, *51*, 271–278.
11. Miederer, M.; Seidl, C.; Beyer, G.J.; Charlton, D.E.; Vranjes-Duric, S.; Comor, J.J.; Huber, R.; Nikula, T.; Apostolidis, C.; Schuhmacher, C.; *et al.* Comparison of the radiotoxicity of two alpha-particle-emitting immunoconjugates, terbium-149 and bismuth-213, directed against a tumor-specific, exon 9 deleted (d9) e-cadherin adhesion protein. *Radiat. Res.* **2003**, *159*, 612–620.
12. Mirzadeh, S.; Kumar, K.; Gansow, O.A. The chemical fate of ^{212}Bi-DOTA formed by β^- decay of ^{212}Pb-DOTA^{2-}. *Radiochim. Acta* **1993**, *60*, 1–10.
13. Schwartz, J.; Jaggi, J.S.; O'Donoghue, J.A.; Ruan, S.; McDevitt, M.; Larson, S.M.; Scheinberg, D.A.; Humm, J.L. Renal uptake of bismuth-213 and its contribution to kidney radiation dose following administration of actinium-225-labeled antibody. *Phys. Med. Biol.* **2011**, *56*, 721–733.
14. Wilbur, D.S. Enigmatic astatine. *Nat. Chem.* **2013**, *5*, 246.
15. Müller, C.; Struthers, H.; Winiger, C.; Zhernosekov, K.; Schibli, R. DOTA conjugate with an albumin-binding entity enables the first folic acid-targeted ^{177}Lu-radionuclide tumor therapy in mice. *J. Nucl. Med.* **2013**, *54*, 124–131.
16. Allen, B.J.; Goozee, G.; Sarkar, S.; Beyer, G.; Morel, C.; Byrne, A.P. Production of terbium-152 by heavy ion reactions and proton induced spallation. *Appl. Radiat. Isot.* **2001**, *54*, 53–58.
17. Köster, U.; Collaboration ISOLDE. Isolde target and ion source chemistry. *Radiochim. Acta* **2001**, *89*, 749–756.
18. Müller, C.; Fischer, E.; Behe, M.; Köster, U.; Dorrer, H.; Reber, J.; Haller, S.; Cohrs, S.; Blanc, A.; Grünberg, J.; *et al.* Future prospects for SPECT imaging using the radiolanthanide terbium-155—Production and preclinical evaluation in tumor-bearing mice. *Nucl. Med. Biol.* **2013**, doi:10.1016/j.nucmedbio.2013.11.002.
19. Mosmann, T. Rapid colorimetric assay for cellular growth and survival: Application to proliferation and cytotoxicity assays. *J. Immunol. Methods* **1983**, *65*, 55–63.
20. Reber, J.; Struthers, H.; Betzel, T.; Hohn, A.; Schibli, R.; Müller, C. Radioiodinated folic acid conjugates: Evaluation of a valuable concept to improve tumor-to-background contrast. *Mol. Pharm.* **2012**, *9*, 1213–1221.
21. Mathias, C.J.; Wang, S.; Lee, R.J.; Waters, D.J.; Low, P.S.; Green, M.A. Tumor-selective radiopharmaceutical targeting via receptor-mediated endocytosis of gallium-67-deferoxamine-folate. *J. Nucl. Med.* **1996**, *37*, 1003–1008.
22. Sanceau, J.; Poupon, M.F.; Delattre, O.; Sastre-Garau, X.; Wietzerbin, J. Strong inhibition of ewing tumor xenograft growth by combination of human interferon-alpha or interferon-beta with ifosfamide. *Oncogene* **2002**, *21*, 7700–7709.
23. Radiation Dose Assessment Resource (RADAR). Avaliable online: www.doseinfo-radar.com (accessed on 7 March 2014).

4

A Bombesin-Shepherdin Radioconjugate Designed for Combined Extra- and Intracellular Targeting

Christiane A. Fischer, Sandra Vomstein and Thomas L. Mindt *

University of Basel Hospital, Clinic of Radiology and Nuclear Medicine,
Division of Radiopharmaceutical Chemistry, Petersgraben 4, 4031 Basel, Switzerland;
E-Mails: christiane.fischer@usb.ch (C.A.F.); Sandra.Vomstein@usb.ch (S.V.)

* Author to whom correspondence should be addressed; E-Mail: Thomas.Mindt@usb.ch

---

Abstract: Radiolabeled peptides which target tumor-specific membrane structures of cancer cells represent a promising class of targeted radiopharmaceuticals for the diagnosis and therapy of cancer. A potential drawback of a number of reported radiopeptides is the rapid washout of a substantial fraction of the initially delivered radioactivity from cancer cells and tumors. This renders the initial targeting effort in part futile and results in a lower imaging quality and efficacy of the radiotracer than achievable. We are investigating the combination of internalizing radiopeptides with molecular entities specific for an intracellular target. By enabling intracellular interactions of the radioconjugate, we aim at reducing/decelerating the externalization of radioactivity from cancer cells. Using the "click-to-chelate" approach, the ^{99m}Tc-tricarbonyl core as a reporter probe for single-photon emission computed tomography (SPECT) was combined with the binding sequence of bombesin for extracellular targeting of the gastrin-releasing peptide receptor (GRP-r) and peptidic inhibitors of the cytosolic heat shock 90 protein (Hsp90) for intracellular targeting. Receptor-specific uptake of the multifunctional radioconjugate could be confirmed, however, the cellular washout of radioactivity was not improved. We assume that either endosomal trapping or lysosomal degradation of the radioconjugate is accountable for these observations.

Keywords: multifunctional radioconjugates; intra- and extracellular targeting; tumor-targeting; ^{99m}Tc-tricarbonyl; bombesin; shepherdin; gastrin releasing peptide receptor; Hsp90; SPECT

---

1. Introduction

Regulatory peptides are known to display high specificity and affinity towards different G-protein coupled receptors (GPCRs) which are overexpressed on the cell membrane of various cancer cells [1]. On this account, a number of radiopharmaceuticals based on these peptides as tumor-targeting vectors are currently under preclinical and clinical evaluation or have already found application in nuclear medicine for the management of cancer [2–4]. However, after receptor-mediated uptake of radiolabeled regulatory peptides into tumors, a rapid washout of a significant fraction of radioactivity is often observed [5–9]. This not only renders the initial targeting efforts in part futile but may also impair imaging quality and the efficacy of radiopharmaceuticals where therapeutic radionuclides are employed. To overcome these limitations, new strategies are needed to enhance the cellular retention of radioactivity inside cancer cells and tumors. A possible approach to achieve this goal is represented by the application of radiolabeled conjugates which combine extra- and intracellular targeting. Such multifunctional radioconjugates have the promise to be recognized first by an extracellular target (e.g., a GPCR) that triggers cell internalization by endocytosis. Once inside the cell, the radioconjugate interacts with its intracellular target (e.g., an organelle or protein) by means of which the radioactive cargo is trapped [10]. Radioconjugates consisting of two molecular moieties, each of which specific for an extra- and intracellular target, respectively, have been reported; however, examples remain scarce. Ginj *et al.* have reported the combination of radiolabeled somatostatin derivatives with a nuclear localization sequence (NLS) to transport Auger electron emitting radionuclides to the cell nucleus. The reported conjugates target specifically the cell nucleus and display a decreased externalization rate *in vitro*; however, no *in vivo* data is available [6]. With the same goal, the groups of Alberto and Santos have combined a ^{99m}Tc-labeled bombesin (BBS) derivative with the DNA intercalator acridine orange, which simultaneously serves as a fluorescent probe for optical imaging. The *in vitro* results reported on the ability of the conjugates to target the cell nucleus are not consistent and data on the externalization of radioactivity from cells is not reported [11,12]. The Garrison group investigated the combination of a radiolabeled BBS derivative with 2-nitroimidazoles, a hypoxia-specific prodrug. Upon enzymatic reduction of the 2-nitroimidazole moiety, the radioconjugate gets covalently linked to intracellular proteins. While an enhancement of the retention of radioactivity in PC-3 cells as a result of 2-nitroimidazole moieties was demonstrated under hypoxic conditions *in vitro*, the effect was less pronounced in a mouse model [13]. Finally, we have recently reported a ^{99m}Tc-tricarbonyl-labeled, dual-targeting radiopeptide conjugate made of a modified amino acid sequence of BBS, [Nle^{14}]BBS(7-14) (QWAVGHLNle), for extracellular targeting of the gastrin-releasing peptide receptor (GRP-r) and a triphenylphosphonium (TPP) entity specific for mitochondria by its ability to accumulate electrophoretically driven in the energized membrane of the organelle [10]. While receptor-specific cell internalization of the conjugate could be confirmed, the cellular washout of radioactivity was not reduced. We tentatively ascribed our observations to the possibility of hindered passage of the TPP moiety through the membrane of mitochondria because of the peptide it is attached to; similar observations have been reported for cell penetrating peptide/TPP conjugates [14]. We therefore set out to investigate the utility of multifunctional radiopeptides which target cytosolic proteins and thus, do not require multiple passages through intracellular membranes, a process considered as a major barrier for targeting intracellular epitopes [15]. With these considerations in mind, we chose the cytosolic chaperone, heat shock protein 90 (Hsp90), as a potential intracellular target for our purpose. Hsp90 is a ubiquitous protein important for, e.g., cell proliferation and survival. As such, it is found overexpressed by nearly all cancer cells in high concentrations [16–18]. Hsp90 assists and controls the non-covalent folding/unfolding of many client proteins, including the peptide survivin [17,19,20]. The group of Altieri has identified the binding sequence of survivin(K79-L87), termed "shepherdin" as an inhibitor of the survivin-Hsp90 interaction and Hsp90 ATPase activity [21]. The high affinity and specificity towards Hsp90 and anticancer activities of shepherdin(79–87) (KHSSGCAFL) and its truncated form shepherdin(79–83) (KHSSG), respectively, have been demonstrated by different approaches [20–24]. However, applications of radiolabeled derivatives of shepherdin or its combination with tumor-targeting peptides for receptor-specific delivery have not yet been described. Herein, we wish to report the synthesis of BBS-shepherdin radioconjugates prepared by the previously reported modular "click-to-chelate" approach [25,26] (Figure 1) and their evaluation *in vitro*.

Figure 1. Assembly of multifunctional, ^{99m}Tc-tricarbonyl-labeled peptide conjugates by amide bond formation, CuAAC, and (radio)metal complexation; residues R^1 and R^2 represent two different entities of biological function (e.g., derivatives of BBS and shepherdin) to be combined in the final radioconjugate.

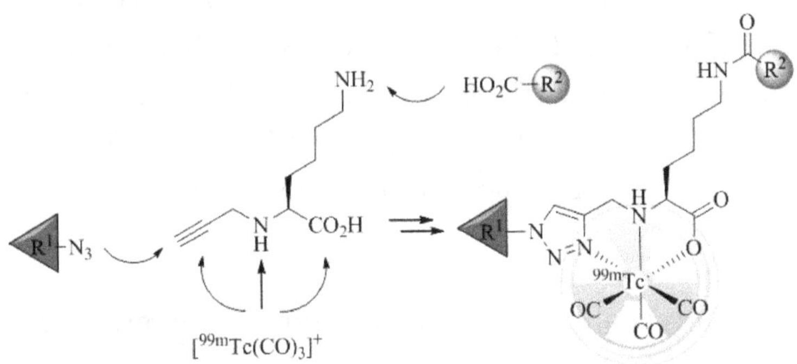

2. Experimental Section

2.1. General Procedures

General procedures, solvents, chemicals, synthesis equipment, analytic instruments (HPLC, MS, NMR, gamma counter) were previously described [10,27]. The "CRS Isolink kit" (Center for Radiopharmaceutical Science, Paul Scherrer Institute, Villigen, Switzerland) was used for the preparation of the precursor $[^{99m}Tc(CO)_3(H_2O)_3]^+$. For analytical separation, a C12 reversed-phase column Phenomenex Jupiter 4u Proteo 90 Å, 4 µm, 250 × 4.6 mm (column A) was used and preparative purification was performed on a Macherey Nagel Nucleodur C18 ISIS, 5 µm, 250 × 16 mm (column B). HPLC solvents were 0.1% trifluoroacetic acid (TFA) in water (A) and 0.1% TFA in acetonitrile (B). Quality control of (radio) metal-labeled peptides was performed using column A and a linear gradient from 80% A to 50% A in 20 min with a flow rate of 1.5 mL/min, or a linear gradient from 80% A to 60% A in 20 min. Peptide purification was performed using column B and different linear gradients with a flow rate of up to 8 mL/min. The observed *m/z* correspond to the monoisotopic ions. Chemical shifts are reported in parts per million (ppm) and coupling constants (*J*) in Hertz (Hz) from high to low field. Standard abbreviations indicating multiplicity are singlet (s), doublet (d), doublet of doublets (dd), triplet (t), and multiplet (m).

2.2. Synthetic Procedures

2.2.1. Organic Synthesis

N(α)Boc-*N*(α)propargyl-Lys(OMe) **1** was synthesized in five steps from commercial BocLysOMe according to published procedures [28]. Subsequently, succinic anhydride (2 equiv. 2.22 mmol) was coupled to *N*(α)Boc-*N*(α)propargyl-Lys(OMe)*HCl (**1**, 370 mg, 1.11 mmol) *via* amide bond formation in CH_2Cl_2 under basic conditions (*i*-Pr_2NEt; 6 equiv.) for two hours at rt (Scheme 1). The reaction mixture was concentrated under reduced pressure and the crude product was dissolved in ethyl acetate. The organic phase was extracted with citric acid (0.1 M) and saturated sodium hydrogen carbonate. The organic layer was disposed. The hydrogen carbonate phase was acidified with hydrogen chloride (5%) under stirring and extracted twice with fresh ethyl acetate. The organic phases were combined, dried over magnesium sulfate, and concentrated under reduced pressure to yield compound **2a** as a pale yellowish oil (435.3 mg, 91%; see Scheme 1). For characterization purposes, the Boc protecting group of **2a** was removed (CH_2Cl_2/TFA, 2:1; 5 h; rt) and the product was analyzed as its TFA salt **2b**; ^{1}H-NMR (400 MHz, MeOH-d_4; recorded after completed H/D exchange): δ = 4.10 (dd, 1H, J = 7.0 Hz, J = 5.0 Hz), 3.96 (dd, 1H, J = 16.6 Hz, J = 2.5 Hz), 3.92 (dd, 1H, J = 16.6 Hz, J = 2.5 Hz), 3.79 (s, 3H), 3.18 (t, 1H, J = 2.5 Hz), 3.12 (m, 2H), 2.52 (t, 2H, J = 6.9 Hz), 2.38 (t, 2H, J = 6.9 Hz), 1.97–1.85 (m, 2H), 1.51–1.44 (m, 2H), 1.43–1.25 (m, 2H) ppm; ^{13}C-NMR (MeOH-d_4): δ = 176.42, 174.81, 170.19, 162.22 (TFA, q, $J_{C\text{-}F}$: 35.7 Hz), 117.86 (TFA, q, $J_{C\text{-}F}$: 290.7 Hz), 79.87, 74.28, 60.07, 54.05, 39.65, 36.61, 31.65, 30.39, 29.99, 29.92, 22.99 ppm; ESI-HRMS ($C_{14}H_{23}N_2O_5$): $[M+H]^+$ *m/z*: 299.16019 (calcd. 299.16013).

Scheme 1. Synthesis of central lysine-based precursor. (a) see reference [28]; (b) succinic anhydride, *i*-Pr_2NEt, CH_2Cl_2, 2 h, rt.

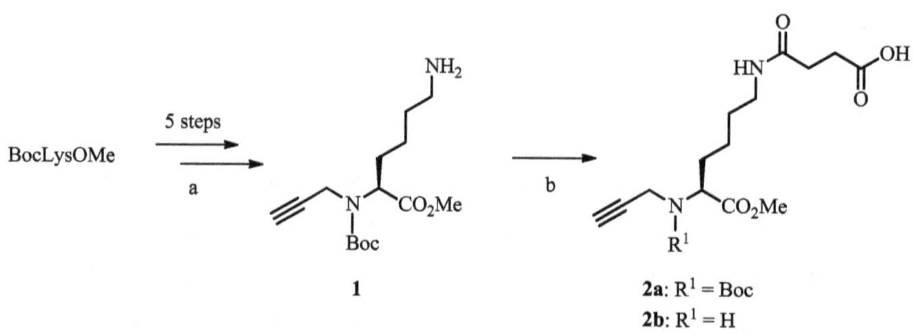

Solid-phase peptide synthesis (SPPS; scale: 0.03–0.25 mmol) was performed as described earlier [10,27]. Side-chain protected Fmoc-amino acids were Cys(Trt), Gln(Trt), His(Trt), Lys(Boc), Ser(tBu), and Trp(Boc). Azide-functionalized bombesin derivative **3** was synthesized according to the literature [10]. The different protected shepherdin peptide sequences [21,24] obtained by SPPS (**4**–**7**; 0.03–0.06 mmol) were subsequently coupled manually *via* selective amide bond formation to the central lysine precursor **2a** on solid support in the presence of HATU (2–3 equiv.) and *i*-Pr_2NEt (5–6 equiv.) in DMF for 2 h at rt. After the coupling was completed, removal of protecting groups and cleavage of the peptides were done with a solution of trifluoroacetic acid, phenol, water, and triisopropylsilane (0.5–1 mL; 87.5/5/5/2.5%) at rt for 2–8 h. The precipitated crude peptides were dissolved in water, purified by preparative HPLC, and lyophilized. Afterwards, selective methyl ester hydrolysis of intermediates was achieved with LiOH (0.5 M; 1–3 h, rt) following a procedure described by Reddy *et al.* [29]. After reactions were completed and the solutions were neutralized with HCl (0.5 M), the crude peptides **8–11** were obtained (see Scheme 2). Finally, the alkyne functionalized shepherdin derivatives **8–11** were reacted with the purified azidoacetic acid-functionalized bombesin sequence **3** according to published procedures [30] *via* the Cu(I)-catalyzed alkyne-azide cycloaddition (CuAAC) [31,32] in solution. In brief, stoichiometric amounts of alkyne-shepherdin peptides **8–11** and azido-BBS peptide **3** (2 μmol) were dissolved in DMSO (400 μL) under an argon atmosphere and a freshly prepared Cu(I) solution was added (60 μL; 3 equiv.), prepared by mixing a $CuSO_4$ pentahydrate solution (0.2 M, 30 μL) with an sodium ascorbate solution (0.4 M, 30 μL) on ice. The reaction was allowed to stir for 1 h at rt and completion of the reaction was checked by analytical HPLC. The click products were purified by preparative HPLC and lyophilized to obtain the final peptide conjugates **12–15** (see Table 1 and Scheme 2). Reference compound **16** (see Scheme 2) was synthesized as described earlier [10].

Scheme 2. Synthesis of peptides and assembly of (radio)metal-labeled, multifunctional conjugates.

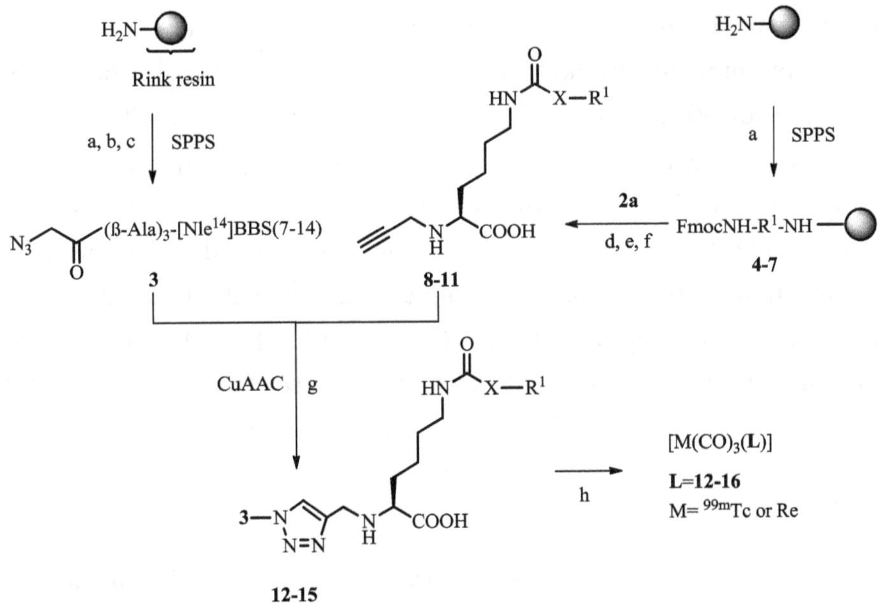

compound (*:protected AA)	X	R^1	
4*,8,12	$-CH_2CH_2CO-$	-KHSSGCAFL	shepherdin[79-87]
5*,9,13	$-CH_2CH_2CO-$	-SKLACFSHG	scrambled shepherdin[79-87]
6*,10,14	$-CH_2CH_2CO-$	-KHSSG	shepherdin[79-83]
7*,11,15	$-CH_2CH_2CO-$	-SGKHS	scrambled shepherdin[79-83]
16	-	CH_3	reference compound

(a) SPPS: (i) piperidine in DMF; (ii) Fmoc-amino acids, TBTU-HOBt, (b) azidoacetic acid, HATU; (c) cleavage solution: trifluoroacetic acid, phenol, water, triisopropylsilane (87.5/5/5/2.5%), 2–5 h, rt; (d) SPPS: **2a**, HATU, (e) cleavage solution, 2–8 h, rt; (f) LiOH (0.5 M), 1–3 h, rt; (g) CuAAC in solution; $CuSO_4$ (0.2 M), Na-ascorbate (0.4 M), 1 h, rt; (h) (radio)metal labeling; for M=^{99m}Tc: **12–16** (0.1 mM, aq.), $[^{99m}Tc(CO)_3(H_2O)_3]^+$, 100 °C, 30 min; for Re complexes: **12–16** (0.4 mM, aq.), $[Et_4N]_2[Re(CO)_3(Br)_3]$, 100 °C, 60 min; AA = amino acid.

Table 1. Analytical data and yields of synthesized peptides and ^{nat}Re-complexes thereof.

Compound	MALDI-MS; *m/z* (observed)	Yield [%]	Purity [%] [c]
12	$[M+H]^+$: 2432.23 (calcd.: 2432.24)	31 [a]	92.9
13	$[M+H]^+$: 2432.18 (calcd.: 2432.24)	10 [a]	95.3
14	$[M+H]^+$: 1998.01 (calcd.: 1998.04)	17 [a]	98.3
15	$[M+H]^+$: 1998.03 (calcd.: 1998.04)	18 [a]	97.5
16	$[M+H]^+$: 1458.75 (calcd.: 1458.80)	23 [a]	97.6
$[Re(CO)_3(12)]$	$[M+H]^+$: 2700.10 (calcd.: 2700.17)	quant. [b]	>98
$[Re(CO)_3(13)]$	$[M+H]^+$: 2700.16 (calcd.: 2700.17)	quant. [b]	>98
$[Re(CO)_3(14)]$	$[M+H]^+$: 2265.95 (calcd.: 2265.97)	quant. [b]	>98
$[Re(CO)_3(15)]$	$[M+H]^+$: 2265.93 (calcd.: 2265.97)	quant. [b]	>98
$[Re(CO)_3(16)]$	$[M+H]^+$: 1712.7 (calcd.: 1712.71)	quant. [b]	>98

[a] overall yield of isolated conjugates; [b] conversion of starting material (HPLC); [c] determined by HPLC; for reference compound **16** see reference [10].

2.2.2. (Radio)Metal Labeling of Peptides

$Na[^{99m}TcO_4]$ was eluted from a Mallinckrodt $^{99}Mo/^{99m}Tc$ generator, and the precursor $[^{99m}Tc(CO)_3(H_2O)_3]^+$ was prepared by adding $[^{99m}TcO_4]^-$ (1.5–2 GBq) to the "CRS Isolink kit for tricarbonyl" and heating for 30 min at 100 °C. Aliquots of 1 mM stock solutions of peptides **12–16** in water (10 μL, 10 nmol) were added to a solution of $[^{99m}Tc(CO)_3(H_2O)_3]^+$ (~100 MBq; 0.1 mM final peptide concentration) and the reaction mixtures were heated at 100 °C for 30 min. Quality controls were performed by radio-HPLC to determine the radiochemical yield and purity of $[^{99m}Tc(CO)_3(\mathbf{L})]$ (L = **12–16**). For characterization purposes, the peptides were labeled with cold ^{nat}Re. In brief, aliquots of aqueous stock solutions of peptides **12–16** (30–100 μL, 1 mM) were added to a solution of $[Et_4N]_2[Re(CO)_3(Br)_3]$ [33] (50–150 μL, 1 mM) and heated for one hour at 100 °C [10]. The rhenium-complexes were purified by HPLC and analyzed by MS (see Table 1).

2.3. LogD Determinations

The hydrophilicity of the radiolabeled peptides **12–16** was evaluated by determination of their partition coefficient between *n*-octanol and phosphate buffered saline (PBS, pH 7.4) using the shake flask method [27]. In brief, 10 μL (1 μM) of radiolabeled peptides **12–16** were added to a pre-saturated solution of *n*-octanol and PBS (1:1, 1 mL) and the tubes were vortexed (1 min) and centrifuged (3,000 rpm, 10 min). Aliquots of 100 μL of each phase were radiometrically measured in a gamma counter and the logD values were calculated by the logarithm of the ratio between the radioactive counts in the octanol fraction and the radioactive counts in the PBS fraction. The experiment was performed 2–3 times, each in quintets, and results are reported by mean values ± standard deviation (SD).

2.4. In Vitro Experiments

Cell culturing of human Caucasian prostate adenocarcinoma (PC-3) cells and *in vitro* assays (internalization, receptor saturation binding, and externalization) were performed as previously described [10,27] and are thus described only in brief.

2.4.1. Internalization Assay

For the determination of cellular uptake, PC-3 cells were incubated with the radiolabeled peptides [^{99m}Tc(CO)$_3$(**L**)] (**L** = **14–16**; 0.25 pmol; 1.5–2.0 kBq/well) for different time points to allow binding and internalization. Non-specific receptor binding and internalization was determined by incubating the cells with excess of natural bombesin(1–14) as a receptor blocking agent. At each time point, the supernatant was collected, representing the free radiopeptide fraction. The cell surface receptor bound fraction was obtained by treating the cells with an acidic saline glycine buffer (100 mM NaCl, 50 mM glycine, pH 2.8; 2 times for 5 min, on ice). The internalized fraction was determined by cell lysis with 1 M NaOH (10 min). Fractions of free, receptor-bound, and internalized radiopeptide were radiometrically measured in the gamma counter and calculated as percentage of applied dose normalized to 10^6 cells for all time points (n = 2–3 in triplicates, reported by means ± SD) [10]. To verify whether specific uptake was influenced by the shepherdin sequence, internalization experiments were also conducted with excess shepherdin(79–87) (AnaSpec Inc., Fremont, CA, USA) as a blocking agent.

2.4.2. Receptor Saturation Binding Assay

PC-3 cells were incubated with increasing concentrations (0.1–100 nM/well) of the radiolabeled peptides [^{99m}Tc(CO)$_3$(**L**)] (L = **14–16**) at 4 °C for 2 h. Non-specific binding was determined in the presence of excess of natural bombesin(1–14) as described above. Fractions of free and receptor-bound radioconjugates were radiometrically measured in the gamma counter for quantification and apparent binding dissociation constants ($K_{d,\,app}$) were calculated (n = 2–4 in triplicates, reported by means ± SD) [10].

2.4.3. Externalization Assay

PC-3 cells were incubated with the radiolabeled peptides [^{99m}Tc(CO)$_3$(**L**)] (**L** = **14–16**; 2.5 pmol; 14–21 kBq/well) for one hour to allow cell internalization. The free and receptor-bound radiopeptide fractions were removed as described above, fresh cell culture medium was added, and the cells were incubated for different time points (10–300 min). At each time-point, the externalized fractions were collected and the medium replaced. The remaining internalized amount of radioactivity was recovered by cell lysis. All fractions were radiometrically measured and calculated as percentage of the total internalized fraction (n = 4–7 in triplicates, reported by means ± SD) [10].

3. Results and Discussion

The syntheses of building blocks and multifunctional conjugates are depicted in Schemes 1 and 2. *N*(α)Boc-*N*(α)propargyl-Lys(OMe) (**1**) was synthesized from commercial BocLysOMe in five steps according to previously published procedures [28]. Reaction of compound **1** with succinic anhydride provided intermediate **2a** appropriately functionalized with a carboxylic acid functionality for conjugation reactions *via* amide bond formation. Shepherdin derivatives **4–7** [21,24] were synthesized by automated solid-phase peptide synthesis (SPPS) using Fmoc-chemistry. Compounds **5** and **7** with a scrambled amino acid sequences were prepared for control experiments. Peptides **4–7** were coupled to the Lys precursor **2a** on solid support, cleaved from the resin, and fully deprotected under standard conditions.

Subsequent hydrolyses of the methyl ester of intermediates with LiOH provided alkyne-derivatized peptides **8–11**. The corresponding CuAAC reaction partner, N-terminally functionalized azido-(βAla)$_3$[Nle^{14}]BBS(7–14) **3**, was obtained by similar SPPS procedures [10]. A (βAla)$_3$ spacer was introduced at the N-terminus of peptide **3** in order to prevent potential interference between the different moieties of the final multifunctional conjugate [9,10]. Reaction of alkyne-bearing shepherdin derivatives **8–11** and azido-BBS **3** by CuAAC in solution afforded final peptide conjugates **12–15**. For a side-by-side comparison, reference conjugate **16**, identical in all respects but lacking a shepherdin moiety (replaced by a methyl group; Scheme 2) was used, the synthesis and characterization of which has been previously described [10]. For analytical data of products see Table 1.

Radiolabeling of the triazole-containing peptide conjugates with ^{99m}Tc-tricarbonyl was achieved following established procedures reported by us and others [10,28,34]. In brief, heating of aqueous solutions of 1,2,3-triazole containing peptide conjugates **12–16** with $[^{99m}Tc(CO)_3(H_2O)_3]^+$ yielded the corresponding radiolabeled compounds [^{99m}Tc(CO)$_3$(**L**)] (**L** = **12–16**) in >95% radiochemical yield and purity and with a specific activity of up to 100 GBq/μmol. As common practice for the identification and characterization of n.c.a. (no carrier added) ^{99m}Tc-labeled compounds, the corresponding non-radioactive analogous compounds [^{nat}Re(CO)$_3$(**L**)] (**L** = **12–16**) were also prepared by reaction of conjugates **12–16** with $[Et_4N]_2[Re(CO)_3(Br)_3]$ [33] (for MS data see Table 1). Direct comparison of the UV-HPLC traces of the rhenium tricarbonyl complexes with the corresponding γ-HPLC traces of ^{99m}Tc-tricarbonyl complexes confirmed in each case their identity (see Supplementary Information).

Already at this stage we recognized a high and persistent unspecific binding of conjugate [^{99m}Tc(CO)$_3$(**12**)] containing the full length shepherdin(79–87) sequence to material used as well as cell surfaces. In particular, the unspecific binding of [^{99m}Tc(CO)$_3$(**12**)] impeded with *in vitro* assays regardless of precautions taken (e.g., using prelubricated disposables, the addition of solvents (e.g., DMSO or EtOH), or varying the composition and ionic strength of the media; data not shown). We therefore focused henceforth on radioconjugates containing the truncated shepherdin(79–83) sequence for which unspecific binding was not an issue. Thus, the physico-chemical properties of compounds [^{99m}Tc(CO)$_3$(**L**)] (**L** = **14,15**) were evaluated in comparison to reference compound [^{99m}Tc(CO)$_3$(**16**)].

The lipophilicity of the conjugates was determined by the shake flask method. LogD values obtained ranged from -1.70 ± 0.13 and -1.68 ± 0.08 for compounds [^{99m}Tc(CO)$_3$(**14**)] and [^{99m}Tc(CO)$_3$(**15**)], respectively, which indicates an improved hydrophilicity in comparison to the reference compound [^{99m}Tc(CO)$_3$(**16**)] (logD = -0.44 ± 0.07).

BBS-shepherdin conjugate [^{99m}Tc(CO)$_3$(**14**)], its analog with the scrambled amino acid sequence [^{99m}Tc(CO)$_3$(**15**)], and reference compound [^{99m}Tc(CO)$_3$(**16**)] exhibited similar cell internalization profiles into GRP-r overexpressing PC-3 cells in terms of extent and rate of uptake (Figure 2). Approximately 25%–30% of the applied radioactivity was internalized within 30–60 min, which is comparable to related bombesin derivatives labeled with the ^{99m}Tc-tricarbonyl core described by us and others [10,35]. Cell internalization was not influenced by the addition of shepherdin(79–87) and receptor-specific uptake was verified for all compounds by blocking experiments in the presence of excess natural bombesin(1-14) (data not shown).

Figure 2. Receptor specific internalization of radiometal conjugates in PC-3 cells, overexpressing GRP-receptor; [^{99m}Tc(CO)$_3$(**14**)] (□, continuous line), [^{99m}Tc(CO)$_3$(**15**)] (Δ, dotted line), [^{99m}Tc(CO)$_3$(**16**)] (○, continuous line); normalized to 10^6 cells per well; n = 2–3 (in triplicates, reported by means ± SD, calculated by non-linear regression using GraphPad Prism 5.0).

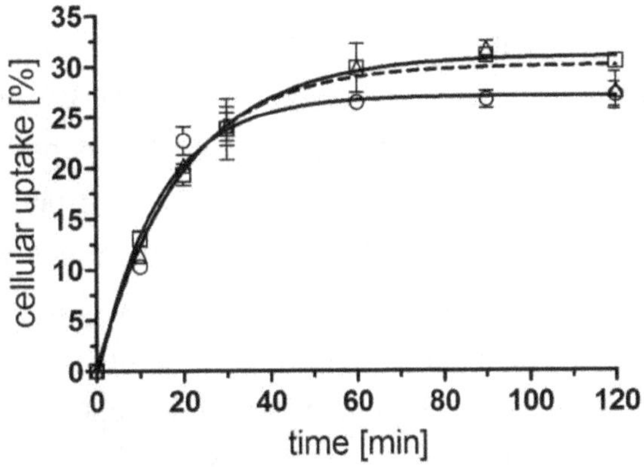

Binding affinities of radiolabeled conjugates [^{99m}Tc(CO)$_3$(**L**)] (**L** = **14**–**16**) towards the GRP-r were investigated by receptor binding saturation assays (Figure 3). All three derivatives showed high affinities towards GRP-r. Compared to reference compound [^{99m}Tc(CO)$_3$(**16**)] with an apparent dissociation constant ($K_{d,\,app}$) of 5.6 ± 0.8 nM, dual-targeting BBS-shepherdin conjugate [^{99m}Tc(CO)$_3$(**14**)] revealed a slightly decreased receptor binding affinity ($K_{d,\,app}$ = 10.9 ± 0.7 nM) as did its scrambled version [^{99m}Tc(CO)$_3$(**15**)] ($K_{d,\,app}$ = 11.3 ± 2.2 nM). K_d values of receptor-specific radiopeptides in the low two-digit nanomolar range are still considered appropriate for applications *in vivo* [36,37].

Figure 3. Specific receptor saturation binding to PC-3 cells; [^{99m}Tc(CO)$_3$(**14**)] (□, continuous line), [^{99m}Tc(CO)$_3$(**15**)] (Δ, dotted line), [^{99m}Tc(CO)$_3$(**16**)] (○, continuous line); normalized to 10^6 cells per well; n = 2–3 (in triplicates, reported by means ± SD, and calculated by non-linear regression using GraphPad Prism 5.0).

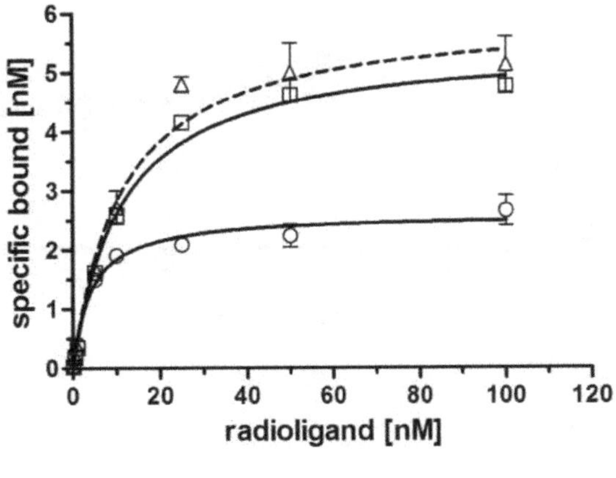

After having verified the specificity and affinity of the radioconjugates for their tumor-specific, extracellular target (GRP-r), we next set out to study the effect of the conjugated shepherdin moiety with regards to the cellular retention of radioactivity. Unexpectedly, the externalization profiles of the three radioconjugates [^{99m}Tc(CO)$_3$(**L**)] (**L** = **14**–**16**) were comparable (Figure 4). A washout of 50% of the initially internalized radioactivity was observed within approximately 90 min for all conjugates. Thus, the additional shepherdin moiety of [^{99m}Tc(CO)$_3$(**14**)] did not lead to an improved cellular retention of radioactivity in comparison to compounds [^{99m}Tc(CO)$_3$(**L**)] (**L** = **15**–**16**). These results were puzzling because of the reported high affinity (80 nM) and specificity of shepherdin(79–83) and peptide conjugates thereof towards Hsp90 [20,21], the expression of which in PC-3 cells was verified by western blot experiments (data not shown). A potential explanation for our findings might include the possibility of endosomal entrapment of the conjugate as a consequence of endocytotic cell internalization, which in turn would prevent interactions of [^{99m}Tc(CO)$_3$(**14**)] with its cytosolic target Hsp90 [12,15,38]. Alternatively, enzymatic degradation of the peptidic radioconjugate within the intracellular endosome-lysosome cascade could result in the destruction of the shepherdin moiety and thus, loss of its specificity towards Hsp90 [15,38,39]. In either case, the intracellular fate of receptor-specific (radio)conjugates after cell internalization by endocytosis is generally not well understood in detail. There are recent reports suggesting solutions to overcome issues of endosomal entrapment including examples of the application of biomimetic peptides [40], cleavable linkers [41,42], and synthetic polymers [15]. In addition, reported non-peptidic inhibitors of Hsp90 [43] could be employed in order to address potential issues of the stability of the Hsp90-specific peptide moieties described herein. To address the challenging goal of improving the cellular retention of radioactivity after receptor-specific delivery to cancer cells by peptidic radiotracers, future research efforts will be directed towards the combination of our conjugates with the strategies outlined above.

Figure 4. Externalization of radiolabeled compounds [^{99m}Tc(CO)$_3$(**L**)] (**L** = **14**–**16**) from PC-3 cells; [^{99m}Tc(CO)$_3$(**14**)] (□, continuous line), [^{99m}Tc(CO)$_3$(**15**)] (Δ, dotted line), [^{99m}Tc(CO)$_3$(**16**)] (○, continuous line); n = 4–7 (in triplicates, reported by means ± SD; calculated by non-linear regression using GraphPad Prism 5.0).

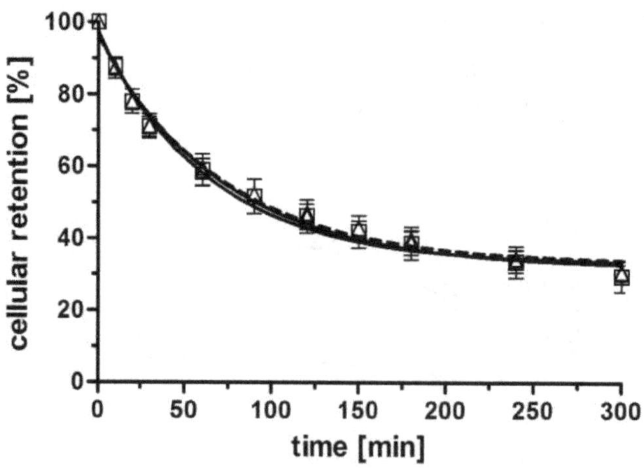

4. Conclusions

We herein report the synthesis and *in vitro* evaluation of bombesin-shepherdin conjugates radiolabeled with the ^{99m}Tc-tricarbonyl core by the "click-to-chelate" strategy. The multifunctional radioconjugates were designed for a combined extra- and intracellular targeting in order to improve the cellular retention of radioactivity after its receptor-specific delivery to cancerous cells. While the specificity of the radioconjugates towards the extracellular target (GRP-r) could be confirmed, the cellular externalization of radioactivity was not improved. The combination of extra- and intracellular targeting entities in a multifunctional radioconjugate represents a novel and innovative approach with potential to improve the efficacy of radiotracers provided that issues such as endosomal entrapment and lysosomal degradation can be addressed.

Acknowledgments

We thank Dieter Staab, Kayhan Akyel, and Ingo Muckenschnabel (Novartis Institutes for Biomedical Research, Basel, Switzerland) for assistance with NMR and MS analysis, Matthias Wymann and Mirjam Zimmermann (Department of Biomedicine, University of Basel, Switzerland), Nicole Hustedt (Friedrich Miescher Institute for Biomedical Research, Basel, Switzerland), Andreas Bauman, and Ibai Valverde (University of Basel Hospital, Radiopharmaceutical Chemistry, Basel, Switzerland) for scientific discussions and technical assistance.

Author Contributions

Christiane A. Fischer carried out the syntheses, characterization, radiolabeling, and *in vitro* evaluations of the conjugates. Sandra Vomstein supported *in vitro* assays. Corresponding author Thomas L. Mindt supervised the project. The manuscript was written by Thomas L. Mindt and Christiane A. Fischer.

References

1. Reubi, J.C. Peptide receptors as molecular targets for cancer diagnosis and therapy. *Endocr. Rev.* **2003**, *24*, 389–427.
2. Correia, J.D.G.; Paulo, A.; Raposinho, P.D.; Santos, I. Radiometallated peptides for molecular imaging and targeted therapy. *Dalton Trans.* **2011**, *40*, 6144–6167.
3. Fani, M.; Mäcke, H.R.; Okarvi, S.M. Radiolabeled peptides: Valuable tools for the detection and treatment of cancer. *Theranostics* **2012**, *2*, 481–501.
4. Schottelius, M.; Wester, H.-J. Molecular imaging targeting peptide receptors. *Methods* **2009**, *48*, 161–177.
5. Raposinho, P.D.; Correia, J.D.G.; Alves, S.; Botelho, M.F.; Santos, A.C.; Santos, I. A $^{99m}Tc(CO)_3$-labeled pyrazolyl-α-melanocyte-stimulating hormone analog conjugate for melanoma targeting. *Nucl. Med. Biol.* **2008**, *35*, 91–99.
6. Ginj, M.; Hinni, K.; Tschumi, S.; Schulz, S.; Mäcke, H.R. Trifunctional somatostatin-based derivatives designed for targeted radiotherapy using auger electron emitters. *J. Nucl. Med.* **2005**, *46*, 2097–2103.
7. García-Garayoa, E.; Bläuenstein, P.; Blanc, A.; Maes, V.; Tourwé, D.; Schubiger, P.A. A stable neurotensin-based radiopharmaceutical for targeted imaging and therapy of neurotensin receptor-positive tumours. *Eur. J. Nucl. Med. Mol. Imaging* **2009**, *36*, 37–47.

8. Kunstler, J.-U.; Veerendra, B.; Figueroa, S.D.; Sieckman, G.L.; Rold, T.L.; Hoffman, T.J.; Smith, C.J.; Pietzsch, H.-J. Organometallic ^{99m}Tc(III) '4+1' bombesin(7–14) conjugates: Synthesis, radiolabeling, and *in vitro/in vivo* studies. *Bioconjug. Chem.* **2007**, *18*, 1651–1661.
9. García-Garayoa, E.; Rüegg, D.; Bläuenstein, P.; Zwimpfer, M.; Khan, I.U.; Maes, V.; Blanc, A.; Beck-Sickinger, A.G.; Tourwé, D.A.; Schubiger, P.A. Chemical and biological characterization of new $Re(CO)_3$/[^{99m}Tc]$(CO)_3$ bombesin analogues. *Nucl. Med. Biol.* **2007**, *34*, 17–28.
10. Kluba, C.A.; Bauman, A.; Valverde, I.E.; Vomstein, S.; Mindt, T.L. Dual-targeting conjugates designed to improve the efficacy of radiolabeled peptides. *Org. Biomol. Chem.* **2012**, *10*, 7594–7602.
11. Esteves, T.; Marques, F.; Paulo, A.; Rino, J.; Nanda, P.; Smith, C.J.; Santos, I. Nuclear targeting with cell-specific multifunctional tricarbonyl M(I) (M is Re, ^{99m}Tc) complexes: Synthesis, characterization, and cell studies. *J. Biol. Inorg. Chem.* **2011**, *16*, 1141–1153.
12. Zelenka, K.; Borsig, L.; Alberto, R. Metal complex mediated conjugation of peptides to nucleus targeting acridine orange: A modular concept for dual-modality imaging agents. *Bioconjug. Chem.* **2011**, *22*, 958–967.
13. Zhou, Z.; Wagh, N.K.; Ogbomo, S.M.; Shi, W.; Jia, Y.; Brusnahan, S.K.; Garrison, J.C. Synthesis and *in vitro* and *in vivo* evaluation of hypoxia-enhanced ^{111}In-bombesin conjugates for prostate cancer imaging. *J. Nucl. Med.* **2013**, *54*, 1605–1612.
14. Ross, M.F.; Filipovska, A.; Smith, R.A.J.; Gait, M.J.; Murphy, M.P. Cell-penetrating peptides do not cross mitochondrial membranes even when conjugated to a lipophilic cation: Evidence against direct passage through phospholipid bilayers. *Biochem. J.* **2004**, *383*, 457–468.
15. Cornelissen, B. Imaging the inside of a tumour: A review of radionuclide imaging and theranostics targeting intracellular epitopes. *J. Label. Compd. Radiopharm.* **2014**, *57*, 310–316.
16. Lindquist, S.; Craig, E.A. The heat-shock proteins. *Annu. Rev. Genet.* **1988**, *22*, 631–677.
17. Whitesell, L.; Lindquist, S.L. HSP90 and the chaperoning of cancer. *Nat. Rev. Cancer* **2005**, *5*, 761–772.
18. Li, Y.; Zhang, T.; Schwartz, S.J.; Sun, D. New developments in Hsp90 inhibitors as anti-cancer therapeutics: Mechanisms, clinical perspective and more potential. *Drug Resist. Update* **2009**, *12*, 17–27.
19. Altieri, D.C. Survivin, cancer networks and pathway-directed drug discovery. *Nat. Rev. Cancer* **2008**, *8*, 61–70.
20. Fortugno, P.; Beltrami, E.; Plescia, J.; Fontana, J.; Pradhan, D.; Marchisio, P.C.; Sessa, W.C.; Altieri, D.C. Regulation of survivin function by Hsp90. *Proc. Natl. Acad. Sci. USA* **2003**, *100*, 13791–13796.
21. Plescia, J.; Salz, W.; Xia, F.; Pennati, M.; Zaffaroni, N.; Daidone, M.G.; Meli, M.; Dohi, T.; Fortugno, P.; Nefedova, Y.; *et al.* Rational design of shepherdin, a novel anticancer agent. *Cancer Cell* **2005**, *7*, 457–468.
22. Xiaojiang, T.; Jinsong, Z.; Jiansheng, W.; Chengen, P.; Guangxiao, Y.; Quanying, W. Adeno-associated virus harboring fusion gene NT4-ant-shepherdin induce cell death in human lung cancer cells. *Cancer Invest.* **2010**, *28*, 465–471.
23. Siegelin, M.D.; Plescia, J.; Raskett, C.M.; Gilbert, C.A.; Ross, A.H.; Altieri, D.C. Global targeting of subcellular heat shock protein-90 networks for therapy of glioblastoma. *Mol. Cancer Ther.* **2010**, *9*, 1638–1646.

24. Gyurkocza, B.; Plescia, J.; Raskett, C.M.; Garlick, D.S.; Lowry, P.A.; Carter, B.Z.; Andreeff, M.; Meli, M.; Colombo, G.; Altieri, D.C. Antileukemic activity of shepherdin and molecular diversity of Hsp90 inhibitors. *J. Natl. Cancer I.* **2006**, *98*, 1068–1077.
25. Mindt, T.L.; Struthers, H.; Brans, L.; Anguelov, T.; Schweinsberg, C.; Maes, V.; Tourwé, D.; Schibli, R. "Click to chelate": Synthesis and installation of metal chelates into biomolecules in a single step. *J. Am. Chem. Soc.* **2006**, *128*, 15096–15097.
26. Kluba, C.A.; Mindt, T.L. Click-to-Chelate: Development of technetium and rhenium-tricarbonyl labeled radiopharmaceuticals. *Molecules* **2013**, *18*, 3206–3226.
27. Valverde, I.E.; Bauman, A.; Kluba, C.A.; Vomstein, S.; Walter, M.A.; Mindt, T.L. 1,2,3-Triazoles as amide bond mimics: Triazole scan yields protease-resistant peptidomimetics for tumor targeting. *Angew. Chem. Int. Ed.* **2013**, *52*, 8957–8960.
28. Mindt, T.L.; Struthers, H.; Spingler, B.; Brans, L.; Tourwé, D.; García-Garayoa, E.; Schibli, R. Molecular assembly of multifunctional ^{99m}Tc radiopharmaceuticals using "clickable" amino acid derivatives. *ChemMedChem.* **2010**, *5*, 2026–2038.
29. Reddy, D.S.; Vander Velde, D.; Aubé, J. Synthesis and conformational studies of dipeptides constrained by disubstituted 3-(aminoethoxy)propionic acid linkers. *J. Org. Chem.* **2004**, *69*, 1716–1719.
30. Valverde, I.E.; Lecaille, F.; Lalmanach, G.; Aucagne, V.; Delmas, A.F. Synthesis of a biologically active triazole-containing analogue of cystatin a through successive peptidomimetic alkyne–azide ligations. *Angew. Chem. Int. Ed.* **2012**, *51*, 718–722.
31. Rostovtsev, V.V.; Green, L.G.; Fokin, V.V.; Sharpless, K.B. A Stepwise huisgen cycloaddition process: Copper(I)-catalyzed regioselective "ligation" of azides and terminal alkynes. *Angew. Chem. Int. Ed.* **2002**, *41*, 2596–2599.
32. Tornøe, C.W.; Christensen, C.; Meldal, M. Peptidotriazoles on solid phase: [1,2,3]-Triazoles by regiospecific copper(I)-catalyzed 1,3-dipolar cycloadditions of terminal alkynes to azides. *J. Org. Chem.* **2002**, *67*, 3057–3064.
33. Alberto, R.; Egli, A.; Abram, U.; Hegetschweiler, K.; Gramlich, V.; Schubiger, P.A. Synthesis and reactivity of $[NEt_4]_2[ReBr_3(CO)_3]$. Formation and structural characterization of the clusters $[NEt_4][Re_3(\mu_3\text{-OH})(\mu\text{-OH})_3(CO)_9]$ and $[NEt_4][Re_2(\mu\text{-OH})_3(CO)_6]$ by alkaline treatment. *J. Chem. Soc. Dalton Trans.* **1994**, *19*, 2815–2820.
34. Alberto, R.; Ortner, K.; Wheatley, N.; Schibli, R.; Schubiger, A.P. Synthesis and properties of boranocarbonate: A convenient in situ CO source for the aqueous preparation of $[^{99m}Tc(OH_2)_3(CO)_3]^+$. *J. Am. Chem. Soc.* **2001**, *123*, 3135–3136.
35. Schweinsberg, C.; Maes, V.; Brans, L.; Bläuenstein, P.; Tourwé, D.A.; Schubiger, P.A.; Schibli, R.; García-Garayoa, E. Novel glycated $[^{99m}Tc(CO)_3]$-labeled bombesin analogues for improved targeting of gastrin-releasing peptide receptor-positive tumors. *Bioconjug. Chem.* **2008**, *19*, 2432–2439.
36. Smith-Jones, P.M.; Bischof, C.; Leimer, M.; Gludovacz, D.; Angelberger, P.; Pangerl, T.; Peck-Radosavljevic, M.; Hamilton, G.; Kaserer, K.; Kofler, A.; *et al.* DOTA-lanreotide: A novel somatostatin analog for tumor diagnosis and therapy. *Endocrinology* **1999**, *140*, 5136–5148.

37. Virgolini, I.; Angelberger, P.; Li, S.; Yang, Q.; Kurtaran, A.; Raderer, M.; Neuhold, N.; Kaserer, K.; Leimer, M.; Peck-Radosavljevic, M.; *et al.* *In vitro* and *in vivo* studies of three radiolabelled somatostatin analogues: ^{123}I-octreotide (OCT), ^{123}I-Tyr-3-OCT and ^{111}In-DTPA-D-Phe-1-OCT. *Eur. J. Nucl. Med.* **1996**, *23*, 1388–1399.

38. Grady, E.F.; Slice, L.W.; Brant, W.O.; Walsh, J.H.; Payan, D.G.; Bunnett, N.W. Direct observation of endocytosis of gastrin releasing peptide and its receptor. *J. Biol. Chem.* **1995**, *270*, 4603–4611.

39. Delom, F.; Fessart, D. Role of phosphorylation in the control of clathrin-mediated internalization of GPCR. *Int. J. Cell Biol.* **2011**, *2011*, 246954.

40. Liang, W.; Lam, J.K.W. Endosomal escape pathways for non-viral nucleic acid delivery systems. In *Molecular Regulation of Endocytosis*; Ceresa, B., Ed., 2012; pp. 421–467.

41. Vlahov, I.R.; Leamon, C.P. Engineering folate–drug conjugates to target cancer: from chemistry to clinic. *Bioconjug. Chem.* **2012**, *23*, 1357–1369.

42. Leriche, G.; Chisholm, L.; Wagner, A. Cleavable linkers in chemical biology. *Bioorg. Med. Chem.* **2012**, *20*, 571–582.

43. Patel, H.J.; Modi, S.; Chiosis, G.; Taldone, T. Advances in the discovery and development of heat-shock protein 90 inhibitors for cancer treatment. *Expert Opin. Drug Discov.* **2011**, *6*, 559–587.

5

Development and Successful Validation of Simple and Fast TLC Spot Tests for Determination of Kryptofix® 2.2.2 and Tetrabutylammonium in ^{18}F-Labeled Radiopharmaceuticals

Matthias Kuntzsch [1], Denis Lamparter [1], Nils Brüggener [1], Marco Müller [2], Gabriele J. Kienzle [1] and Gerald Reischl [1,*]

[1] Department of Preclinical Imaging and Radiopharmacy, Eberhard Karls University Tübingen, Röntgenweg 15, Tübingen D-72076, Germany;
E-Mails: matthias.kuntzsch@med.uni-tuebingen.de (M.K.); lamparter_d@ukw.de (D.L.); nils.brueggener@med.uni-tuebingen.de (N.B.); gabriele.kienzle@med.uni-tuebingen.de (G.J.K.)

[2] Department of Radiochemistry, ABX GmbH, Heinrich-Gläser-Straße 10, Radeberg D-01454, Germany; E-Mail: marco.mueller@abx.de

* Author to whom correspondence should be addressed; E-Mail: gerald.reischl@uni-tuebingen.de

---

Abstract: Kryptofix® 2.2.2 (Kry) or tetrabutylammonium (TBA) are commonly used as phase transfer catalysts in ^{18}F-radiopharmaceutical productions for positron emission tomography (PET). Due to their toxicity, quality control has to be performed before administration of the tracer to assure that limit concentration of residual reagent is not reached. Here, we describe the successful development and pharmaceutical validation (for specificity, accuracy and detection limit) of a simplified color spot test on TLC plates. We were able to prove its applicability as a general, time and resources saving, easy to handle and reliable method in daily routine analyzing ^{18}F-tracer formulations for Kry (in [^{18}F]FDG or [^{18}F]FECh) or TBA contaminations (in [^{18}F]FLT) with special regard to complex matrix compositions.

Keywords: Kryptofix® 2.2.2; tetrabutylammonium; fluorine-18; quality control; thin layer chromatography (TLC) spot test

---

1. Introduction

Production of ^{18}F-radiopharmaceuticals is most commonly done by labeling the respective precursor with [^{18}F]fluoride via nucleophilic substitution. [^{18}F]Fluoride is a cyclotron produced radionuclide (nuclear reaction: $^{18}O(p,n)^{18}F$) from [^{18}O]water. To assure reactivity of the [^{18}F]fluoride, it is regularly dried azeotropically and phase transfer catalysts need to be added to enhance nucleophilicity of the anion. Most prominent example for this approach is the synthesis of 2-deoxy-2-[^{18}F]fluoro-*D*-glucose ([^{18}F]FDG) introduced by Hamacher *et al.* [1].

Kryptofix® 2.2.2 (Kry), a crown ether, is one of the most widely used among the phase transfer reagents, another one is tetrabutylammonium (TBA; added e.g., as hydroxide, carbonate or hydrogen carbonate). Radiopharmaceutical formulations have to be analyzed for residual contaminations with these reagents before human application, due to their toxicity (e.g., Kry: LD_{50} (i.v.) in rodents = 32–35 mg/kg [2]). For Kry, limit in European Pharmacopoeia (Ph. Eur.) is 2.2 mg/V (*i.e.*, patient dose; see monograph for [^{18}F]FDG {#1325; fludeoxyglucose (^{18}F) injection} and other ^{18}F-radiopharmaceuticals: [^{18}F]FLT {#2460; 3'-deoxy-3'-[^{18}F]fluorothymidine}, [^{18}F]FMISO {#2459; [^{18}F]fluoromisonidazole} [3]), in US Pharmacopoeia (USP) limit is <50 µg/mL [4]. For TBA in ^{18}F-radiopharmaceuticals a limit of 2.6 mg/V is defined in Ph. Eur. (see same monographs as for Kry). Ph. Eur. suggests a color spot test on a thin layer chromatography (TLC) plate for Kry and a HPLC method for TBA in ^{18}F-radiopharmaceutical monographs (see above).

In the past, various procedures have been described in the literature for identification and quantification of Kry, with the aim of providing specific and fast methods. TLC procedures are the most widespread, as they do not require sophisticated instrumental equipment. A color spot test on a TLC plate as used in monographs with iodoplatinate [5] for staining was described by Mock *et al.* [6]. To increase specificity and avoid false positive (e.g., from other amines) or false negative results (from stabilizers) thin layer chromatography systems were developed [7–10]. But also gas chromatography (GC; [11]), high-performance liquid chromatography (HPLC; [12]) or liquid chromatography-tandem mass spectrometry (LC/MS/MS; [13]) and even NMR or IR spectroscopy [14] were applied. More recently, a very fast (<1 min) and highly sensitive (lower limit = 0.5 ng/mL) rapid-resolution liquid chromatography MS/MS coupled system for analysis of Kry was published [15]. Still, these methods suffer from certain disadvantages. The latter (GC, LC, MS, NMR, IR) need high-quality instrumental equipment combined with a higher effort for validation. On the other hand, TLC tests are more time consuming due to development of plates or require the expensive reagent iodoplatinate. In addition, in our opinion to prove that in a certain radiopharmaceutical formulation the Kry (or TBA) content is below a defined limit—without the necessity of exact quantification, the test should be as simple and quick as possible, but nevertheless meeting pharmaceutical requirements. This particularly holds true in view of the fact that all literature data agree that, when synthesis and purification were performed successfully, Kry or TBA residues were extremely low and far from limits. When any test for Kry (or TBA) is applied to a newly produced radiopharmaceutical, it will always need some kind of validation, no matter how specific the test proved to be so far. Matrix effects may play an important role, pH as well. The important factor is how much time and effort it will take in daily routine.

After first promising results with the TLC spot tests as will be described below for Kry and TBA, we set up validations regarding specificity, accuracy and detection limit for [^{18}F]FDG (Kry) and, to demonstrate a more general applicability, for 2-[^{18}F]fluoroethylcholine ([^{18}F]FECh; also Kry), where residual *N,N*-dimethylaminoethanol (DMAE) may interfere [16]. As the HPLC procedure for TBA analysis described in the monographs appeared to be challenging, the spot test was also to be validated for this reagent, with [^{18}F]FLT as example [17]. As an additional important parameter, the stability of the necessary standard solutions containing the limit concentrations of Kry or TBA should also be investigated.

2. Experimental

2.1. General

All reagents were of highest purity available or of pharmaceutical grade, where necessary (article numbers in brackets) and were used as received. From Merck (Darmstadt, Germany) were purchased: Ethanol (1.00983), hydrochloric acid (1.09137), iodine (1.04761), Kryptofix 2.2.2 (8.14925), methanol (1.06007), NaCl (1.06404), $NaH_2PO_4 \cdot 2H_2O$ (1.06345), NaOH (1.06482), NH_4OH (25% in water; 1.05432) and trisodium-citrate (1.06448). TLC silica plates were from Macherey-Nagel (Düren, Germany, 805021), water for injection (WFI) was from Fresenius Kabi (Bad Homburg, Germany, 1636065), disodium-hydrogencitrate (35,908-4) and DMAE (391263) from Aldrich (Steinheim, Germany) and tetrabutylammonium hydroxide 30-hydrate from Sigma (Steinheim, Germany, 86859). Sterile phosphate buffered saline (PBS) was provided from the University pharmacy.

2.2. Syntheses of [^{18}F]FDG, [^{18}F]FECh and [^{18}F]FLT

N.c.a. [^{18}F]fluoride was produced at the PETtrace cyclotron (GE Healthcare, Uppsala, Sweden), via the $^{18}O(p,n)^{18}F$ nuclear reaction by irradiating 2.5 mL of >95% enriched [^{18}O]water (Rotem, Be'er Sheva, Israel) with 16.5 MeV protons in a niobium target body with Havar® foils. Products from automated syntheses were used as samples in the described validations. [^{18}F]FDG was produced on a TRACERlab MX synthesizer (GE Healthcare), cassettes were from Rotem (Israel) and reagent kits from ABX (Radeberg, Germany) with the standard method supplied from GE except that the final volume was increased to 20 mL by addition of water for injection and 90 µL of ethanol for stabilization. The final matrix of the [^{18}F]FDG formulation was a citrate buffer (specification limits pH 5.0–8.0; normally a pH value of 5.5–6.0 is found) containing a specified amount of ethanol with limits of 2000–5000 mg/L. [^{18}F]FECh was produced on a modified TRACERlab FX F_N synthesizer (GE Healthcare) yielding 13 mL of [^{18}F]FECh in a PBS buffer (pH 7.4). Synthesis of [^{18}F]FLT was performed on TRACERlab MX with cassettes, synthesis software sequence and reagent kits from ABX. Here, the final formulation was again a citrate buffer (21 mL; nominal pH 5.0), containing 10% of ethanol.

2.3. Solutions for the Validation of Kryptofix 2.2.2 in [^{18}F]FDG

(a) Matrix buffers: The buffers contained salt concentrations as in [^{18}F]FDG formulations, *i.e.*, 0.6% NaCl and 0.7% disodium-hydrogencitrate in water for injection. pH was 5.0 ± 0.2 or was adjusted to pH 6.0 ± 0.2 with 1 N NaOH. Solutions were stored at 2.0–8.0 °C for a maximum of one week.

(b) [^{18}F]FDG solutions were stored at 2.0–8.0 °C for a maximum of 2 days.
(c) Kry stock solutions: An appropriate amount of Kry was added to either matrix buffer pH 5.0 or pH 6.0 to give Kry concentrations of 100 mg/L Kry (pH 5.0), 1000 mg/L (pH 5.0) and 1000 mg/L (pH 6.0). These 3 stock solutions were stored at room temperature.
(d) Kry standard solutions: From the stock solutions 1000 mg/L Kry (either pH 5.0 or pH 6.0) series of standard solutions were prepared with Kry concentrations of 3.1, 6.25, 12.5, 25, 50, 75, 100 and 125 mg/L.
(e) To 900 µL of [^{18}F]FDG solution 100 µL of the 1000 mg/L (pH 5.0) Kry solution were added to obtain a standard of 100 mg/L Kry in [^{18}F]FDG.

Solutions (c)–(e) had a shelf life of 1 day.

2.4. Solutions for the Validation of Kryptofix 2.2.2 in [^{18}F]FECh

As matrix buffer PBS was used (pH 7.4). When necessary, pH was adjusted to pH 6.5 using a 10% solution of NaH_2PO_4. Solutions of Kry in PBS or [^{18}F]FECh solution were prepared similarly to the ones in the [^{18}F]FDG validation, containing 100 mg/L Kry (pH 7.4 or 6.5) as well as solutions of 200 mg/L DMAE in PBS or [^{18}F]FECh solution. Series of standard solutions were prepared with Kry concentrations of 3.1, 6.25, 12.5, 25, 50, 75, 100 and 125 mg/L in PBS (pH 7.4 or 6.5).

2.5. Solutions for the Validation of Tetrabutylammonium in [^{18}F]FLT

(a) Matrix buffer: The buffer was prepared to obtain salt concentrations as in [^{18}F]FLT formulations, *i.e.*, 1.10 g disodium-hydrogencitrate-1.5-hydrate, 6.28 g trisodium-citrate-2-hydrate, 3.78 g NaCl, 8.69 mL of 1 N HCl and 100 mL of ethanol (absolute) were dissolved in water for injection to give a volume of 1000 mL, resulting in pH 5.0 ± 0.2.
(b) From a stock solution of 10,000 mg/L tetrabutylammonium hydroxide 30-hydrate in matrix buffer, standard solutions were prepared with concentrations of 40, 45, 55, 70, 85, 100 and 115 mg/L of TBA.
(c) Solutions for validation of pH dependence (pH: 4.5, 5.0, 6.0, 7.0, 8.0) were prepared from solutions (b) (pH 5.0) adding either 1 N NaOH or 1 N HCl.
(d) [^{18}F]FLT solutions were used as synthesized or tetrabutylammonium hydroxide 30-hydrate was added to give concentrations of 45 mg/L or 100 mg/L TBA.
(e) MeOH and NH_4OH (25% in water) were mixed in a relation of 90:10 (v/v).

2.6. TLC Procedure for Analysis of Kry

Spots of 2 µL samples were applied on silica plates by means of an Eppendorf micro pipette. It proved to be mandatory that the tip slightly touched the plate and allowed the liquid to drain slowly and penetrate the silica material without any active pressure from the pipette. Plates were immediately placed on a holder inside a glass chamber for 10 min above iodine (*ca.* 5 g) covering the complete bottom of the vessel, homogenously saturating the whole chamber with iodine vapor. Plates were photographed for documentation (PowerShot SX110 IS, macro mode; jpg files, Canon, Krefeld, Germany) and visually analyzed. All experiments were $n = 3$.

2.7. TLC Procedure for Analysis of TBA

Spots of 2 μL samples were applied on silica plates by means of an Eppendorf micro pipette, in analogy to Kry analysis, in addition it was essential that only two spots per plate were applied. Otherwise time was to long between first and last spot application and results were invalid. Spots needed to be ca. 10 mm from the edges of the plate. After drying of spots with a cool air stream (hair dryer) 10 μL of the MeOH/NH_4OH solution were applied on each spot. Plates were then placed in the same iodine containing chamber as for Kry, for exactly 1 min. Afterwards, plates were photographed immediately for documentation and visually analyzed (before discoloration). All experiments were $n = 3$.

3. Results and Discussion

TLC spot tests were validated as quality control methods to assure that residual contaminations of Kry ([^{18}F]FDG, [^{18}F]FECh) or TBA ([^{18}F]FLT) in ^{18}F-radiopharmaceutical formulations were below the limits required by e.g., Ph. Eur. Objectives of the validation experiments were specificity, accuracy and detection limit. Moreover, stability of standard solutions for routine quality control was evaluated. Validations had to be performed individually for each radiopharmaceutical, taking into account that determination of either Kry or TBA may be matrix dependent. All experiments were performed in triplicate.

3.1. Validation of Kry in [^{18}F]FDG Formulation

Concentrations of 100 mg/L of Kry were used either in matrix or [^{18}F]FDG solutions, in accordance with requirements of current Ph. Eur. [3]. The limit defined in the Pharmacopoeia is 2.2 mg/V, *i.e.*, per patient. The maximum volume in our case that could theoretically be injected in one patient is 20 mL, resulting in a calculated limit concentration of 110 mg/L. Our specification of <100 mg/L is more narrowly defined. For determination of the detection limit of the method additional solutions with concentrations from 3.1 to 125 mg/L were used. After staining with iodine, background on the plates showed an orange, light brown color. Spots of solutions containing Kry were dark brown with a diameter of 1–2 mm. In first experiments, the standard solution was prepared in WFI instead of citrate buffer. But it could be shown that as result spots were darker and of a smaller diameter. Therefore, Kry standard solutions are always prepared using buffer, to have most comparable conditions. Also, in preliminary tests it was shown that the intensity of the color of the Kry spot was dependent on the pH value of the test solution. At pH 5.0, intensity was lower than at higher pH. Therefore, buffers of standard solutions were adjusted to pH 5.0, representing the most unfavorable case. In general, content of residual Kry in [^{18}F]FDG solutions (>100 productions) was far below the limit of 100 mg/L. Only in cases where pH of a solution was 6.0 or higher and the spot of the batch sample was of similar or higher intensity than the standard solution (100 mg/L; pH 5.0) there would be uncertainty. Then, the standard solution would need to be adjusted to the pH of this batch sample and the test to be repeated, to prove that Kry concentration of the batch solution was below the specified limit.

To test for the specificity of the method, [^{18}F]FDG solutions and plain matrix buffers (pH 5.0 and 6.0) were investigated. With matrix buffers no coloration of the spots was visible, with [^{18}F]FDG a very weak, diffuse, light brown spot developed that was completely different from Kry spots from standard solutions (Figure 1a,b). Comparison of standard solutions of 100 mg/L of Kry in either [^{18}F]FDG solution or matrix buffer (pH 6.0) showed small, dark spots of comparable intensity (Figure 1b). Third, the two series of standard solutions (pH 5.0 and pH 6.0) with Kry concentrations of 3.1, 6.25, 12.5, 25, 50, 75, 100 and 125 mg/L were investigated (Figure 1c). Within both series spots differing in concentrations by a factor of 2 could be distinguished. As already shown in the preliminary tests, spots from a certain concentration at pH 6.0 corresponded to spots from the series at pH 5.0 with twice the concentration.

Figure 1. Validation of the TLC spot test for Kry in [^{18}F]FDG: **(a)** Test for specificity. TLC plate after iodine staining, samples (n = 3) are without Kry. 1. row: [^{18}F]FDG solution; 2. row: citrate matrix buffer (pH 5.0); 3. row: citrate matrix buffer (pH 6.0); **(b)** Test for Specificity. Samples (n = 3) of 100 mg/L Kry in either [^{18}F]FDG solution (1. row) or citrate buffer matrix (pH 6.0; 2. row); **(c)** Test for specificity and detection limit. Samples of Kry standard solutions with concentrations of 3.13, 6.25, 12.5, 25, 50, 75, 100 and 125 mg/L in buffer matrix (from left to right; 1. row: pH 5.0; 2. row: pH 6.0; n = 3; one example shown); **(d)** Test for Accuracy. Comparison of samples (n = 3) of 100 mg/L Kry in matrix (pH 5.0; 1. row); [^{18}F]FDG solution and 100 mg/L Kry added (pH 5.0; 2. row) and pure [^{18}F]FDG solution (3. row).

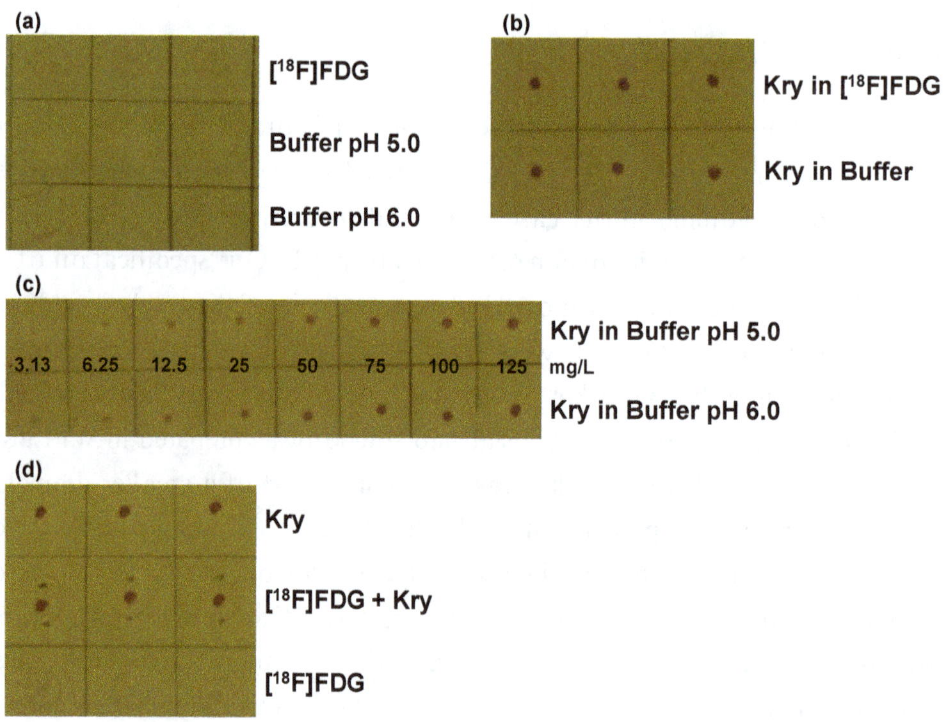

From the same set of experiments the detection limit of the method was identified to be 6.25 mg/L, from a clearly visible spot. For proving the accuracy of the method, three types of spots were compared (Figure 1d): Kry in buffer (100 mg/L; spot 1), spot 2 was from 2 μL of [^{18}F]FDG solution, after drying for 10 s with a hair dryer 2 μL of Kry in buffer (100 mg/L) were added on top and spot 3 was from pure [^{18}F]FDG solution. On one TLC plate buffer of pH 5.0 was used (spots 1 and 2), on a second plate buffer of pH 6.0 was applied. Independent from pH value spots 3 were hardly visible, whereas spots 1 and 2 showed same shape and intensity. The results from these validations met the defined specifications from the respective validation plan, proving the applicability of the described TLC method as test for residual Kry in [^{18}F]FDG formulations, regarding specificity, accuracy and detection limit.

For routine quality control it was decided to use a standard solution containing 100 mg/L of Kry in matrix buffer pH 5.0, which then is tested against the individual [^{18}F]FDG batch. This standard solution is prepared as large batch and stored in portions of 1 mL in small glass vials at <−15 °C. In frame of the validation the stability of the standard solution was evaluated after 2 weeks, 1 month, 3 months and 6 months by comparison with a freshly mixed solution. 3 different batches of standard solution were prepared. These stability studies demonstrated that spots from stored solutions showed no difference to spots from fresh solutions. Consequently, the shelf life of the Kry standard solution was specified to be 6 months.

3.2. Validation of Kry in [^{18}F]FECh Formulation

Validation was performed in a similar way as for [^{18}F]FDG, regarding specificity, accuracy, detection limit and stability of standard solutions. Kry standard solutions had the same concentration of 100 mg/L as limit, as there is no monograph for [^{18}F]FECh yet available. Calculating from our batch volume of 13 mL that might be injected in a patient, a limit concentration of 169 mg/L would result (2.2 mg/V). Like for [^{18}F]FDG, our limit is narrower. Besides the difference in matrix buffer ([^{18}F]FDG: citrate, ethanol as stabilizer *vs.* [^{18}F]FECh: PBS), [^{18}F]FECh formulations may also contain residual DMAE (specified limit: 200 mg/L), which may interfere with the test and indeed preliminary experiments showed light brownish coloration of spots from DMAE. Secondly, as in the [^{18}F]FDG validation a pH dependence of the test was shown (lower pH values resulted in spots of a less intense color) and here, the specifications for [^{18}F]FECh are pH 6.5–8.5 (PBS has a pH of 7.4) the same effect might occur here as well. Consequently, in a comparative study solutions at pH of 6.5 and pH 7.4 needed to be validated as well.

In general, coloration of plates and spots was similar to the [^{18}F]FDG validation. Specificity of the test was proven comparing matrix buffer, [^{18}F]FECh solution, 200 mg/L DMAE in buffer and 200 mg/L DMAE in [^{18}F]FECh solution *vs.* 100 mg/L Kry in matrix buffer standard solution. All spots from samples without Kry were much less intensive (Figure 2a), demonstrating especially that the disturbing effect of DMAE is negligible. Secondly, spots from solutions of 100 mg/L Kry in matrix buffer or [^{18}F]FECh solution were dark brown and of same intensity (Figure 2b). Thirdly, using the solutions from the second experiment, but adjusted to pH 6.5 gave again for 100 mg/L Kry in buffer or [^{18}F]FECh solution, spots of same intensity (plates not shown). And finally, two series of standard solutions (pH 6.5 and 7.4) with Kry concentrations of 3.1, 6.25, 12.5, 25, 50, 75, 100 and 125 mg/L in PBS were investigated (Figure 2c). In both series differences in concentration by a factor of 2 were clearly visible. Intensities of spots were similar for same concentrations, showing that at least at the investigated pH values no pH dependence of the test could be observed. pH 8.5 (upper specification limit of [^{18}F]FECh formulation) was not investigated, as (if at all) spots should be more intensive at higher pH (see [^{18}F]FDG), resulting in a false result of a Kry concentration higher than the real value, which is uncritical from a pharmaceutical point of view.

Figure 2. Validation of the TLC spot test for Kry in [^{18}F]FECh: (**a**) Test for specificity. 1. row: PBS buffer (pH 7.4); 2. row: [^{18}F]FECh solution; 3. row: 200 mg/L DMAE in PBS; 4. row: 200 mg/L DMAE in [^{18}F]FECh solution; 5. row: 100 mg/L Kry in PBS (n = 3); (**b**) Test for specificity. Samples (n = 3) of 100 mg/L Kry in either [^{18}F]FECh solution (1. row) or PBS (2. row); (**c**) Test for specificity and detection limit. Samples of Kry standard solutions with concentrations of 3.13, 6.25, 12.5, 25, 50, 75, 100 and 125 mg/L in PBS (from left to right; 1. row: pH 7.4; 2. row: pH 6.5; n = 3; one example shown); **(d)** Test for Accuracy. Comparison of samples (n = 3) of 100 mg/L Kry in PBS (pH 7.4; 1. row); [^{18}F]FECh solution with 100 mg/L Kry added (pH 7.4; 2. row) and pure [^{18}F]FECh solution (3. row).

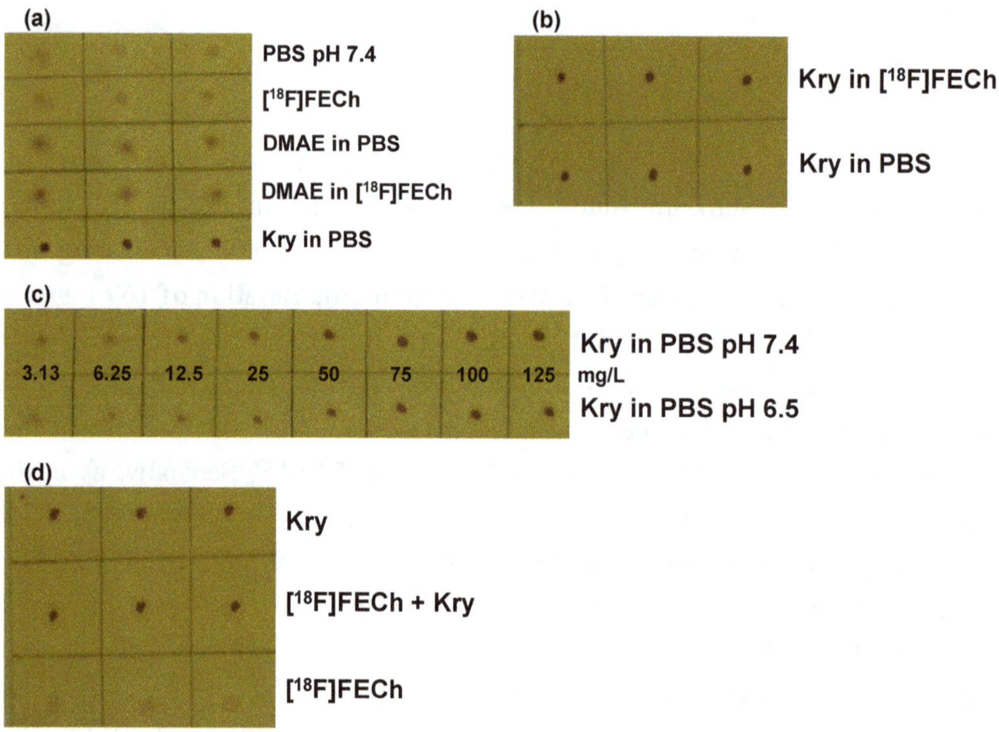

For defining the detection limit the series of Kry concentrations (Figure 2c) were analyzed. The spot from the Kry concentration of 12.5 mg/L was clearly visible, detection limit was therefore well below the specified nominal value of "≤50 mg/L". Compared to the [^{18}F]FDG validation, detection limit was higher for Kry in [^{18}F]FECh solutions.

Accuracy of the method was again proven by comparing spots of 100 mg/L Kry in matrix buffer (1); [^{18}F]FECh solution, drying, addition of 100 mg/L Kry in buffer (2) and as spot 3 [^{18}F]FECh solution was applied. Experiments were again performed at pH 6.5 and 7.4, showing no pH dependence. In both cases spots 3 showed minimum coloration, spots 1 and 2 were of same intensity (Figure 2d). Overall, validation was performed successfully, clearly demonstrating the feasibility of this TLC spot test.

Stability of the standard solution to be used in routine quality control (100 mg/L Kry in PBS matrix buffer, pH 7.4), stored in 1 mL portions at <−15 °C was proven to be 6 months (three different batches; performance as in [^{18}F]FDG validation).

3.3. Validation of TBA in [^{18}F]FLT Formulation

After the successful application of the TLC spot test for detection of Kry in [^{18}F]FDG or [^{18}F]FECh solution, now it was investigated, if this test was also valid for detection of TBA in [^{18}F]FLT formulation. From first tests it was obvious that before staining with iodine, 10 µL of MeOH/NH_4OH (90:10 *v/v*) must be applied on each spot to detect TBA and development times in the iodine chamber had to be 1 min. [^{18}F]FLT solution was a citrate buffer like [^{18}F]FDG formulation, but containing ca. 10% of ethanol (*v/v*) in contrast to [^{18}F]FDG with only *ca.* 0.3% of ethanol (*v/v*). Preliminary experiments showed no influence of ethanol content on the test. Again, pH dependence needed to be tested, as the TBA standard solution was planned to have a pH of 5.0, specification for [^{18}F]FLT formulation is pH 4.5–8.0.

To meet Ph. Eur. requirements for the limit of TBA impurities in ^{18}F-radiopharmaceuticals (2.6 mg/V) the general standard solution contained 100 mg/L TBA, as the maximum volume in our case is 21 mL, *i.e.*, the calculated limit from Ph. Eur. would be 124 mg/L. For determination of the detection limit and to see what differences in concentrations could be differentiated, series of solutions were prepared with TBA concentrations of 40, 45, 55, 70, 85, 100 and 115 mg/L. After iodine staining, plates showed a yellow-grey color, spots of solutions containing TBA were dark brown (diameter of 1–2 mm surrounded by grey concentric circles). For validation of specificity matrix buffer solutions (pH 5.0 and pH 6.0), [^{18}F]FLT solutions and standard solutions containing 45 mg/L TBA (pH 5.0 and pH 6.0) were compared. Spots from matrix gave almost no coloration as well as [^{18}F]FLT solutions; but from standard solutions spots were clearly visible (Figure 3a). No pH dependence was observed. Standard solutions containing 45 mg/L TBA and [^{18}F]FLT solutions containing 45 mg/L TBA gave spots of same intensity (Figure 3b). Comparison of spots from the series of concentrations showed that only differences in concentrations of ≥60 mg/L could be visualized definitely and also that only spots on the same plate were comparable due to plate individual results of staining (Figure 3c). The spot from the standard solution of 40 mg/L of TBA was clearly visible and therefore this concentration was defined as detection limit (Figure 3c). Accuracy of the method could be demonstrated by comparing spots from TBA solutions (45 mg/L), spots from [^{18}F]FLT solutions (pure) and spots from [^{18}F]FLT solutions with TBA standard (45 mg/L) added. This set of experiments was performed with solutions at pH 5.0 and pH 6.0. No pH dependence was visible. Spots from [^{18}F]FLT solutions were hardly visible. Spots from solutions containing TBA were clearly visible and of same intensity (see examples in Figure 3a–c. To check for the pH dependence over the whole range of specification, standard solutions with 100 mg/L of TBA and pH 4.5, 5.0, 6.0, 7.0, 8.0 were tested. No difference in intensity was visible at any pH value (plates not shown). These results demonstrated the applicability of the TLC spot test also for TBA in [^{18}F]FLT formulation. In analogy to [^{18}F]FDG and [^{18}F]FECh validations, stability of the standard solution for routine quality control (100 mg/L TBA in matrix buffer, pH 5.0), stored in 1 mL portions at <−15 °C was verified so far for up to 1 month.

Figure 3. Validation of the TLC spot test for TBA in [^{18}F]FLT: **(a)** Test for specificity (2 spots per plate; n = 3; one example shown). Upper plate: citrate buffer matrix (pH 5.0); middle plate: [^{18}F]FLT solution; lower plate: 45 mg/L TBA (left pH 5.0; right pH 6.0); **(b)** Test for specificity. Samples (example shown) of 45 mg/L TBA in either citrate buffer matrix (pH 5.0; left) or [^{18}F]FLT solution (right); **(c)** Test for specificity and detection limit. Examples for the comparison of samples of TBA standard solutions with concentrations of 40, 55, 70 and 100 mg/L in citrate buffer matrix (pH 5.0).

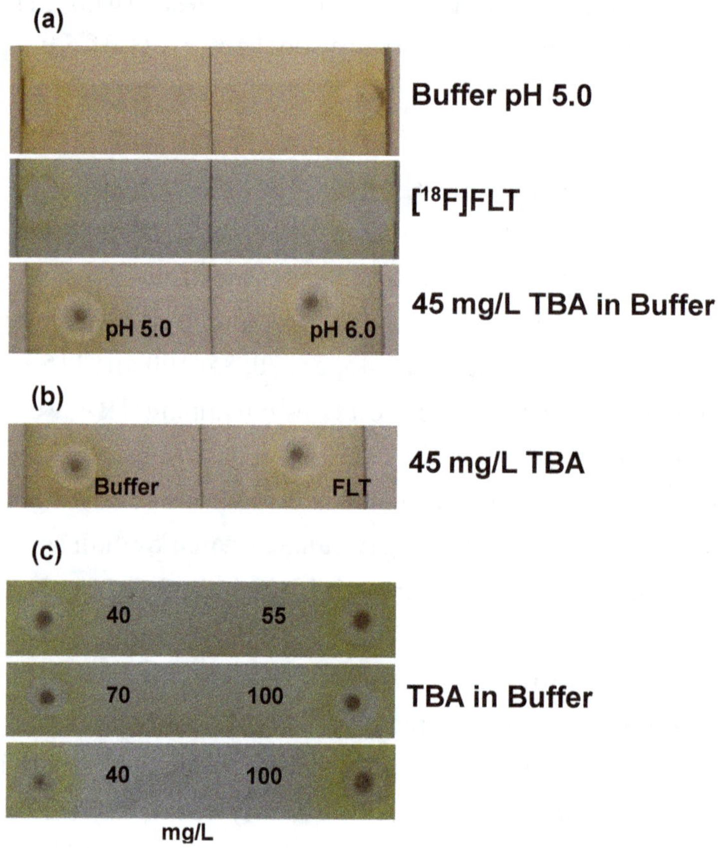

3.4. General Discussion

Overall, the presented and validated TLC spot test proved its capability for determination of residual Kry in [^{18}F]FDG and [^{18}F]FECh formulations with the perspective to become a general method. Indeed, validations have to be carried out for each tracer formulation and its individual matrix, as organic impurities (e.g., amines) might give false positive or stabilizers false negative results. So far, our results never showed disturbing interferences of major concern. No problems arose from neither ethanol nor residual DMAE (in [^{18}F]FECh solutions) or pH dependencies of spot intensities. Latter effect would lead to the necessity of pH adjustments of standard solutions for valid results of each batch in daily routine, but on the one hand residual Kry and also TBA concentrations close to the specified limits were never observed, normally they are not detectable—and detection limits are low. On the other hand, in the investigated radiopharmaceuticals (all in buffered solutions) alterations in pH values were minimal (Table 1).

Table 1. Compilation of parameters investigated and results in the described validations regarding specificity, accuracy and detection limit of the TLC spot test for residual Kry in [^{18}F]FDG and [^{18}F]FECh as well as TBA in [^{18}F]FLT.

Parameters	Kry in FDG	Kry in FECh	TBA in FLT
Nominal limit/mg/V [1] mg/L [2]	<2.2 <100	<2.2 <100	<2.6 <100
Specificity			
Color of spots for:			
Product solution	minimal	minimal	minimal
Matrix buffer	minimal	minimal	minimal
100 mg/L reagent solution	clearly visible	clearly visible	clearly visible
Intensity of spots of reagent in buffer or product solution comparable	YES	YES	YES
Distinguishability of spots with concentration difference of	Factor 2	Factor 2	≥60 mg/L
pH dependence	not relevant	NO	NO
Effect of ethanol	NO (0.3%) [3]	n. a.	NO (10%) [3]
Effect of DMAE	n. a.	minimal	n. a.
Accuracy			
Addition of reagent to product gives comparable spots to reagent in buffer	YES	YES	YES
Detection limit/mg/L	6.25	12.5	40
Reagent in matrix standard used in routine	100 mg/L pH 5.0	100 mg/L pH 7.4	100 mg/L pH 5.0
Stability (months at <−15°C)	6	6	1

[1] Ph. Eur.; [2] our institution; [3] ethanol concentration in brackets; n. a. = not applicable.

Whereas the test for Kry proved its robustness, the test for TBA reacted more sensitively to variations and instructions for performance of the test had to be followed strictly, like fast administration on plate, drying, time of development *etc.* Only two spots could be administered on one plate, to minimize time before iodine staining, otherwise results were erroneous. Only spots on one plate were comparable, which made validation laborious, but gives no problem in routine analysis, when only sample and standard solution are applied. Detection limit was higher for TBA than for Kry and concentrations of TBA spots that were to be compared needed to differ by 60 mg/L to give valid results. Still, these aspects are no problem for routine analysis, as TBA concentrations in [^{18}F]FLT formulations from routine production were found to be very low (see Figure 3a), and then determination of a concentration of "<100 mg/L" is reliably assured (Table 1).

This TLC spot test is designed to determine required limits to be met and not to absolutely quantify the concentration of Kry or TBA present, although this was possible for [^{18}F]FDG or [^{18}F]FECh. Nevertheless, in routine quality control for chemical impurities the specification "below limit" (e.g., "<100 mg/L") is absolutely sufficient and in conformity with Pharmacopoeia norms.

4. Conclusions

A TLC spot test for determination of residual Kry or TBA in ^{18}F-radiopharmaceutical formulations was successfully developed and formally validated for specificity, accuracy and detection limit for [^{18}F]FDG, [^{18}F]FECh (Kry) and [^{18}F]FLT (TBA). Interference with various matrix effects was negligible; the test is adequate, easy to handle, very fast and resources saving (no expensive reagents or HPLC system necessary). Now, it is already implemented in routine quality control of these three tracers in our institution, in case of [^{18}F]FDG it was formally accepted by authorities within our marketing license. With these positive results, the test is now under validation for further ^{18}F-radiopharmaceuticals.

Author Contributions

G.J.K. and G.R. designed the research. M.M. developed the TBA test. G.J.K. prepared the validation plans. M.K., D.L. and N.B. performed validations and summarized the validation reports. G.R. wrote the manuscript. All authors edited the manuscript.

References

1. Hamacher, K.; Coenen, H.H.; Stöcklin, G. Efficient stereospecific synthesis of no-carrier-added 2-[^{18}F]-fluoro-2-deoxy-D-glucose using aminopolyether supported nucleophilic substitution. *J. Nucl. Med.* **1986**, *27*, 235–238.
2. Baudot, P.; Jacque, M.; Robin, M. Effect of a diaza–polyoxa–macrobicyclic complexing agent on the urinary elimination of lead in lead poisoned rats. *Toxicol. Appl. Pharmacol.* **1977**, *41*, 113–118.
3. *The European Pharmacopoeia*, 8.0; European Directorate for the Quality of the Medicines (EDQM): Strassbourg, France, 2014.
4. *The United States Pharmacopoeia, USP-37, NF-32*; United States Pharmacopoeial Convention Inc.: Rockville, MD, USA, 2014.
5. Zweig, G.; Sherma, J. *CRC Handbook of Chromatography*; CRC Press: Cleveland, OH, USA, 1972; Volume II, p. 113.
6. Mock, B.H.; Winkle, W.; Vavrek, M.T. A color spot test for the detection of Kryptofix 2.2.2 in [^{18}F]FDG preparation. *Nucl. Med. Biol.* **1997**, *24*, 193–195.
7. Moerlein, S.M.; Brodack, J.W.; Siegel, B.A.; Welch, M.J. Elimination of contaminant Kryptofix 2.2.2 in the routine production of 2-[^{18}F]fluoro-2-deoxy-D-glucose. *Appl. Radiat. Isot.* **1989**, *40*, 741–743.
8. Chaly, T.; Dahl, J.R. Thin layer chromatographic detection of Kryptofix 2.2.2 in the routine synthesis of [^{18}F]2-fluoro-2-deoxy-D-glucose. *Int. J. Rad. Appl. Instrum. B* **1989**, *16*, 385–387.
9. Alexoff, D.L.; Fowler, J.S.; Gatley, S.J. Removal of the 2.2.2 Cryptand (Kryptofix 2.2.2^{TM}) from ^{18}FDG by cation exchange. *Appl. Radiat. Isot.* **1991**, *42*, 1189–1193.

10. Scott, P.J.; Kilbourn, M.R. Determination of residual Kryptofix 2.2.2 levels in [^{18}F]-labeled radiopharmaceuticals for human use. *Appl. Radiat. Isot.* **2007**, *65*, 1359–1362.
11. Ferrieri, R.A.; Schlyer, D.J.; Alexoff, D.L.; Fowler, J.S.; Wolf, A.P. Direct analysis of Kryptofix 2.2.2 in ^{18}FDG by gas chromatography using a nitrogen-selective detector. *Nucl. Med. Biol.* **1993**, *20*, 367–369.
12. Nakao, R.; Ito, T.; Yamaguchi, M.; Suzuki, K. Simultaneous analysis of FDG, ClDG and Kryptofix 2.2.2 in [^{18}F]FDG preparation by high-performance liquid chromatography with UV detection. *Nucl. Med. Biol.* **2008**, *35*, 239–244.
13. Ma, Y.; Huang, B.X.; Channing, M.A.; Eckelman, W.C. Quantification of Kryptofix 2.2.2 in 2-[^{18}F]FDG and other radiopharmaceuticals by LC/MS/MS. *Nucl. Med. Biol.* **2002**, *29*, 125–129.
14. Coenen, H.H.; Pike, V.W.; Stöcklin, G.; Wagner, R. Recommendation for a practical production of 2-[^{18}F]fluoro-2-deoxy-D-glucose. *Appl. Radiat. Isot.* **1987**, *38*, 605–610.
15. Lao, Y.; Yang, C.; Zou, W.; Gan, M.; Chen, P.; Su, W. Quantification of Kryptofix 2.2.2 in [^{18}F]fluorine-labelled radiopharmaceuticals by rapid-resolution liquid chromatography. *Nucl. Med. Commun.* **2012**, *33*, 498–502.
16. Kienzle, G.J.; Kuntzsch, M.; Reischl, G. Successful validation of a simple and fast determination of Kryptofix 2.2.2 in fludeoxyglucose(^{18}F) injection. *J. Labelled Compd. Radiopharm.* **2011**, *54*, S384.
17. Lamparter, D.; Kienzle, G.J.; Müller, M.; Reischl, G. Validation of a fast TLC determination of tetrabutylammonium (TBA) in fludeoxythymidine(^{18}F) injection. *J. Labelled Compd. Radiopharm.* **2013**, *56*, S484.

6

Synthesis and Preliminary Evaluation of a 2-Oxoquinoline Carboxylic Acid Derivative for PET Imaging the Cannabinoid Type 2 Receptor

Linjing Mu [1,*], Roger Slavik [2], Adrienne Müller [2], Kasim Popaj [1], Stjepko Čermak [2], Markus Weber [3], Roger Schibli [1,2], Stefanie D. Krämer [2] and Simon M. Ametamey [2]

[1] Center for Radiopharmaceutical Sciences of ETH-PSI-USZ, Department of Nuclear Medicine, University Hospital Zürich, CH-8091 Zürich, Switzerland

[2] Center for Radiopharmaceutical Sciences of ETH-PSI-USZ, Institute of Pharmaceutical Sciences, Department of Chemistry and Applied Biosciences, ETH Zurich, CH-8093 Zürich, Switzerland

[3] Neuromuscular Diseases Unit/ALS Clinic, Kantonsspital St. Gallen, CH-9007 St. Gallen, Switzerland

* Author to whom correspondence should be addressed; E-Mail: linjing.mu@usz.ch.

Abstract: Cannabinoid receptor subtype 2 (CB2) has been shown to be up-regulated in activated microglia and therefore plays an important role in neuroinflammatory and neurodegenerative diseases such as multiple sclerosis, amyotrophic lateral sclerosis and Alzheimer's disease. The CB2 receptor is therefore considered as a very promising target for therapeutic approaches as well as for imaging. A promising 2-oxoquinoline derivative designated KP23 was synthesized and radiolabeled and its potential as a ligand for PET imaging the CB2 receptor was evaluated. [^{11}C]KP23 was obtained in 10%–25% radiochemical yield (decay corrected) and 99% radiochemical purity. It showed high stability in phosphate buffer, rat and mouse plasma. In vitro autoradiography of rat and mouse spleen slices, as spleen expresses a high physiological expression of CB2 receptors, demonstrated that [^{11}C]KP23 exhibits specific binding towards CB2. High spleen uptake of [^{11}C]KP23 was observed in dynamic *in vivo* PET studies with Wistar rats. In conclusion, [^{11}C]KP23 showed promising *in vitro* and *in vivo* characteristics. Further evaluation with diseased animal model which has higher CB2 expression levels in the brain is warranted.

Keywords: cannabinoid receptor type 2 ligand; CB2 receptor; neurodegeneration; radiolabeling; autoradiography; small-animal PET

1. Introduction

The use of cannabis as a therapeutic agent dates back about 5,000 years with descriptions of its numerous effects including alterations in mood, cognitive functions, memory and perception of the user [1]. The plant cannabis sativa, commonly known as marijuana contains over 60 compounds. The major psychoactive constituent is delta-9-tetrahydrocannabinol (Δ^9-THC). Cannabinoids exert their effects through an endogenous cannabinoid system in the central and peripheral nervous system. Currently two subtypes of cannabinoid receptors have been isolated and cloned: CB1 and CB2. There is also some evidence that other cannabinoid receptors GPR18 and GPR55 may exist [2,3]. Not much is known about GPR18 and GPR55 subtypes and current research efforts in the field of cannabinoid receptors are directed towards exploring their pharmacology and physiological roles. The CB1 receptor is the most studied receptor of the endocannabinoid system and is densely expressed in the CNS by many classes of neurons [4,5]. The CB2 receptor on the other hand is found predominantly in cells of the immune system, spleen, lymph nodes but has very low or undetectable expression levels in the CNS under basal conditions [6,7]. Under pathological conditions, however, the CB2 receptor can be up-regulated on activated microglia (macrophages of the brain). It is well known that cannabinoid receptors are involved in a broad range of processes including appetite, anxiety, memory, cognition, immune regulation and inflammation [8], however, the function of CB2 in neuroinflammation, microglia activation and intrusion of immune cells is not yet fully understood. Visualization and quantification of CB2 receptor expression by non-invasive PET imaging provides a high potential for understanding the role of CB2 in the development and progression of neuroinflammatory and neurodegenerative diseases.

In the past decade, substantial progress has been made in the synthesis and evaluation of radiotracers for PET imaging of the CB1 receptor [9–11]. [^{18}F]MK-9470 has been used in the clinical setting to support CB1 receptor drug development for measuring receptor occupancy, to investigate CB1 receptor variability with gender and normal ageing and in studying pathophysiological conditions [12–14]. Although the pharmacological and therapeutic potential of selective CB2 ligands has been studied and reviewed extensively in the literature [15,16], the field of non-invasive CB2 imaging remains largely unexplored. Only a limited number of CB2 radioligands have been synthesized and tested as PET tracers [17–21], among them the 2-oxoquinoline-3-carboxamide derivative, [^{11}C]NE40, which has been evaluated in healthy volunteers. [^{11}C]NE40 exhibited the expected uptake in lymphoid tissue and appropriate brain kinetics [22]. Herein, we report the radiolabeling, *in vitro* and *in vivo* evaluation of a 2-oxoquinoline containing structure, [^{11}C]KP23, as a potential PET radiotracer for imaging cannabinoid type 2 receptors.

2. Experimental Section

2.1. Materials and Methods

Animal experiments were in accordance with the Swiss Animal Welfare legislation and were approved by the Veterinary Office of the Canton Zurich. Six week old female NMRI mice and male Wistar rats were purchased from Charles River (Sulzfeld, Germany) and kept under standard conditions.

All chemicals, unless otherwise stated, were purchased from Sigma-Aldrich (Zug, Switzerland) or Merck (Buchs, Switzerland) and used without further purification. Solvents for extractions, column chromatography and thin layer chromatography (TLC) were purchased as commercial grade. Organic reactions were monitored by TLC analysis using Sigma-Aldrich silica gel 60 plates (2−25 μm). Mobile phase for TLC was a mixture of pentane and ethyl acetate at suitable ratios. Developed TLCs were visualized under UV light at 254 nm. Nuclear magnetic resonance (NMR) spectra (^{1}H and ^{13}C-NMR) were recorded in Fourier transform mode at the field strength specified on Bruker Avance FT-NMR spectrometers. The measured chemical shifts are reported in δ (ppm) and the residual signal of the solvent was used as the internal standard. Multiplicities in the ^{1}H-NMR spectra are described as: s = singlet, d = doublet, t = triplet, m = multiplet, b = broad; coupling constants are reported in Hz. High resolution mass spectrometry (HRMS) was performed with a Bruker FTMS 4.7 T BioAPEXII spectrometer.

High-performance liquid chromatography (HPLC) analyses were performed using a reversed phase column (ACE column, C18, 3 μm). The mobile phase consisted of 0.1% TFA in water and acetonitrile. The acetonitrile gradient from 30% to 95% over 10 min at 1 mL/min flow rate was applied. Analytical radio-HPLC was performed on an Agilent 1100 series system equipped with a Raytest Gabi Star radiodetector (Agilent Technologies, Morges, Switzerland). Semi-preparative HPLC purifications were carried out using a reversed phase column (ACE column, Symmetry C8 5μm; 7.8 × 50 mm) under the following conditions: 0.1% H_3PO_4 in H_2O (solvent A), MeCN (solvent B); 0.0–1.0 min, 30% B; 1.1–12.0 min, 30%–90% B; 12.1–20 min, 90% B; 20.1–40 min, 30% B; flow rate: 4 mL/min. A Merck-Hitachi L2130 system equipped with a radiation detector VRM 202 (Veenstra Instrument, Joure, the Netherlands) was used for semi-preparative HPLC. Specific activity was calculated by comparing ultraviolet peak intensity of the final formulated products with calibration curves of corresponding non-radioactive standards of known concentrations. For the *in vitro* and *ex vivo* stability studies, an Ultra-performance liquid chromatography (UPLC™) system from Waters with a Waters Acquity UPLC BEH C18 column (2.1 × 50 mm, 1.7 μm) and an attached Berthold co-incidence detector (FlowStar LB513, Berthold Technologies, Bad Wildbad,) was used. The mobile phase consisted of a gradient of acetonitrile in water with 0.1% TFA from 10% to 95% over 2 min, flow rate 0.6 mL/min.

2.2. Chemistry

2.2.1. Synthesis of Compound **7** as Precursor for ^{18}F-Radiolabeling

To a solution of 8-butoxy-*N*-(2-hydroxy-2-phenylethyl)-7-methoxy-2-oxo-1,2-dihydroquinoline-3-carboxamide (**6**, 615 mg, 1.5 mmol) in dichloromethane (DCM, 5 mL) was added triethylamine

(300 mg, 3.0 mmol). The mixture was cooled to 0 °C in an ice-bath and a solution of methanesulfonyl chloride (205 mg, 1.8 mmol) in DCM (3 mL) was added dropwise. The mixture was stirred over night at RT. The reaction mixture was diluted with EtOAc (200 mL) and washed with 0.2 M aq. HCl (3 × 20 mL) and brine (2 × 10 mL). The organic layer was dried over Na_2SO_4 and solvents were removed under reduced pressure. The crude was purified over 100 g silica gel using EtOAc/Hexan 1:1 afforded 8-butoxy-*N*-(2-chloro-2-phenylethyl)-7-methoxy-2-oxo-1,2-dihydroquinoline-3-carboxamide (7, 263 mg, 0.614 mmol, 41% yield), but not the expected mesylated product. ^{1}H-NMR (400 MHz, $CDCl_3$): δ 10.00 (t, J = 5.7 Hz, 1H), 9.30 (s, 1H), 8.85 (s, 1H), 7.48–7.44 (m, 3H), 7.40–7.31 (m, 3H), 6.94 (d, J = 4.5 Hz, 1H), 5.15 (dd, J_1 = 5.4 Hz, J_2 = 8.5 Hz, 1H), 4.18–4.07 (m, 3H), 3.97 (s, 3H), 3.94–3.87 (m, 1H), 1.83–1.76 (m, 2H), 1.55–1.46 (m, 2H), 0.99 (t, J = 7.4 Hz, 3H). HRMS: calculated for $[M+H]^+$ $C_{23}H_{26}ClN_2O_4$ is 429.1581; found 429.1576; Purity by HPLC: 98%.

2.2.2. Synthesis of Compound KP26 as Precursor for ^{11}C-Radiolabeling

To a solution of 8-butoxy-*N*-(2-fluoro-2-phenylethyl)-7-methoxy-2-oxo-1,2-dihydroquinoline-3-carboxamide (KP23, 660 mg, 1.6 mmol) in DMF (15 mL) was added lithium chloride (1.36 g, 32 mmol). The mixture was heated to reflux for 4 hours. After cooling to RT, the mixture was diluted with EtOAc (400 mL) and washed with aq. HCl (0.2 M, 3 × 30 mL) and brine (2 × 30 mL) and dried over Na_2SO_4. Solvents were removed under reduced pressure and column chromatography of the crude over 200 g silica gel using EtOAc/hexane/EtOH 1:1:0.1 gave pure 8-butoxy-*N*-(2-fluoro-2-phenylethyl)-7-hydroxy-2-oxo-1,2-dihydroquinoline-3-carboxamide (KP26, 458 mg, 1.150 mmol, 71.8% yield). ^{1}H-NMR (400 MHz, $CDCl_3$): δ 9.91 (s, 1H), 9.23 (s, 1H), 8.84 (s, 1H), 8.50 (br. s, 1H), 7.34 (d, J = 8.7 Hz, 1H), 7.28–7.22 (m, 1H), 7.05–7.00 (m, 2H), 6.98–6.95 (m, 1H), 6.90 (dt, J_1 = 2.1 Hz, J_2 = 8.4 Hz, 1H), 4.13 (t, J = 6.9 Hz, 2H), 3.77–3.71 (m, 2H), 2.95 (t, J = 7.2 Hz, 2H), 1.83–1.76 (m, 2H), 1.52–1.43 (m, 2H), 0.96 (t, J = 7.4 Hz, 3H). ^{13}C-NMR (100 MHz, $CDCl_3$): δ 164.3, 162.1, 145.4, 133.9, 131.0, 130.0, 129.9, 125.9, 124.5, 124.4, 115.8, 115.5, 114.3, 113.58, 113.5, 113.3, 73.8, 41.0, 35.5, 32.2, 19.1, 13.8. HRMS: calculated for $[M + H]^+$ $C_{22}H_{24}N_2O_4$ is 399.1715; found 399.1711; Purity by HPLC: 98%.

2.3. Radiochemistry

2.3.1. Radiosynthesis of [^{18}F]KP23

No-carrier-added (n.c.a) [^{18}F]fluoride was produced via the ^{18}O(p,n)^{18}F nuclear reaction using an IBA Cyclone 18/9 cyclotron (IBA, Ottignies-Louvain-la-Neuve, Belgium). For this, >98% isotopically enriched ^{18}O-water (Nukem GmbH, city, Germany) was irradiated by 18 MeV proton beams. Produced [^{18}F]fluoride/[^{18}O]water solution was transferred using a helium stream from the target to a shielded hot cell equipped with a manipulator where radiosynthesis was performed. The activity was trapped on a QMA cartridge (preconditioned with 0.5 M aq. K_2CO_3 (1 × 5 mL) and then H_2O (1 × 5 mL) and dried in air. The trapped [^{18}F]fluoride was eluted from the cartridge and eluted with a solution of Kryptofix ($K_{2.2.2}$, 5 mg) and K_2CO_3 (1 mg) in acetonitrile (1.4 mL) and water (0.6 mL) or tetrabutylammonium hydroxide (0.6 mL, 0.18 mM) into a 10 mL sealed reaction vessel. The [^{18}F]fluoride (*ca.* 10−15 GBq) was dried by azeotropic distillation of acetonitrile at 110 °C under vacuum with a stream of nitrogen. The azeotropic drying process was repeated 3 times with 1 mL of acetonitrile. To the dried $K_{2.2.2}$/K[^{18}F]F complex was added the chlorinated compound **7** (*ca.* 2 mg) in different anhydrous solvents such as DMF, DMSO or acetonotrile (0.3 mL), and the reaction mixture was heated and analyzed by HPLC.

2.3.2. Radiosynthesis of [^{11}C]KP23

Carbon-11 was produced via the ^{14}N(p,α)^{11}C nuclear reaction at a Cyclone 18/9 cyclotron (18 MeV, IBA) in the form of [^{11}C]CO_2. [^{11}C]Methyl iodide ([^{11}C]MeI) was generated in a 2-step reaction sequence involving the catalytic reduction of [^{11}C]CO_2 to [^{11}C]methane and subsequent gas phase iodination. [^{11}C]KP23 was prepared by reaction of the desmethyl precursor compound (0.5–1 mg) with [^{11}C]MeI (*ca.* 40–50 GBq) in DMF solution in the presence of Cs_2CO_3 (5 mg) at 120 °C for 3 min. The crude product was diluted with water (1.3 mL) and injected onto a semi-preparative HPLC. The radiolabeled product was collected, diluted with water (10 mL), passed through a preconditioned C18 cartridge (Waters, Boston, MA, USA, preconditioned with 5 mL EtOH and 10 mL water), washed with water (5 mL), and eluted with EtOH (0.5 mL). After adding 9.5 mL of water, the 5% ethanol solution containing [^{11}C]KP23 was then passed through a sterile filter (0.2 μm) and used for all *in vitro*/*in vivo* studies.

2.4. In Vitro *Characterization*

2.4.1. Competition Binding Assay

Frozen membrane preparations from CHO-K1 cells transfected with human CB1 (hCB1) and CB2 (hCB2), respectively (PerkinElmer, Waltham, MA, USA), were thawed on ice and diluted to a final protein concentration of 1 μg/mL in assay buffer (50 mM TRIS/HCl, 1 mM EDTA (Applichem, Darmstadt, Germany), 3 mM $MgCl_2$, pH 7.4, containing 0.05% bovine serum albumin, BSA). Membrane dilutions (0.5 μg protein in 550 μL final volume) were incubated at 30 °C with KP23 at concentrations between 10^{-5} and 10^{-11} M and 1.4 nM [^{3}H]CP-55,940 (PerkinElmer, Waltham, MA, USA), a hCB1 and hCB2 agonist with K_i values of 0.58 and 0.68 nM, respectively. Nonspecific binding of [^{3}H]CP-55,940 was determined after addition of 5 μM hCB1/hCB2 agonist WIN-55212-2 (K_i 1.89 and 0.28 nM, respectively) [23]. All samples were prepared in triplicates. After 90 min, 3 mL ice cold assay buffer was added and samples were immediately filtered through Whatman GF/C filters (pre-soaked in 0.05% polyethylenimine) and washed twice with 3 mL ice cold assay buffer. Bound [^{3}H]CP-55,940 was quantified in a Beckman LS 6500 Liquid Scintillation Counter (Beckman™, Brea, CA, USA) and IC_{50} values were determined by non-linear regression analysis [24]. K_i values were determined with the equation from Cheng-Prusoff and are means from three independent experiments (K_D values of 0.14 and 0.11 nM from PerkinElmer were used for [^{3}H]CP-55,940 binding to hCB1 and hCB2 receptors, respectively).

2.4.2. *In Vitro* Stability Studies

To test the plasma stability of the radioligand, 10 μL (4 MBq) of [^{11}C]KP23 solution were added to phosphate buffer (300 μL, 4 mM NaH_2PO_4/Na_2HPO_4, 155 mM NaCl, pH 7.4), mouse and rat plasma

(300 µL), respectively. The mixture was vortexed and four aliquots of 70 µL were incubated at 37 °C. Ice cold acetonitrile (100 µL) was added to stop the enzymatic reactions at different time points (0, 10, 20 and 40 min). After centrifugation (10,000 *g*, 3 min), the supernatant was passed through a filter (0.45 µm, Minisart SRP 4, Sartorius Stedim Biotech, Goettingen, Germany) and analyzed by UPLC.

2.4.3. *In Vitro* Autoradiography

In vitro autoradiography with [^{11}C]KP23 was performed on 20 µm tissue slices (rat/mouse spleen) adsorbed to SuperFrost Plus slides. Slices were thawed (10 min) on ice before pre-incubation with incubation buffer (50 mM TRIS/HCl, pH 7.4, containing 5% BSA) at 4 °C for 10 min. Excess solution was carefully removed and the tissue slices were dried in a ventilated hood for 10 min. Then slides were incubated with 0.6 or 0.2 nM [^{11}C]KP23 alone or together with specific CB2 agonist (GW405833, 1 µM) in incubation buffer. After incubation for 15 min at RT in a humid chamber, slides were washed twice with ice cold washing buffer (50 mM TRIS/HCl, pH 7.4, 1% BSA, 5% EtOH) for 2 min each and dipped twice in water. Dried slides were exposed to a phosphor imager plate for 30 min and the plate was scanned in a BAS5000 reader (Fujifilm, Dielsdorf, Switzerland).

2.5. In Vivo *Characterization*

2.5.1. *In Vivo* PET Imaging

PET scanning was performed with the GE VISTA eXplore PET/CT tomograph (Sedecal, Madrid, Spain). The scanner is characterized by high sensitivity (absolute central point source sensitivity of 4% for the 250–700 eV energy windows) and an axial field of view of 4.8 cm [25]. Male Wistar rats (278 ± 2 g, n = 2) were immobilized by isoflurane inhalation and the tracer was injected into a tail vein on the tomographic bed [26]. Tracer accumulation in the spleen or brain were recorded by dynamic one-bed position PET scans over 60 min starting with the injection of 13 respectively 40 MBq (0.05 to 0.15 nmol) of [^{11}C]KP23. PET data was reconstructed by 3-dimensional FORE/2-dimensional OSEM in user-defined time frames with a voxel size of 0.3875 × 0.3875 × 0.775 mm. Singles and random corrections but no attenuation correction were applied. Image files were evaluated with the software PMOD v3.4 (PMOD Technologies Inc., Zurich, Switzerland). Time activity curves (TACs) of brain regions were generated with the implemented rat brain region of interest (ROI) template and TACs of the abdominal region with the respective ROIs generated by the PMOD segmentation tool. Spleen, liver and background TACs were confirmed by analysis of manually drawn regions of interest. Standardized uptake values (SUV) were calculated as tissue activities (Bq/cm^3), normalized to the injected dose per body weight (Bq/g).

2.5.2. Metabolite Studies

[^{11}C]KP23 was administered intravenously to a restrained Wistar rat (413 g) by tail vein injection (*ca.* 160 MBq). The animal was sacrificed by decapitation 30 min p.i. and blood and urine were collected. Whole blood was collected in heparin-coated tubes (BD Vacutainers, Plymouth, UK) and centrifuged at 5,000 *g* for 5 min, 4 °C. The proteins of the supernatant plasma and urine were precipitated by addition of an equal volume of acetonitrile and centrifuged at 5,000 *g* for another

5 min. The supernatants were filtered and analyzed by UPLC. For the determination of *in vivo* radiometabolites at 15 min p.i. blood samples were withdrawn from the tail vein opposite to the injection site.

3. Results and Discussion

3.1. Chemistry and Radiochemistry

The non-radioactive standard reference compound KP23 was synthesized based on the modified procedure described by Turkman [27]. Compound **2** was obtained in 30% yield by the aromatic nitration of 3-hydroxy-4-methoxybenzaldehyde (**1**) with nitric acid. Then *O*-alkylation with 1-bromobutane afforded compound **3** in 89% yield. Reduction of compound **3** using iron powder followed by reaction *in situ* with dimethyl malonate yielded compound **4**. The acid compound **5** was produced quantitatively by saponification reaction of the methyl ester compound **4** under basic conditions. Amide bond formation using the acid compound **5** with either 2-amino-1-phenylethanol or 2-fluoro-2-phenylethanamine free base led to compound **6** and KP23, respectively. Compound **6** was reacted with mesylchloride to afford chloro derivative **7**, which was used as supposed to be a precursor for fluorine-18 labeling. Demethylation of compound KP23 was performed with LiCl to afford the precursor compound KP26 for carbon-11 labeling. The newly synthesized compounds were characterized by mass spectrometry and NMR and their chemical purities were assessed by HPLC.

The structure of compound KP23 (Scheme 1) is amenable to radiolabeling with either fluorine-18 or carbon-11 (Scheme 2), therefore, the corresponding chloro and phenolic precursor compounds 7 and KP26 were prepared and tested for radiolabeling. For the fluorine-18 radiolabeling of KP23, it was originally planned to synthesize a precursor with a sulfonate leaving group. Initial attempts to tosylate compound **6** to afford a precursor with a tosyl leaving group were unsuccessful. Mesylation, however, exclusively afforded chloro analog **7** in 41% yields. This result has also been observed for other similar compounds in the literature [28,29]. It is suggested that this conversion occurs via spontaneous displacement of the sulfonate group by nitrogen (anchimeric assistance) with formation of reactive aziridinium ion intermediate. Consequent collapse of the aziridinium ion pair to the more stable chloride then occurs, upon exchange of the mesylate counterion with chloride [30]. ^{18}F-radiolabeling was unsuccessful even using different solvents e.g., MeCN, DMF or DMSO and combined with different [^{18}F]-reagents such as $K_{2.2.2}$/K[^{18}F]F or [^{18}F]TBAF. Neither increasing the reaction temperature, duration of the radiolabeling reaction nor precursor concentrations had any positive influence on the outcome of radiolabeling yield. This can be explained by the fact that chloride is a poor leaving group.

KP23 was successfully labeled with carbon-11 in a one-step reaction by reacting the phenolic precursor with [^{11}C]methyl iodide (Scheme 2). [^{11}C]KP23 (*ca.* 1–3 GBq) was obtained in 99% radiochemical purity after semi-preparative HPLC purification. The total radiolabeling time was around 40 min after delivery of [^{11}C]CO_2 from the cyclotron to the hot-cell. Specific activity was high and ranged from 80 to 240 GBq/μmol at the end of synthesis. The radiochemical yield was 10%–25% (decay corrected).

Scheme 1. Synthesis of the standard reference KP23 and precursors **7** and KP26 for radiolabeling.

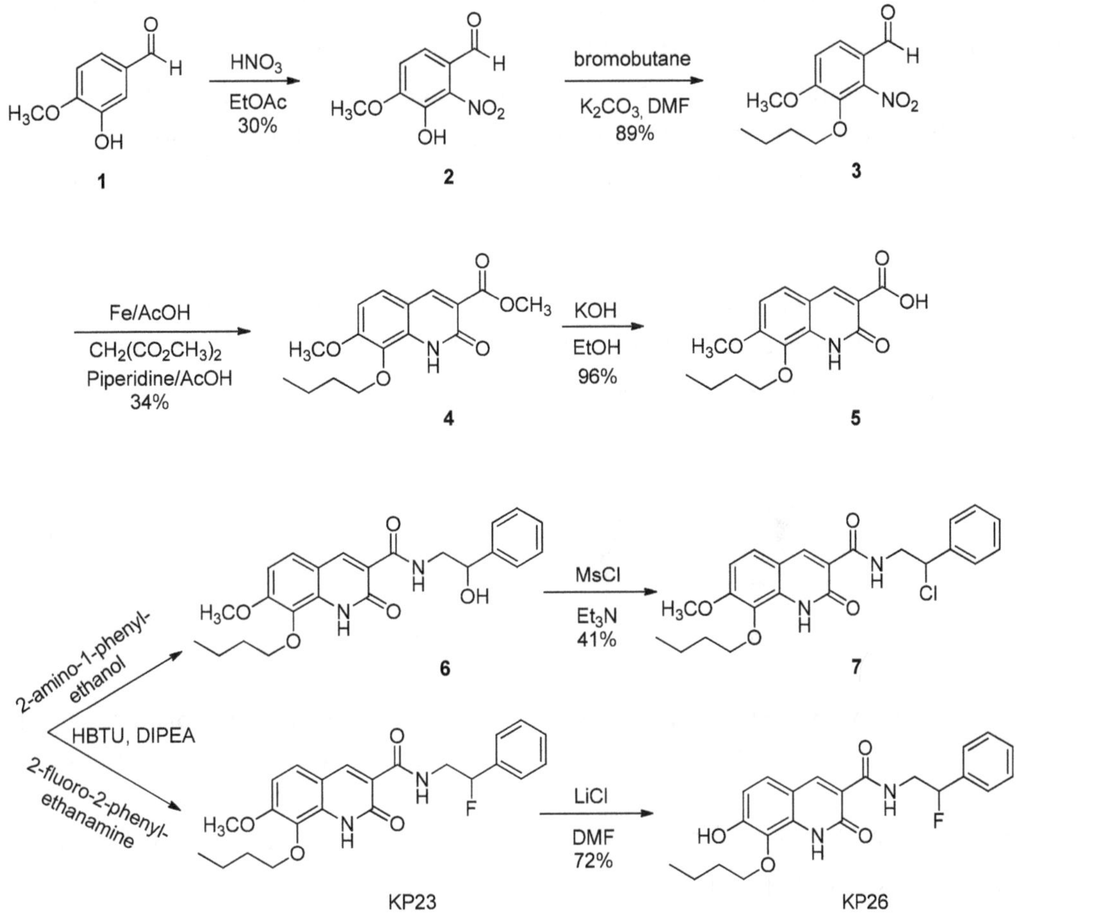

Scheme 2. Radiosyntheses of compounds [^{18}F]KP23 and [^{11}C]KP23.

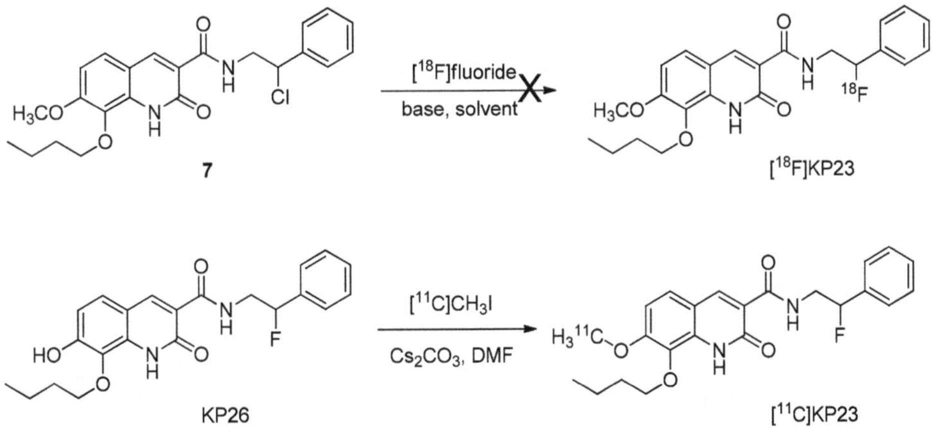

3.2. In Vitro *Characterization*

In vitro competitive binding assays were performed with membranes obtained from CHO-K1 cells stably transfected with human CB1 and CB2, respectively, using [^{3}H]-CP-55940. The binding affinity of the nonradioactive KP23 obtained from three independent experiments was 6.8 ± 5.8 nM towards human CB2 and > 10,000 nM towards CB1, slightly lower affinity than the reported data of 0.8 ± 0.3 nM towards human CB2 and >10,000 nM towards CB1 [27]. The affinity and selectivity of KP23 towards

CB2 are the highest among the known 2-oxoquinoline carboxylic acid derivatives including $[^{11}C]$NE40, the first CB2 PET tracer evaluated in healthy human subjects which exhibits a K_i value of 9.6 nM. Autoradiography with slices from rat and mouse spleen, an organ with high CB2 levels [31], demonstrated high binding which was blocked by excess GW4058233 (CB2 specific agonist), indicating specific binding of $[^{11}C]$KP23 to CB2 (Figure 1) in both cases. However, relatively high non-specific binding was observed in the spleen tissue (Figures 1 A2 and B2) which is not surprising considering the calculated LogP value of 3.81.

Figure 1. Autoradiography of rat (**A**) and mouse (**B**) spleen sections incubated with 0.6 nM $[^{11}C]$KP23 in the absence of blocking agent (A1 and B1) or in the presence of excess blocking agent 1 μM GW4058233 (A2 and B2).

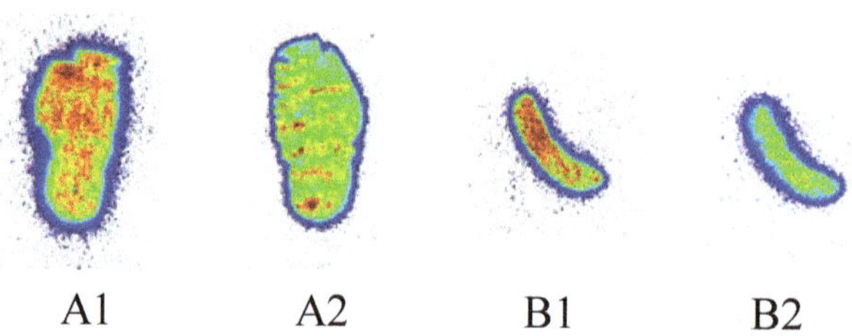

In vitro plasma stability tests were carried out in PBS, mouse and rat plasma over a period of 40 min at 37 °C. No radioactive degradation products of $[^{11}C]$KP23 were detected (Figure 2).

Figure 2. Radio-UPLC profiles of $[^{11}C]$KP23 (t_R = 2.1 min) after 2 h in PBS and after 40 min in mouse and rat plasma.

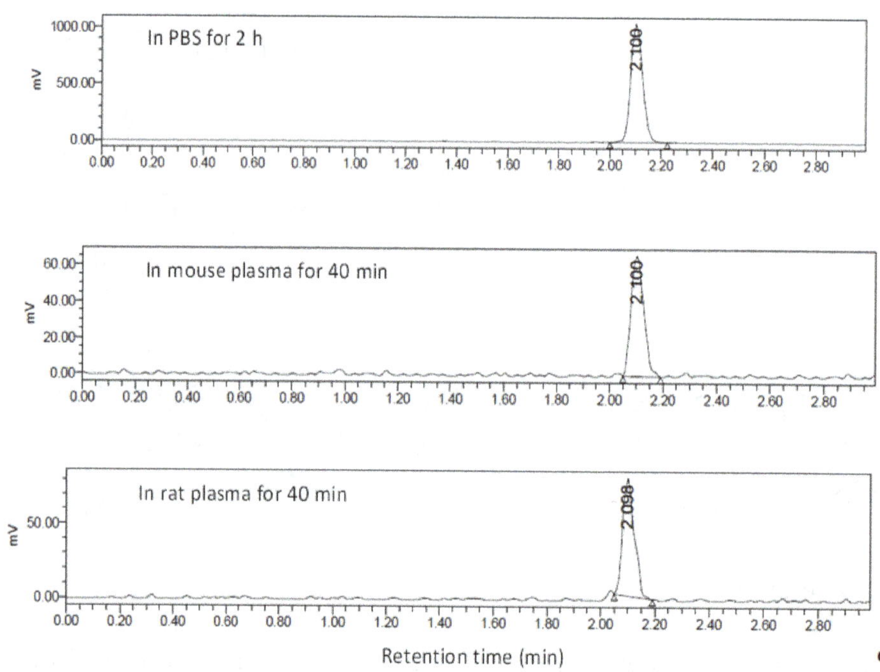

3.3. In Vivo *PET Imaging of $[^{11}C]$KP23*

Figure 3A shows PET images of a coronal section and maximal intensity projection (MIP) of the abdominal region of a rat fused to the respective CT, and averaged from 6 to 15 min p.i. $[^{11}C]$KP23 accumulated in spleen, liver and intestines. The high spleen uptake is in accordance with the expression pattern of CB2 while the high accumulation in liver suggests a hepatobiliary elimination pathway. Background radioactivity in muscle tissue was relatively low. The TACs of liver, spleen and peripheral tissue outside the rips are shown in Figure 3B. Radioactivity peaked around 4 min p.i. for liver; the level of activity concentration steadily increased during the initial 8 min p.i. in spleen and then slowly washed out. During the whole data acquisition, the level of activity concentration was higher in the spleen region than in the background (flank).

Figure 3. PET/CT images of [^{11}C]KP23 in the spleen-liver region in rat. (**A**) Coronal section and maximal intensity projection (MIP) averaged from 6 to 15 min p.i. (**B**) TACs of [^{11}C]KP23 in spleen, liver and flank.

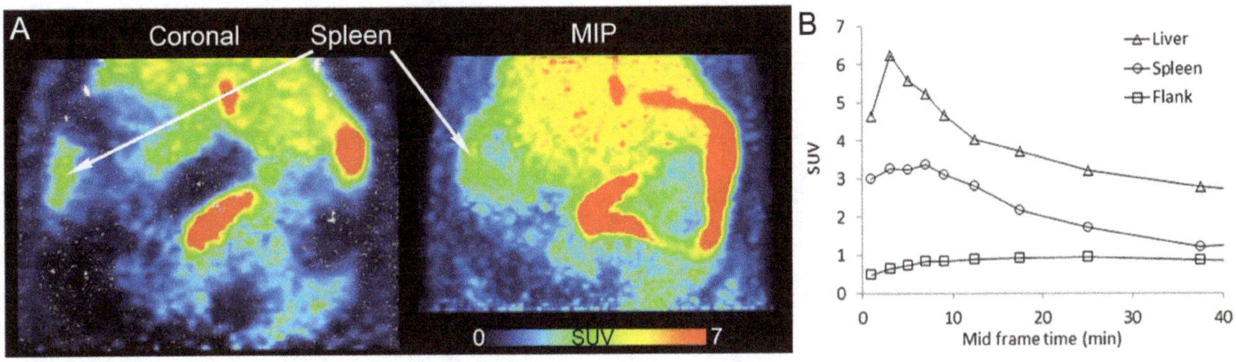

Distribution of the tracer in rat brain was evaluated by PET (Figure 4A). Region of interest TAC analysis showed low uptake in healthy rat brain which is in line with the low expression level of CB2 receptor (Figure 4B). Radioactivity levels in brain were lower than in peripheral tissues in general. The expression profile of CB2 provides great opportunities for PET imaging with low background in the brain region, whereas under inflammation conditions a 10-100-fold higher CB2 receptor density is expected in activated microglia [32].

Figure 4. [^{11}C]KP23 PET images of a rat brain superimposed on an MRI template . A: From left, axial, sagittal and coronal sections. In the last coronal image, regions of interest are encircled and used for TAC analysis shown in B. a, cortex; b, cerebellum; c, caudate putamen; d, hippocampus. Images are averaged from 2–60 min p.i. B TACs of rat brain regions of [^{11}C]KP23.

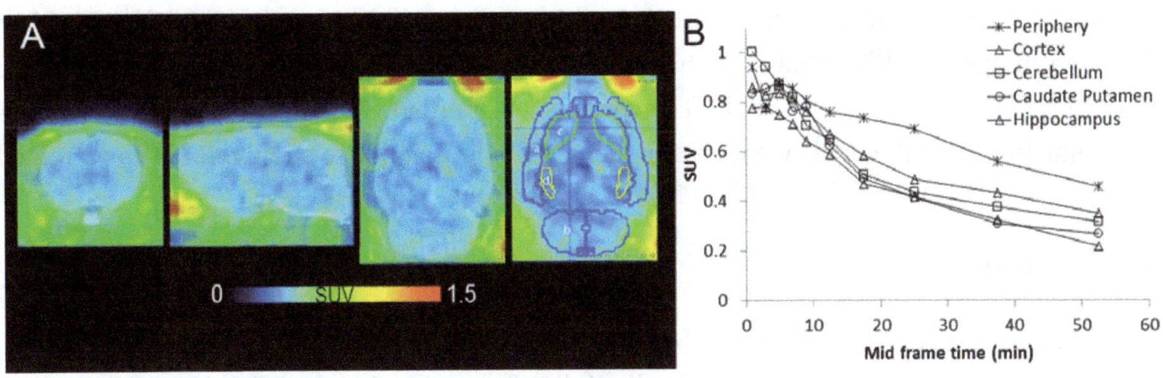

3.4. In Vivo *Metabolic Studies*

The metabolic fate of [^{11}C]KP23 was studied using blood and urine samples of a Wistar rat. In blood plasma samples, two to three radiometabolites which were more hydrophilic than the parent tracer, [^{11}C]KP23, were detected. As illustrated in Figure 5, one major radiometabolite slightly more polar than the parent compound was generated in blood plasma samples. The percentage of parent tracer radioactivity decreased to 40% at 15 min p.i., 25% at 30 min p.i. No intact compound could be found in the urine sample after 30 min p.i.

Figure 5. Radio-UPLC profiles of [^{11}C]KP23 metabolites in blood plasma samples obtained at 15 min and 30 min p.i. and in the urine sample obtained at 30 min p.i.

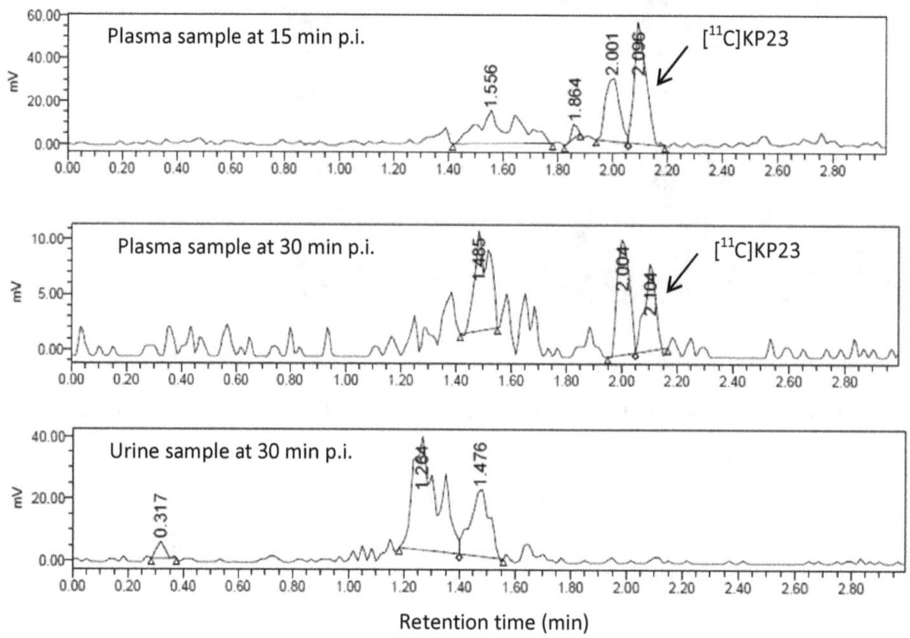

4. Conclusions

[^{11}C]KP23 showed promising *in vitro* characteristics. Its affinity and selectivity for CB2 is the highest among the known 2-oxoquinoline carboxylic acid derivatives. In vitro autoradiography with slices from rat and mouse spleen demonstrated specific binding. High spleen uptake of [^{11}C]KP23 was also observed in dynamic PET studies with Wistar rats. As expected, distribution to healthy rat brain was relatively low in the *in vivo* PET experiments. Further evaluation of [^{11}C]KP23 using neuroinflammation animal models which has higher CB2 expression levels in the brain is warranted.

Acknowledgments

This work was partially funded by the Swiss ALS Foundation. We thank Bruno Mancosu for his support with carbon-11 radiolabeling and Claudia Keller for performing the PET/CT scans.

Author Contributions

L.M. planned and organized the whole study, responsible for radiolabeling, quality control, radiotracer stability studies both *in vitro*/*in vivo* and manuscript writing; R.S. Analyzed organic compounds ^{1}H-NMR, ^{13}C-NMR, HRMS and performed the *in vitro* evaluation of KP-23 and [^{11}C]KP-23 including competitive binding assays and autoradiography; A.M. analyzed the PET data, helped writing the manuscript; K.P. Organic synthesis the precursor and reference compounds; S.Č. Involved in spleen tissue preparation and autoradiography experiments; M.W. Revision of the manuscript, final approval of the version to be published; R.S. Involved in the results discussion, final approval of the version to be published; S.D.K. supervision of and involved in the planning and interpretation of *in vivo* experiments; S.M.A. Involved in the experiments planning, revision of the manuscript.

References

1. Vincent, B.J.; McQuiston, D.J.; Einhorn, L.H.; Nagy, C.M.; Brames, M.J. Review of cannabinoids and their antiemetic effectiveness. *Drugs* **1983**, *25* (Suppl. 1), 52–62.
2. Console-Bram, L.; Marcu, J.; Abood, M.E. Cannabinoid receptors: Nomenclature and pharmacological principles. *Prog. Neuropsychopharmacol. Biol. Psychiatry* **2012**, *38*, 4–15.
3. Pertwee, R.G.; Howlett, A.C.; Abood, M.E.; Alexander, S.P.; di Marzo, V.; Elphick, M.R.; Greasley, P.J.; Hansen, H.S.; Kunos, G.; Mackie, K.; *et al.* International Union of Basic and Clinical Pharmacology. LXXIX. Cannabinoid receptors and their ligands: Beyond CB(1) and CB(2). *Pharmacol. Rev.* **2010**, *62*, 588–631.
4. Matsuda, L.A.; Lolait, S.J.; Brownstein, M.J.; Young, A.C.; Bonner, T.I. Structure of a cannabinoid receptor and functional expression of the cloned cDNA. *Nature* **1990**, *346*, 561–564.
5. Herkenham, M.; Lynn, A.B.; Johnson, M.R.; Melvin, L.S.; de Costa, B.R.; Rice, K.C. Characterization and localization of cannabinoid receptors in rat brain: A quantitative *in vitro* autoradiographic study. *J. Neurosci.* **1991**, *11*, 563–583.
6. Maresz, K.; Carrier, E.J.; Ponomarev, E.D.; Hillard, C.J.; Dittel, B.N. Modulation of the cannabinoid CB2 receptor in microglial cells in response to inflammatory stimuli. *J. Neurochem.* **2005**, *95*, 437–445.
7. Chin, C.L.; Tovcimak, A.E.; Hradil, V.P.; Seifert, T.R.; Hollingsworth, P.R.; Chandran, P.; Zhu, C.Z.; Gauvin, D.; Pai, M.; Wetter, J.; *et al.* Differential effects of cannabinoid receptor agonists on regional brain activity using pharmacological MRI. *Br. J. Pharmacol.* **2008**, *153*, 367–379.
8. Pertwee, R.G. Pharmacology of cannabinoid CB1 and CB2 receptors. *Pharmacol. Ther.* **1997**, *74*, 129–180.
9. Burns, H.D.; van Laere, K.; Sanabria-Bohorquez, S.; Hamill, T.G.; Bormans, G.; Eng, W.S.; Gibson, R.; Ryan, C.; Connolly, B.; Patel, S.; *et al.* [18F]MK-9470, a positron emission

tomography (PET) tracer for *in vivo* human PET brain imaging of the cannabinoid-1 receptor. *Proc. Natl. Acad. Sci. USA* **2007**, *104*, 9800–9805.

10. Liu, P.; Lin, L.S.; Hamill, T.G.; Jewell, J.P.; Lanza, T.J., Jr.; Gibson, R.E.; Krause, S.M.; Ryan, C.; Eng, W.; Sanabria, S.; *et al.* Discovery of *N*-{(1S,2S)-2-(3-cyanophenyl)-3-[4-(2-[18F]fluoroethoxy)phenyl]-1-methylpropyl}-2-methyl-2-[(5-methylpyridin-2-yl)oxy]propanamide, a cannabinoid-1 receptor positron emission tomography tracer suitable for clinical use. *J. Med. Chem.* **2007**, *50*, 3427–3430.
11. Horti, A.G.; van Laere, K. Development of radioligands for *in vivo* imaging of type 1 cannabinoid receptors (CB1) in human brain. *Curr. Pharm. Des.* **2008**, *14*, 3363–3383.
12. Van Laere, K.; Casteels, C.; Lunskens, S.; Goffin, K.; Grachev, I.D.; Bormans, G.; Vandenberghe, W. Regional changes in type 1 cannabinoid receptor availability in Parkinson's disease *in vivo*. *Neurobiol. Aging* **2012**, *33*, 620.e1–8.
13. Van Laere, K.; Goffin, K.; Casteels, C.; Dupont, P.; Mortelmans, L.; de Hoon, J.; Bormans, G. Gender-dependent increases with healthy aging of the human cerebral cannabinoid-type 1 receptor binding using [(18)F]MK-9470 PET. *Neuroimage* **2008**, *39*, 1533–1541.
14. Van Laere, K.; Koole, M.; Sanabria Bohorquez, S.M.; Goffin, K.; Guenther, I.; Belanger, M.J.; Cote, J.; Rothenberg, P.; de Lepeleire, I.; Grachev, I.D.; *et al.* Whole-body biodistribution and radiation dosimetry of the human cannabinoid type-1 receptor ligand 18F-MK-9470 in healthy subjects. *J. Nucl. Med.* **2008**, *49*, 439–445.
15. Muccioli, G.G.; Lambert, D.M. Current knowledge on the antagonists and inverse agonists of cannabinoid receptors. *Curr. Med. Chem.* **2005**, *12*, 1361–1394.
16. Raitio, K.H.; Salo, O.M.; Nevalainen, T.; Poso, A.; Jarvinen, T. Targeting the cannabinoid CB2 receptor: Mutations, modeling and development of CB2 selective ligands. *Curr. Med. Chem.* **2005**, *12*, 1217–1237.
17. Evens, N.; Muccioli, G.G.; Houbrechts, N.; Lambert, D.M.; Verbruggen, A.M.; Van Laere, K.; Bormans, G.M. Synthesis and biological evaluation of carbon-11- and fluorine-18-labeled 2-oxoquinoline derivatives for type 2 cannabinoid receptor positron emission tomography imaging. *Nucl. Med. Biol.* **2009**, *36*, 455–465.
18. Vandeputte, C.; Evens, N.; Toelen, J.; Deroose, C.M.; Bosier, B.; Ibrahimi, A.; van der Perren, A.; Gijsbers, R.; Janssen, P.; Lambert, D.M.; *et al.* A PET brain reporter gene system based on type 2 cannabinoid receptors. *J. Nucl. Med.* **2011**, *52*, 1102–1109.
19. Mu, L.; Bieri, D.; Slavik, R.; Drandarov, K.; Muller, A.; Cermak, S.; Weber, M.; Schibli, R.; Kramer, S.D.; Ametamey, S.M. Radiolabeling and *in vitro*/*in vivo* evaluation of *N*-(1-adamantyl)-8-methoxy-4-*oxo*-1-phenyl-1,4-dihydroquinoline-3-carboxamide as a PET probe for imaging cannabinoid type 2 receptor. *J. Neurochem.* **2013**, *126*, 616–624.
20. Evens, N.; Vandeputte, C.; Coolen, C.; Janssen, P.; Sciot, R.; Baekelandt, V.; Verbruggen, A.M.; Debyser, Z.; van Laere, K.; Bormans, G.M. Preclinical evaluation of [11C]NE40, a type 2 cannabinoid receptor PET tracer. *Nucl. Med. Biol.* **2012**, *39*, 389–399.
21. Turkman, N.; Shavrin, A.; Paolillo, V.; Yeh, H.H.; Flores, L.; Soghomonian, S.; Rabinovich, B.; Volgin, A.; Gelovani, J.; Alauddin, M. Synthesis and preliminary evaluation of [18F]-labeled 2-oxoquinoline derivatives for PET imaging of cannabinoid CB2 receptor. *Nucl. Med. Biol.* **2012**, *39*, 593–600.

22. Ahmad, R.; Koole, M.; Evens, N.; Serdons, K.; Verbruggen, A.; Bormans, G.; van Laere, K. Whole-body biodistribution and radiation dosimetry of the cannabinoid type 2 receptor ligand [11C]-NE40 in healthy subjects. *Mol. Imaging Biol.* **2013**, *15*, 384–390.
23. Showalter, V.M.; Compton, D.R.; Martin, B.R.; Abood, M.E. Evaluation of binding in a transfected cell line expressing a peripheral cannabinoid receptor (CB2): Identification of cannabinoid receptor subtype selective ligands. *J. Pharmacol. Exp. Ther.* **1996**, *278*, 989–999.
24. Ruhl, T.; Deuther-Conrad, W.; Fischer, S.; Gunther, R.; Hennig, L.; Krautscheid, H.; Brust, P. Cannabinoid receptor type 2 (CB2)-selective N-aryl-oxadiazolyl-propionamides: Synthesis, radiolabelling, molecular modelling and biological evaluation. *Org. Med. Chem. Lett.* **2012**, *2*, 32.
25. Wang, Y.; Seidel, J.; Tsui, B.M.; Vaquero, J.J.; Pomper, M.G. Performance evaluation of the GE healthcare eXplore VISTA dual-ring small-animal PET scanner. *J. Nucl. Med.* **2006**, *47*, 1891–900.
26. Honer, M.; Bruhlmeier, M.; Missimer, J.; Schubiger, A.P.; Ametamey, S.M. Dynamic imaging of striatal D2 receptors in mice using quad-HIDAC PET. *J. Nucl. Med.* **2004**, *45*, 464–470.
27. Turkman, N.; Shavrin, A.; Ivanov, R.A.; Rabinovich, B.; Volgin, A.; Gelovani, J.G.; Alauddin, M.M. Fluorinated cannabinoid CB2 receptor ligands: Synthesis and *in vitro* binding characteristics of 2-oxoquinoline derivatives. *Bioorg. Med. Chem.* **2011**, *19*, 5698–5707.
28. Bacherikov, V.A.; Chou, T.C.; Dong, H.J.; Zhang, X.G.; Chen, C.H.; Lin, Y.W.; Tsai, T.J.; Lee, R.Z.; Liu, L.F.; Su, T.L. Potent antitumor 9-anilinoacridines bearing an alkylating N-mustard residue on the anilino ring: Synthesis and biological activity. *Bioorg. Med. Chem.* **2005**, *13*, 3993–4006.
29. Savle, P.S.; Medhekar, R.A.; Kelley, E.L.; May, J.G.; Watkins, S.F.; Fronczek, F.R.; Quinn, D.M.; Gandour, R.D. Change in the mode of inhibition of acetylcholinesterase by (4-nitrophenyl)sulfonoxyl derivatives of conformationally constrained choline analogues. *Chem. Res. Toxicol.* **1998**, *11*, 19–25.
30. Boeckman, R.K.; Miller, Y.; Savage, D.; Summerton, J.E. Total synthesis of a possible specific and effective acid-targeted cancer diagnostic, a camphor derived bis-*N*-oxide dimer. *Tetrahedron Lett.* **2011**, *52*, 2243–2245.
31. Gong, J.P.; Onaivi, E.S.; Ishiguro, H.; Liu, Q.R.; Tagliaferro, P.A.; Brusco, A.; Uhl, G.R. Cannabinoid CB2 receptors: Immunohistochemical localization in rat brain. *Brain Res.* **2006**, *1071*, 10–23.
32. Evens, N.; Bormans, G.M. Non-invasive imaging of the type 2 cannabinoid receptor, focus on positron emission tomography. *Curr. Top. Med. Chem.* **2010**, *10*, 1527–1543.

7

In Vivo Monitoring of the Antiangiogenic Effect of Neurotensin Receptor-Mediated Radiotherapy by Small-Animal Positron Emission Tomography

Simone Maschauer [1], Tina Ruckdeschel [1], Philipp Tripal [1], Roland Haubner [2], Jürgen Einsiedel [3], Harald Hübner [3], Peter Gmeiner [3], Torsten Kuwert [1] and Olaf Prante [1,*]

[1] Department of Nuclear Medicine, Laboratory of Molecular Imaging and Radiochemistry, Friedrich Alexander University, Schwabachanlage 6, 91054 Erlangen, Germany; E-Mails: simone.maschauer@uk-erlangen.de (S.M.); tina_ruckdeschel@gmx.de (T.R.); philipp.tripal@uk-erlangen.de (P.T.); torsten.kuwert@uk-erlangen.de (T.K.)

[2] Department of Nuclear Medicine, Innsbruck Medical University, Anichstr. 35, 6020 Innsbruck, Austria; E-Mail: roland.haubner@i-med.ac.at

[3] Department of Chemistry and Pharmacy, Medicinal Chemistry, Emil Fischer Center, Friedrich Alexander University, Schuhstraße 19, 91052 Erlangen, Germany; E-Mails: Jürgen.einsiedel@fau.de (J.E.); harald.huebner@fau.de (H.H.); peter.gmeiner@fau.de (P.G.)

* Author to whom correspondence should be addressed; E-Mail: olaf.prante@uk-erlangen.de

---

Abstract: The neurotensin receptor (NTS1) has emerged as an interesting target for molecular imaging and radiotherapy of NTS-positive tumors due to the overexpression in a range of tumors. The aim of this study was to develop a ^{177}Lu-labeled NTS1 radioligand, its application for radiotherapy in a preclinical model and the imaging of therapy success by small-animal positron emission tomography (μPET) using [^{68}Ga]DOTA-RGD as a specific tracer for imaging angiogenesis. The ^{177}Lu-labeled peptide was subjected to studies on HT29-tumor-bearing nude mice *in vivo*, defining four groups of animals (single dose, two fractionated doses, four fractionated doses and sham-treated animals). Body weight and tumor diameters were determined three times per week. Up to day 28 after treatment, μPET studies were performed with [^{68}Ga]DOTA-RGD. At days 7–10 after treatment with four fractionated doses of 11–14 MBq (each at days 0, 3, 6 and 10), the tumor growth was slightly decreased in comparison with untreated animals. Using a single high dose of 51 MBq, a significantly decreased tumor diameter of about 50% was observed with the beginning of treatment. Our preliminary PET imaging data suggested decreased tumor uptake values of [^{68}Ga]DOTA-RGD in treated animals compared to controls at day 7 after treatment. This pilot study suggests that early PET imaging with [^{68}Ga]DOTA-RGD in radiotherapy studies to monitor integrin expression could be a promising tool to predict therapy success *in vivo*. Further successive PET experiments are needed to confirm the significance and predictive value of RGD-PET for NTS-mediated radiotherapy.

Keywords: neurotensin receptor; positron emission tomography; radiotherapy; lutetium-177; RGD peptide; angiogenesis

---

1. Introduction

Neurotensin (NT) is a peptide consisting of 13 amino acids (pGlu-Leu-Tyr-Glu-Asn-Lys-Pro-Arg-Arg-Pro-Try-Ile-Leu) that has been originally isolated in 1973 by Carraway and Leeman from calf hypothalamus [1]. The biologically active sequence is the C-terminal part NT(8–13) (Arg-Arg-Pro-Tyr-Ile-Leu) [2] which binds to the three neurotensin receptor subtypes NTS1, NTS2, NTS3 [3] and has therefore been selected as a lead structure for medicinal chemists [4–13]. The NTS1 is upregulated in various tumor types including prostate, pancreas, mamma, lung and colon carcinoma [14–16]. In addition, NTS1 shows negligible expression in healthy tissues where these tumors arise from, making it a very specific molecular target for imaging and targeted cancer therapy [16]. NT(8–13) is rapidly degraded by endogenous peptidases *in vivo*, therefore a variety of studies addressed this issue by modifying the amino acid sequence of NT(8–13) [17–23].

Up to now, only a few NT(8–13) analogs have been radiolabeled with an isotope suitable for endoradiotherapy [24–27]. Among these rare examples, the ^{188}Re-labeled peptide "NT-XIX" with the amino acid sequence (N$^{\alpha}$His)Ac-Arg-(*N*-CH_3)-Arg-Pro-Dmt-Tle-Leu has been used for radiotherapy studies on tumor-bearing nude mice [24]. This radiopeptide showed promising effects, as the tumor growth in the animals was decreased at day 6 after begin of treatment. However, this study did not use successive diagnostic imaging experiments, such as positron emission tomography (PET) imaging, in a longitudinal setup for the prediction of therapy outcome.

Lutetium-177 is a β-emitter with a maximum energy of 0.5 MeV and a half-life of 6.7 days, displaying favorable physical properties compared to rhenium-188 (E_{max} = 2.1 MeV, $t_{½}$ = 17 h). Lutetium-177 has a maximal tissue penetration of 2 mm, making it an optimal radionuclide for the irradiation of small tumors. Therefore, we aimed at developing a ^{177}Lu-labeled NT-derivative, based on our previously reported metabolically stable amino acid sequence NLys-Lys-Pro-Tyr-Tle-Leu [28,29], and studied the applicability of this radiopeptide ([^{177}Lu]**NT127**, Figure 1) for endoradiotherapy in NTS1-positive HT29-tumor-bearing nude mice.

The various integrin-specific PET tracers, all derived from pentacyclic RGD peptides [30,31], should be excellent molecular tools for monitoring early response of tumors to (radio)therapy, since antiangiogenic effects should occur at early stages after successful treatment [32–34]. Consequently, we studied the suitability of [^{68}Ga]DOTA-RGD (Figure 1, [35]) for the noninvasive monitoring of tumor response to radiotherapy with [^{177}Lu]**NT127** in a pilot study by successive PET imaging experiments, including days 7, 14, 21 and 28 after treatment and varying the administration of the dose from four fractionated doses (4 × 11–14 MBq, $n = 4$ mice) to a single high dose (1 × 50 MBq, $n = 3$ mice).

Figure 1. Chemical structures of [^{68}Ga]DOTA-RGD [35] (**top**) and [^{177}Lu]**NT127** (**bottom**).

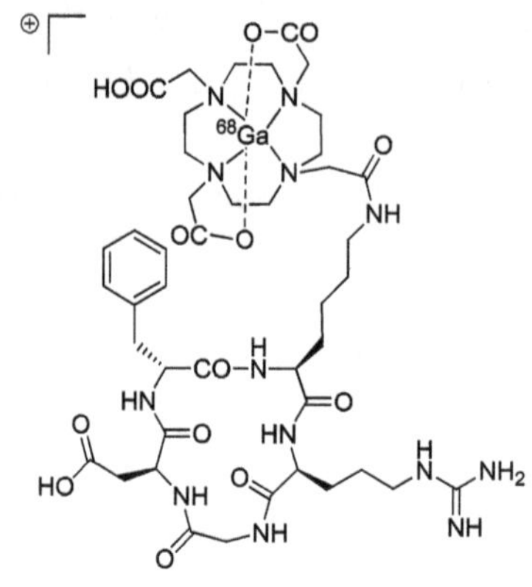

[^{68}Ga]DOTA-RGD
K_i ($\alpha_v\beta_3$) = 5.5 nM

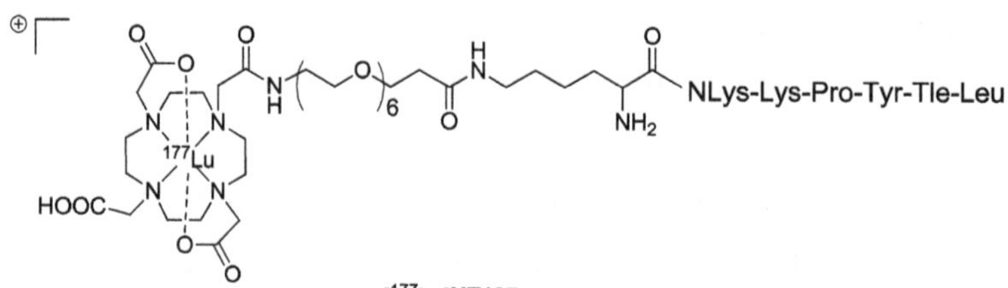

[^{177}Lu]**NT127**
K_i (NTS1) = 30 nM
K_i (NTS2) = 220 nM

2. Experimental

2.1. General

Reagents, building blocks and dry solvents were obtained from commercial sources and were used as received. Analytical radio-HPLC was performed on an Agilent 1100 system (Agilent Technologies, Böblingen, Germany) equipped with a quaternary pump and variable wavelength detector and radio-HPLC detector D505TR (Canberra Packard, Schwadorf, Austria). Computer analysis of the HPLC data was performed using FLO-One software (Canberra Packard).

*2.2. Synthesis of **NT127***

Unless otherwise noted, reactions were conducted without inert atmosphere. Microwave assisted (Discover® microwave oven, CEM Corp., Kamp-Lintfort, Germany) peptide synthesis was carried out in glass tubes loosely sealed with a silicon septum. Remark: the development of overpressure was avoided by using DMF as the solvent. In between each irradiation step, intermittent cooling of the reaction mixture to a temperature of −10 °C was achieved by sufficient agitation in an ethanol-ice bath. Preparative RP-HPLC was performed using Agilent 1100 preparative series (column: Zorbax Eclipse XDB-C8, 21.2 × 150 mm, 5 µm particles [C8], flow rate. 10 mL /min, detection wavelength: 220 nm) and solvent systems as specified below. Purity and identity were assessed by analytical RP-HPLC

(Agilent 1100 analytical series, column: Zorbax Eclipse XDB-C8 analytical column, 4.6 × 150 mm, 5 µm, flow rate: 0.5 mL/min, detection wavelength: 220 nm) coupled to a Bruker Esquire 2000 mass detector equipped with an ESI-trap. Solvent systems are specified below.

The peptide synthesis was achieved starting from commercially available Fmoc-Leu-Wang resin (Novabiochem®, Merck KGaA, Darmstadt, Germany, loading 0.64 mmol/g). Amino acids were incorporated as their commercially available derivatives in the following order: Fmoc-Tle-OH (a), Fmoc-Tyr(*t*Bu)-OH (b), Fmoc-Pro-OH (c), Fmoc-Lys(Boc)-OH (d), *N*-Fmoc-*N*-(4-Boc-aminobutyl)-Gly-OH (e, Aldrich, Taufkirchen, Germany), Boc-Lys(Fmoc)-OH (f), Fmoc-21-amino-4,7,10,13,16,19-hexaoxaheneicosanoic acid (g, Novabiochem) and 4,7,10-tris-*tert*-butoxycarbonylmethyl-1,4,7,10-tetraaza-cyclododec-1-yl)-acetic acid (DOTA-tri-*t*-Bu-ester, h, Chematech, Dijon, France). Elongation of the peptide chain was done by repetitive cycles of Fmoc deprotection applying 20% piperidine in DMF (microwave irradiation: 5× 5 s, 100 W), followed by 5 washings with DMF and subsequent peptide couplings using the following conditions: AA/PyBOP/diisopropylethylamine HOBt (5 eq/5 eq/5 eq/7.5 eq for a,b,c,d and 4 eq/4 eq/4 eq/6 eq for g) or AA/HATU/DIPEA (4 eq/4 eq/4 eq for e, 5 eq/5 eq/5 eq for f performing the coupling twice and 2.6 eq/2.6 eq/2.6 eq for h). The building blocks and reagents were dissolved in a minimum amount of DMF and the irradiation was performed 15× 10 s employing 50 W. After the last acylation step, the resin was 10× rinsed with CH_2Cl_2 and dried *in vacuo*. The on resin cleavage of *t*-Bu and Boc groups was achieved by stirring in a mixture of 10% v/v conc. H_2SO_4 in dioxane at 8 °C for 2 h and subsequent washing with 30% v/v DIPEA in CH_2Cl_2, followed by CH_2Cl_2 (2×). The cleavage from the resin was performed using a mixture of TFA/phenol/H_2O/triisopropylsilane 88:5:5:2 for 2 h. After evaporation of the solvent and precipitation in *tert*-butylmethyl ether, the crude peptide was purified using preparative RP-HPLC (eluent: CH_3CN (A) + 0.1% HCO_2H in H_2O (B) applying a linear gradient 3%–20% A in 97%–80% B in 16 min, t_R: 13.9 min) and subsequent lyophilization to afford the peptide as the formate salt. Peptide purity and identity was assessed by analytical HPLC. System 1:10%–40% CH_3OH in 90%–60% H_2O + 0.1% HCO_2H in 18 min, purity: 92% (t_R: 17.3 min); system 2:3%–30% CH_3CN in 97%–70% H_2O + 0.1% HCO_2H in 26 min, purity: 93% (t_R: 17.4 min). $[M+H]^+$; calcd for $C_{75}H_{132}N_{15}O_{23}$: 1611.0, found: 1611.0.

2.3. Synthesis of [^{175}Lu]NT127

NT127 (3.6 mg, 2 µmol) was dissolved in HEPES (0.5 M, 600 µL, pH 5) and $Lu(NO_3)_3$ (1.5 mg, 4 µmol) was added. After 10 min at 98 °C [^{175}Lu]**NT127** was purified by semipreparative HPLC (Kromasil C8, 125 × 8 mm, 10%–50% acetonitrile (0.1% TFA) in water (0.1% TFA) in a linear gradient over 25 min, 4 mL/min, t_R = 9.8 min). Peptide purity and identity was assessed by analytical HPLC. System 1: 10%–40% CH_3OH + 0.1% HCO_2H in 90%–60% H_2O in 18 min, Purity: >99% (t_R: 16.8 min). $[M]^+$; calcd for $C_{75}H_{129}N_{15}O_{23}Lu$: 1782.9, found: 1782.8.

2.4. Neurotensin Receptor Binding Experiments

Receptor binding data were determined according to protocols as described previously [6,36]. In detail, NTS1 binding was measured using homogenates of membranes from CHO cells stably expressing human NTS1 at a final concentration of 2 µg/well and the radioligand [^{3}H]neurotensin (specific activity 116 Ci/mmol; PerkinElmer, Rodgau, Germany) at a concentration of 0.50 nM.

Specific binding of the radioligand was determined at a K_D value of 0.69 nM and a B_{max} of 6200 fmol/mg protein. Nonspecific binding was determined in the presence of 10 μM neurotensin. NTS2 binding was done using homogenates of membranes from transiently transfected HEK 293 cells at a concentration of 20 μg/well together with 0.50 nM of [^{3}H]NT(8-13) (specific activity 136 Ci/mmol; custom synthesis by GE Healthcare, Freiburg, Germany) at a K_D value of 1.3 nM and a B_{max} of 800 fmol/mg protein. Nonspecific binding was determined in the presence of 10 μM NT(8–13). Protein concentration was generally determined by the method of Lowry using bovine serum albumin as standard [37]. Data analysis of the competition curves from the radioligand binding experiments was accomplished by non-linear regression analysis using the algorithms in PRISM5.0 (GraphPad Software, San Diego, CA, USA). EC_{50} values derived from the resulting dose response curves were transformed into the corresponding K_i values according to the equation of Cheng and Prusoff [38].

*2.5. Synthesis of [^{177}Lu]**NT127***

NT127 (4 nmol) was dissolved in 5 μL of metal-free water and HEPES (0.5 M, 200 μL, pH 5) and n.c.a. [^{177}Lu]$LuCl_3$ (20–50 μL, 50–100 MBq, Isotope Technologies Garching (ITG) GmbH, Garching, Germany) was added. After 10 min at 98 °C the reaction mixture was diluted with isotonic saline (0.9%) and [^{177}Lu]**NT127** was used without further purification for *in vitro* and *in vivo* experiments. The radiochemical yield and radiochemical purity was determined from an aliquot taken from the reaction mixture by radio-HPLC (t_R = 2.20 min; Chromolith RP-18e, 10 × 4.6 mm, 10%–50% acetonitrile (0.1% TFA) in water (0.1% TFA) in a linear gradient over 5 min, 4 mL/min) and was determined >98%.

2.6. Synthesis of [^{68}Ga]DOTA-RGD

To the DOTA-conjugated precursor c(RGDfK(DOTA)) [35] (10 nmol) in acetate buffer (2.5 M, 140 μL) was added an aliquot of [^{68}Ga]$GaCl_3$ (200 MBq in 500 μL, 0.6 M HCl), freshly eluted from a ^{68}Ge/^{68}Ga generator (IDB Holland BV (Baarle-Nassau, The Netherlands)/iThemba LABS (Cape Town, South Africa)), resulting in a final pH of 4.0. After incubation for 10 min at 98°C, the solution was neutralized by the addition of sodium bicarbonate (1 M, 120 μL). The radiochemical yield was >98% as determined by radio-HPLC (t_R = 1.30 min; Chromolith RP-18e, 10 × 4.6 mm, 10%–50% acetonitrile (0.1% TFA) in water (0.1% TFA) in a linear gradient over 5 min, 4 mL/min) and the specific activity was determined to be 10–15 GBq/μmol. The resulting solution was used for small animal PET studies without further purification.

*2.7. Stability of [^{177}Lu]**NT127***

An aliquot of [^{177}Lu]**NT127** (30 μL, about 2 MBq) was added to human serum (200 μL) and incubated at 37 °C. Aliquots (25 μL) were taken at various time intervals (5–210 min) and quenched in ethanol/water (1:1, 100 μL). The samples were centrifuged, and the supernatants were analyzed by radio-HPLC (t_R = 2.20 min; Chromolith RP-18e, 10 × 4.6 mm, 10%–50% acetonitrile (0.1% TFA) in water (0.1% TFA) in a linear gradient over 5 min, 4 mL/min).

2.8. Cell Culture

The human NTS1-expressing cell line HT29 (ECACC NO 91072201) [39], was grown in culture medium (McCoy's 5a medium containing glutamine (2 mM) supplemented with fetal bovine serum (FBS, 10%)) at 37 °C in a humidified atmosphere of 5% CO_2. Cells were routinely subcultured every 3–4 days. Viability of the cells was determined by staining with trypan blue and was >90% for all cells used in *in vitro* and *in vivo* studies.

*2.9. Internalization and Efflux Studies with [^{177}Lu]**NT127***

Three days before experimental use, approximately 250,000 HT29 cells were seeded in 24-multiwell plates. The medium was changed to binding buffer (culture medium supplemented with 1% bovine serum albumin (BSA), HEPES (10 mM), chymostatin (2 mg/L) and soybean trypsin inhibitor (100 mg/L), 0.5 mL) and [^{177}Lu]**NT127** (0.3 MBq, 10 μL) was added to each well. Cells were incubated for different time intervals (5, 15, 30, 60, 90 and 120 min) at 37 °C, before the incubation was terminated by placing the cells on ice, aspirating the incubation buffer and washing the cell layer twice with ice-cold PBS. The cell layers were washed twice with an acidic washing buffer (20 mM sodium acetate, pH 5) to remove non-sequestered radioactivity. Cells were harvested with NaOH (0.1 M, 1 mL) and counted in a gamma counter (Wizard Wallac, Perkin Elmer). Nonspecific binding was determined in the presence of neurotensin (1 μM). Two independent experiments were performed in quadruplicate.

For efflux studies HT29 cells were seeded in 24-multiwell plates and incubated with [^{177}Lu]**NT127** as described above. After an incubation time of 30 min at 37 °C the plates were placed on ice and the cells were washed with ice-cold PBS (500 μL), acidic wash buffer (500 μL, 1 min) and again with ice-cold PBS (500 μL). Subsequently, fresh binding buffer (500 μL) was added to each well and the plates were incubated at 37 °C. After 5 min, 15 min, 30 min, 45 min, 60 min and 90 min the plates were placed on ice, the supernatant was transferred to a counting tube, the cells were washed once with ice-cold PBS (500 μL) and this washing PBS was combined with the respective supernatant in the counting tubes. Cells were harvested with NaOH (0.1 M, 1 mL) and cell suspensions and washing solutions were counted in a gamma counter (Wizard Wallac). The experiment was performed twice in quadruplicate.

2.10. Animal Model (Nude Mice Bearing HT29 Xenografts)

All animal experiments were performed in compliance with the protocols approved by the local animal protection authorities (Regierung Mittelfranken, Ansbach, Germany, No. 54-2532.1-22/10). Female athymic nude mice (nu/nu) were obtained from Harlan Winkelmann GmbH (Borchen, Germany) at 4 weeks of age and were kept under standard conditions (12 h light/dark) with food and water available ad libitum. HT29 cells were harvested and suspended in sterile PBS at a concentration of 10^7 cells/mL. Each mouse was injected subcutaneously in the lower region of the left shoulder on the back with viable cells (2×10^6) in PBS (200 μL).

2.11. Biodistribution Studies

10–14 days after inoculation of the HT29 cells (tumor weight: 200–700 mg), the mice (about 10–12 weeks old with about 35–40 g body weight) were used for biodistribution studies. HT29 xenografted mice were injected with [^{177}Lu]**NT127** (1–3 MBq/mouse) intravenously into the tail vein. They were sacrificed by cervical dislocation 1 h, 4 h and 24 h after injection. Tumors and other tissues (blood, lung, liver, kidneys, heart, spleen, brain, muscle, femur and intestine) were rapidly removed and weighed. Radioactivity of the dissected tissues was measured using a gamma counter (Wallac Wizard, Perkin Elmer). Results were expressed as percentage of injected dose per gram of tissue (% ID/g), and tumor-to-organ ratios were calculated. Two randomly chosen mice were used for the determination of nonspecific tracer uptake *in vivo*. These blocking experiments were carried out by intravenous coinjection of mice with [^{177}Lu]**NT127** together with NT4 [28] (100 µg/animal). These mice were sacrificed by cervical dislocation at 4 h post injection (p.i.) and organs and tissue were removed, weighed and counted as described above.

2.12. Radiotherapy Studies with [^{177}Lu]NT127 and Small Animal PET Imaging

5–6 days after inoculation of the HT29 cells (tumor diameter: 4–5 mm), the mice (about 10–12 weeks old with about 35–40 g body weight) were divided into four groups. The control group (n = 8) received i.v. the vehicle (0.5 nmol **NT127** in 100 µL saline) with no activity at the same days as the treated animals. Treated group 1 (n = 4) received i.v. 28–38 MBq/mouse [^{177}Lu]**NT127** in two fractionated doses of 11–15 MBq (at days 0) and 17–23 MBq at day 6, treated group 2 (n = 3) received a single dose of 49–51 MBq/mouse [^{177}Lu]**NT127** (at day 0) and treated group 3 (n = 4) received 50–51 MBq/mouse [^{177}Lu]**NT127** in four fractionated doses of 11–14 MBq/mouse (at days 0, 3, 6 and 10). Each dose contained between 0.3–0.7 nmol **NT127**. The body weight of the mice was determined three times a week and the diameter of the tumors was measured with a calliper three times a week for 30–33 days starting the day of the first injection (day 0). An additional group of three animals was injected with a single low dose of 21 MBq/mouse. These were also used for histological staining of tissue samples from kidney and liver.

PET scans and image analysis were performed using a microPET rodent model scanner (Inveon, Siemens Healthcare, Erlangen, Germany). About 3–8 MBq of [^{68}Ga]DOTA-RGD was intravenously injected into each mouse at day 7, 14, 21 and 28 after the first [^{177}Lu]**NT127**-treatment under isoflurane anesthesia (4%). Animals were subjected to a 15 min scan starting from 45 min p.i. After 3D-OSEM iterative image reconstruction with decay and attenuation correction, regions of interest (ROIs) were drawn over the tumor region, and the mean within a tumor was converted to standard uptake values (SUV) considering the injected activity and body weight.

2.13. Histology of Tissue Samples from Kidney and Liver

28 days after first treatment the mice were sacrificed by cervical dislocation and kidneys and liver were dissected and immediately fixed in 4% neutral buffered formalin at room temperature overnight and then stored in phosphate buffered saline at 4 °C. For histological examinations the tissue was paraffin-embedded, cut in four-micrometer sections and stained with Masson-Goldner trichrome.

Quantification of tissue inflammation was done using a digital light microscope (Axioplan 2 imaging, Zeiss) with the software Metafer 4 (v. 3.9.1) and VSlide (v. 1.0.125). A virtual grid was placed over the sections and the quantitative detection of inflammation per visual field was carried out according to the following scheme: none (0), low (1), moderate (2), much (3).

3. Results and Discussion

Our plan of synthesis was based on our previous publications on metabolically stabilized NT(8–13) derivatives (Scheme 1) [7,28,29].

Scheme 1. (Radio)synthesis of [^{175}Lu]**NT127** and [^{177}Lu]**NT127**.

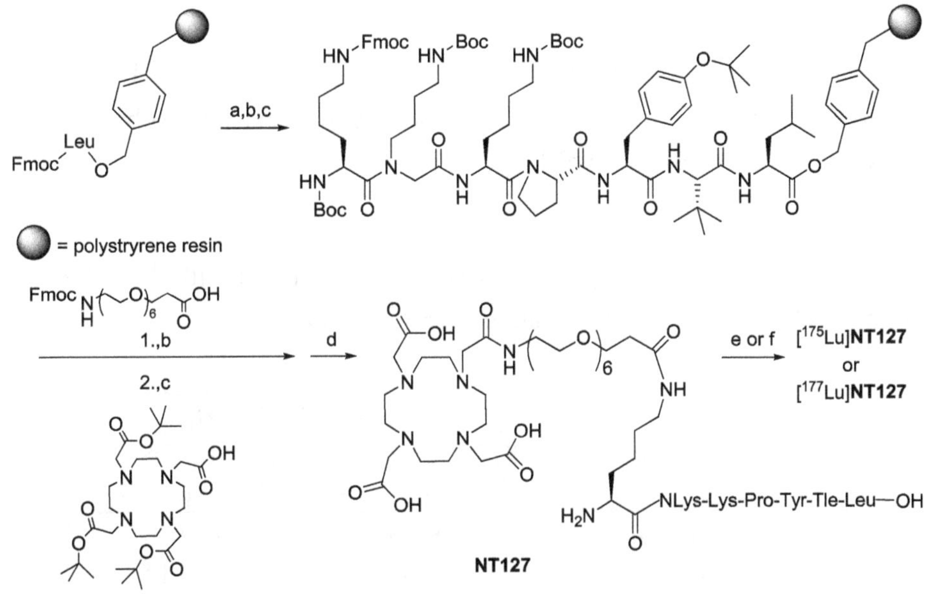

Reagents and conditions: (**a**) Fmoc-deprotection: piperidine/DMF (1:4), μ~: 5× 5 s, 100 W, 5 × cooling to −10 °C; (**b**) peptide coupling for Fmoc-Tle-OH, Fmoc-Tyr(*t*Bu)-OH, Fmoc-Pro-OH, Fmoc-Lys(Boc)-OH, Fmoc-21-amino-4,7,10,13,16,19-hexaoxaheneicosanoic acid: Fmoc-AA-OH, PyBOP, DIPEA, HOBt, DMF, μ~, 15× 10 s, 50 W, 15× cooling to −10 °C; (**c**) for *N*-Fmoc-*N*-(4-Boc-aminobutyl)-Gly-OH, Boc-Lys(Fmoc)-OH, DOTA-tri-*t*-Bu-ester: Fmoc-AA-OH, HATU, DIPEA, DMF, μ~-assisted coupling (see **b**); (**d**) deprotection/cleavage of the peptide: (1) H_2SO_4/dioxane (1:9), 8 °C, 2 h; (2) DIPEA/CH_2Cl_2 (3:7); (3) TFA, phenol, H_2O, triisopropylsilane 88:5:5:2, 2 h, followed by RP-HPLC; (**e**) $Lu(NO_3)_3$, 0.5 M HEPES pH 5, 98 °C, 10 min or (**f**) n.c.a. [^{177}Lu]$LuCl_3$, 0.5 M HEPES pH 5, 98 °C, 10 min.

In detail, we applied solid-phase methods with repetitive cycles of Fmoc deprotection with piperidine and acylation with the respective Fmoc-protected amino acids. Amino acid activation was done in the presence of PyBOP/HOBt, thus allowing us to incorporate *t*-leucine, tyrosine, proline, lysine, and amino-4,7,10,13,16,19-hexaoxaheneicosanoic acid. The more powerful coupling agent HATU was employed for the attachment of *N*-(4-aminobutyl)-glycine, for the lysine linker as well as for the chelator 1,4,7,10-tetraazacyclododecane-1,4,7,10-tetraacetic acid (DOTA), which was coupled as the commercially available tri-*t*-butyl ester derivative. Microwave acceleration proved to be advantageous for both Fmoc deprotection and acylation reactions. For a safe peptide cleavage without concomitant *t*-butylation of the peptide side chains, we decided to apply our recently published two step protocol removing the *t*-butyl-based protective groups by a pre-treatment with 10% sulfuric acid in dioxane at 8 °C at first [10]. Thereafter, final cleavage from the resin with TFA resulted in the formation of crude peptide with acceptable amounts of *t*-butylated byproduct, sufficiently pure to allow successful high-performance liquid chromatography (HPLC) purification. The synthesis of the lutetium complex [^{175}Lu]**127** was accomplished by stirring **NT127** for 10 min with an excess of $Lu(NO_3)_3$ (2 equiv) in 0.5 M HEPES buffer (pH 5) at 98 °C, followed by RP-HPLC purification (Scheme 1). Electrospray ionization-mass spectrometry revealed the $[M]^+$ peak of [^{175}Lu]**127**, confirming previous studies on DOTA-conjugated peptides with one free deprotonated carboxylate group at physiological pH that does not participate with the pseudo-octahedral geometry of the Ga-DOTA complex of the peptide [40].

After verification of the purity of **NT127** (⩾92%) and of the reference compound [^{175}Lu]**NT127** (>99%), the lutetium complex [^{175}Lu]**NT127** was subjected to receptor binding studies for the neurotensin receptor subtypes NTS1 and NTS2. The results revealed substantial NTS1 subtype selectivity with a K_i value for NTS1 of 30 nM (Table 1).

Table 1. Receptor binding data of [^{175}Lu]**NT127** in comparison with the reference ligands neurotensin and NT(8-13) employing human NTS1 and NTS2 [a].

Compound	K_i value ± SEM [nM]	
	K_i [nM] NTS1 [b] [^{3}H]neurotensin	K_i [nM] NTS2 [c] [^{3}H]NT(8-13)
Neurotensin	0.51 ± 0.06 [d]	4.9 ± 0.3
NT(8-13)	0.29 ± 0.03	1.4 ± 0.1 [d]
[^{175}Lu]**NT127**	30 ± 6	220 ± 93

[a] K_i values ± SEM are the means of three individual experiments each done in triplicate; [b] Membranes from CHO cells stably expressing human NTS1; [c] Homogenates from HEK cells transiently expressing human NTS2; [d] K_d values ± SEM are the means of 13–20 individual saturation experiments each done in quadruplicates.

Starting from **NT127**, the radiosynthesis of [^{177}Lu]**NT127** was performed in HEPES buffer at 98 °C to give [^{177}Lu]**NT127** in high radiochemical yield and high radiochemical purity (> 98%) without the need for further purification (Scheme 1). The stability of the tracer in human serum *in vitro* was 89% after incubation at 37 °C for 3.5 h (Figures S1 and S2).

The amount of internalization [^{177}Lu]**NT127** was determined *in vitro* using HT29 cells. [^{177}Lu]**NT127** revealed an internalization rate of 82% ± 9% after 15 min which remained constant over 120 min (Figure 2). To determine the efflux from the cells, [^{177}Lu]**NT127** was allowed to internalize for 30 min into HT29 cells, then the cells were washed with acid buffer to remove surface bound radioactivity, and fresh media was added. After 90 min there was still a high amount of internalized [^{177}Lu]**NT127** of 42% ± 5% (Figure 2).

Figure 2. Internalization and efflux of [^{177}Lu]**NT127** in human HT29 cells. Each data point represents the mean ± standard deviation of two experiments performed in quadruplicate.

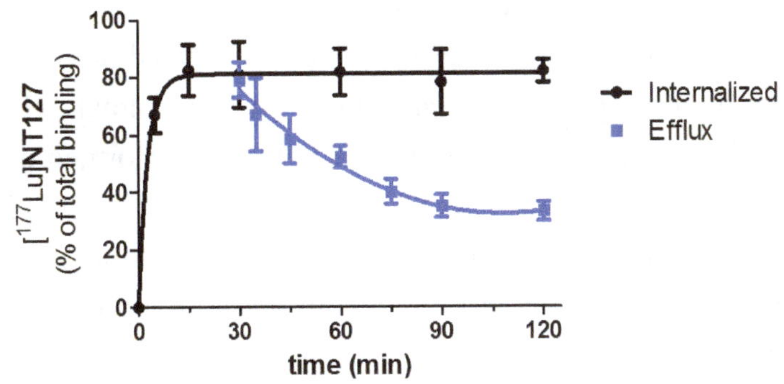

The biodistribution studies of [^{177}Lu]**NT127** were carried out with HT29 tumor-bearing nude mice and showed a strong accumulation of the tracer in the kidney with 38 ± 1% ID/g at 1 h post-injection (p.i.), which was reduced to 20% ± 5% ID/g at 24 h p.i. (Figure 3). [^{177}Lu]**NT127** showed the second highest accumulation in the HT29 tumor at 1 h p.i. (1.5% ± 0.2% ID/g), whereas after 24 h the tracer was partially washed out again (0.6% ID/g). In the liver the radioactivity concentration was 0.7% ± 0.1% ID/g after 1 h and 0.4% ID/g after 24 h. The clearance from blood was very fast, resulting in 0.05% ID/g in blood at 1 h p.i. which was reduced to 0.01% ID/g at 24 h p.i., providing an excellently high tumor-to-blood ratio of 30 (60 min p.i.) and 60 (24 h p.i.), respectively.

Figure 3. Biodistribution of [^{177}Lu]**NT127** in HT29 xenografted nude mice 1 h , 4 h and 24 h after injection and 4 h after injection of [^{177}Lu]**NT127** together with **NT4** (100 μg/mouse, "blocking"). Each data point represents the mean ± standard deviation of tissue samples from two mice.

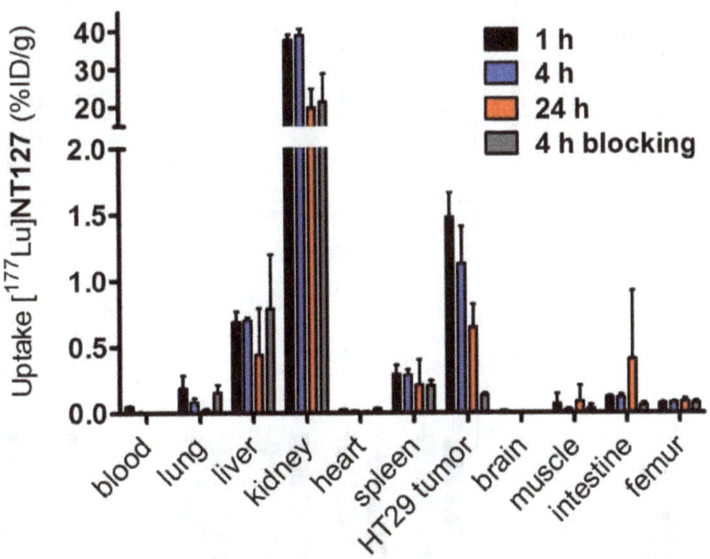

In order to determine the specific binding of [^{177}Lu]**NT127** *in vivo*, two HT29 tumor-bearing nude mice were co-injected with [^{177}Lu]**NT127** and the high-affinity NTS1 ligand **NT4** [28]. In the HT29 tumor the accumulation of [^{177}Lu]**NT127** was significantly reduced at 4 h p.i. by the co-injection of **NT4** from 1.1% ID/g to 0.1% ID/g, indicating the specificity of tracer uptake in the HT29 tumors.

To study the effect of [^{177}Lu]**NT127** as a radiotherapeutical agent, HT29 tumor-bearing nude mice were injected with different doses of [^{177}Lu]**NT127** and the tumor growth as well as the body weight was measured every third day over a 30 day-period and compared with mice injected with vehicle only. In all experiments, the course of the body weight of the treated animals during therapy did not reveal a static decrease, indicating the physical fitness of the animals (Figure S3). However, a statistical analysis of the differences in body weight has not been performed due to the low number of animals used in this initial study. In group 1 that received two doses of 11–15 MBq and 17–23 MBq for each animal at day 0 and day 6, respectively, no change in tumor growth was observed when compared to the control group (Figure 4a). The animals in treatment group 2, receiving four fractionated doses of 11–14 MBq/mouse at days 0, 3, 6 and 10, also did not show any significant change in the mean tumor growth (Figure 4b). It is worth mentioning that two of the four treated mice of this group showed reduced tumor growth, however, the mean value over all four animals did not reveal any significant difference in the relative tumor growth. In contrast to the fractionated administration, the animals in treatment group 3 received a single high dose of 50 MBq per animal at the beginning of radiotherapy. These animals showed a significant reduction of about 50% in the mean tumor growth for all treated animals compared to the sham-treated controls (Figure 4c).

Figure 4. (a,b,c) Change in tumor growth after a single high **(c)** dose or a two-time **(a)** or four-time **(b)** sequential dose of [^{177}Lu]**NT127**. **(d,e,f)** Standard uptake values (SUVmean) of [^{68}Ga]DOTA-RGD in HT29 tumor-bearing nude mice at day 7, 14, 21 and 28 after injection of a single **(f)**; two-time **(d)**; or four-time **(e)** dose of [^{177}Lu]**NT127**. *$p < 0.05$, $n = 8$ (sham-treated animals) *vs.* $n = 3$ (treated animals).

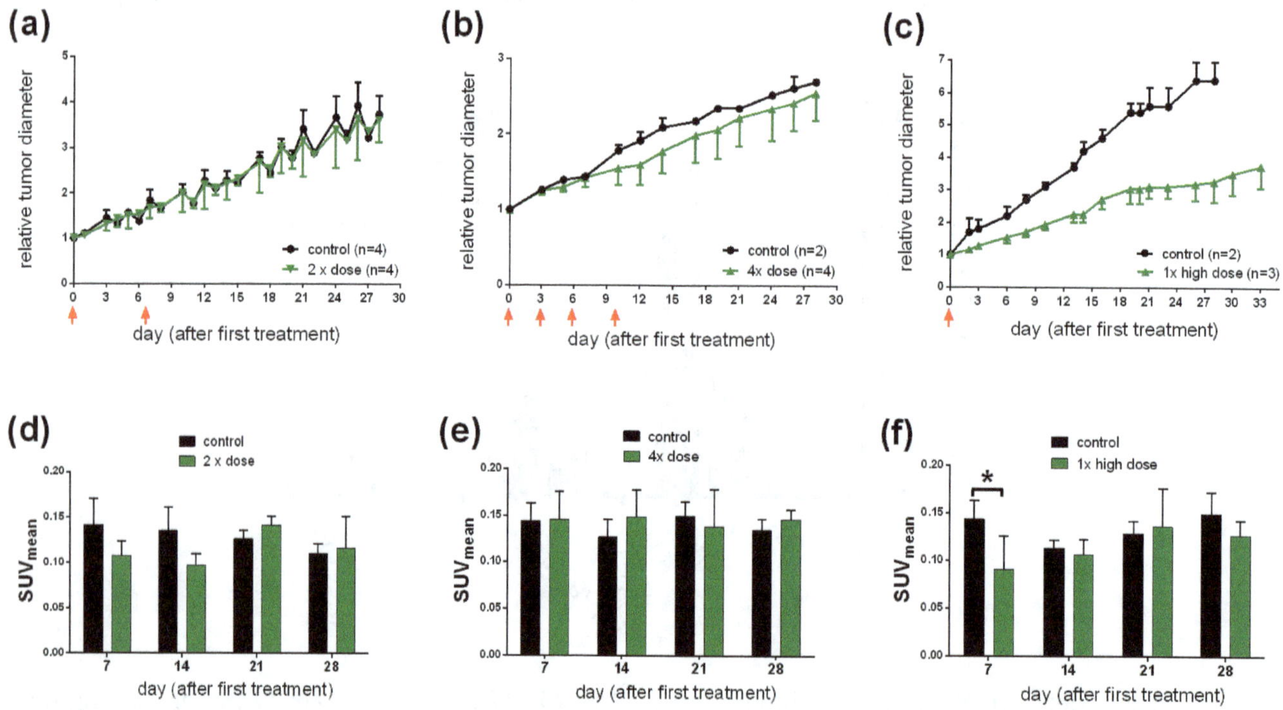

Next, we investigated the use of [^{68}Ga]DOTA-RGD to monitor the response of tumors to the radiotherapy with [^{177}Lu]**NT127** in the four nude mice groups. Therefore, PET scans with [^{68}Ga]DOTA-RGD were performed at day 7, 14 21 and 28 after first treatment. As shown in

Figure 4d–f the only significant change in tumor uptake values (SUV_{mean}) can be observed at day 7 after treatment by the single high dose of 50 MBq (Figure 4f, $p < 0.05$, $n = 8$ (sham-treated animals) *vs.* $n = 3$ (treated animals)). The decreased uptake of the RGD tracer indicated a lower degree of $\alpha_v\beta_3$ integrin expression in the tumor region at day 7 after treatment. The difference between control and treated animals was also confirmed by the μPET image analysis of a representative pair of animals, when the treated animal indicated a significantly lower uptake of [^{68}Ga]DOTA-RGD in the HT29 tumor region compared to the corresponding sham-treated animal, as shown in Figure 5. However, we could not detect any significant changes in the tumor uptake of [^{68}Ga]DOTA-RGD between treated and untreated animal groups at later time points of more than seven days after treatment (Figure 4f). This result might reflect the response of HT29 tumors toward radiation, resulting in regeneration of maximal integrin expression in the tumor region that did not differ significantly any more from the level that was found in sham-treated animals at day 7 and later after treatment. Noteworthy, HT29 are well-known to show a radiation-induced increase in radioresistance at low doses [41], so this phenomenon could account for the weak response of HT29 tumors toward fractionated therapy by administration of four equal doses (group 3, Figure 4b).

Figure 5. Representative PET scans at 45–60 min p.i. of [^{68}Ga]DOTA-RGD obtained from HT29 tumor-bearing nude mice **(a)** at day 7 after radiotherapy with [^{177}Lu]**NT127** (1× high dose, 50 MBq) *vs.* **(b)** sham-treated at day 7 after begin of treatment. Both images are normalized to the same standard uptake value (SUV_{mean}) scale. Red arrows indicate the HT29 tumor.

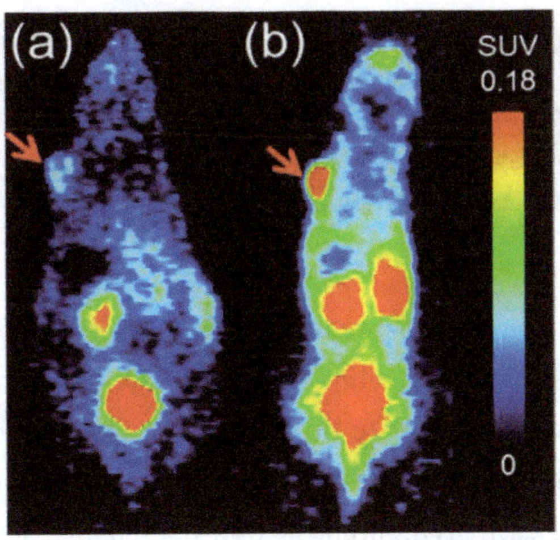

Taken together, the single high-dose endoradiotherapy with 50 MBq [^{177}Lu]**NT127** showed a substantial mean effect of 50% reduced tumor diameter, which is comparable to the result reported by Schubiger and coworkers for the rhenium-labeled peptide analog [24]. Moreover, preliminary μPET experiments identified day 7 after treatment as a potential time point for the analysis of integrin expression by RGD-PET, trying to identify an anti-angiogenic effect as an early predictor of response to endoradiotherapy with [^{177}Lu]**NT127**.

The clearance of [^{177}Lu]**NT127** predominantly occurred through the kidney and to a lower portion through the liver (Figure 3), so that these organs received the highest radiation dose during tumor therapy. Therefore, we performed histological staining to study potential tissue damage, e.g., fibrotic lesions, in kidney and liver. In particular, both the glomeruli and the tubules in the kidney sections from animals that received a two-time consecutive dose show strong fibrosis compared to sham-treated control animals (Figure 6). In the corresponding liver sections, both the singular and the sequential dose led to increased tissue damage (Figure 6). This finding might hamper the translation of the NTS1-mediated radiotherapy approach with [^{177}Lu]**NT127** into human application in the future.

Figure 6. Histological examinations of kidney (**upper row**) and liver (**lower row**). Masson-goldner trichrome staining of liver and kidney sections from mice which received a single low dose of 21 MBq (1× dose) or two fractionated doses of 13 MBq and 19 MBq (2× dose) in comparison with sham-treated animals (control). Red arrows indicate fibrotic lesions in kidney. White arrows indicated fibrotic lesions in liver. All images are representative photographs captured at a magnification of ×10 (the scale bar represents 800 μm). Bar charts: The number of fibrotic tissue damages was quantified for whole sections of each tissue at comparable position and evaluated according to the following classification: 0/no fibrosis, 1/few fibrosis, 2/medium fibrosis, 3/many fibrosis. The asterisk indicated a significant difference ($p < 0.05$, one-way Anova test).

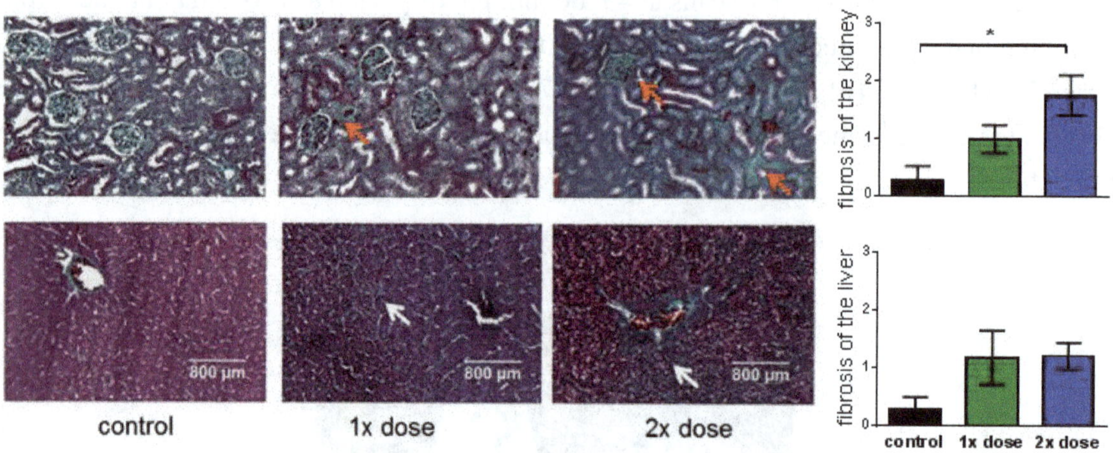

In medical oncology, it is desirable to predict as early as possible whether an individual tumor responds to treatment. Structural imaging techniques such as X-ray computerized tomography (CT) or magnetic resonance imaging (MRI) capitalize on changes in tumor size for this purpose. However, a treatment-induced decrease of tumor size does often not occur until weeks to months after institution of treatment; furthermore, e.g., in lymphomas, non-neoplastic scar tissue may persist despite eradication of the tumor cells, leading to false-negative CT or MRI results. Therefore, the possible value of the molecular imaging modality PET for this purpose has been subject of considerable research efforts in the last decade (for a review, see [42]). The PET measurement of glucose consumption using [^{18}F]fluorodeoxyglucose has, indeed, been proven to be of some value in this regard and, in particular, for establishing proof of treatment response in lymphomas, colorectal carcinomas, and gastrointestinal stroma tumors.

Changes in tumor vasculature are thought to have an important role in determining tumor response to radiotherapy [43]. Furthermore, radiation treatment does not only destroy the neoplastic cells, but also the vascular bed of the tumor as endothelial cells are even more sensitive to radiation than most cancer cells. Therefore, in this study, in addition to tumor volume, we analysed integrin expression to predict treatment effect. In the single-dose group that responded by significant tumor shrinkage to therapy radioreceptor treatment produced also an early decrease in RGD tracer uptake as measured by PET. However, this was only short-lived, although the treated animals consistently had lower tumor volumes than those in the control group until the end-point of treatment at day 28. One possible explanation for this phenomenon is provided by inflammatory changes occurring after initial radiation damage to the vascular bed of the tumors and to the tumor cells themselves. Indeed, some evidence for that could be seen in our histopathological specimens. To date, literature is scarce with regard to alterations of integrin tissue expression caused by radiation treatment. Therefore, this interpretation of our results must remain speculative, awaiting confirmation by future research.

4. Conclusions

With [^{177}Lu]**NT127** in our hands, we offer an agonist radiopeptide with high-affinity to NTS1, providing the option to study endoradiotherapy with that radiopeptide in preclinical animal models. In NTS1-positive HT29-tumor-bearing nude mice, we observed decreased tumor progression after administration of a single high-dose of the radiopeptide. In the sequentially treated animals, the decreased tumor progression was less pronounced visible when analyzing the tumor diameter. However, our preliminary PET imaging data at day 7 after treatment with a single high dose of [^{177}Lu]**NT127** suggested decreased uptake values of [^{68}Ga]DOTA-RGD compared to sham-treated controls. Further longitudinal PET imaging studies are needed to confirm the statistical significance and predictive value of RGD-PET for NTS1-mediated radiotherapy.

Acknowledgments

The authors thank Iris Torres and Manuel Geisthoff for expert technical support and Udo Gaipl (Department of Radiation Oncology, University Hospital, Erlangen) for assistance and support in digital light microscopy. ITG Garching is acknowledged for delivering n.c.a. Lu-177. This work was supported by the Deutsche Forschungsgemeinschaft (DFG, grants MA 4295/1-2).

Author Contributions

S.M. designed and coordinated the study, performed the radiosyntheses, supervised the data analyses and interpretations and contributed to writing of the manuscript. T.R. performed the *in vitro* and *in vivo* experiments and analyzed the data. P.T. was involved in the animal experiments and supervised the cell culture, histology, and microscopic analyses. R.H. synthesized the RGD peptide and critically reviewed the manuscript. J.E. designed and synthesized the NT peptides and contributed to writing of the manuscript. H.H. performed the neurotensin receptor binding assays and analyzed the data. P.G. and T.K. contributed to writing of the manuscript and critically reviewed the manuscript. O.P. designed and supervised all aspects of the current study and contributed to writing of the manuscript. All authors approved the final manuscript.

References

1. Carraway, R.; Leeman, S.E. The isolation of a new hypotensive peptide, neurotensin, from bovine hypothalami. *J. Biol. Chem.* **1973**, *248*, 6854–6861.
2. Tyler-McMahon, B.M.; Boules, M.; Richelson, E. Neurotensin: Peptide for the next millennium. *Regul. Pept.* **2000**, *93*, 125–136.
3. Vincent, J.P.; Mazella, J.; Kitabgi, P. Neurotensin and neurotensin receptors. *Trends Pharmacol. Sci.* **1999**, *20*, 302–309.
4. Bittermann, H.; Boeckler, F.; Einsiedel, J.; Gmeiner, P. A highly practical RCM approach towards a molecular building kit of spirocyclic reverse turn mimics. *Chem. Eur. J.* **2006**, *12*, 6315–6322.
5. Bittermann, H.; Einsiedel, J.; Hübner, H.; Gmeiner, P. Evaluation of lactam-bridged neurotensin analogues adjusting psi(Pro(10)) close to the experimentally derived bioactive conformation of NT(8-13). *J. Med. Chem.* **2004**, *47*, 5587–5590.
6. Einsiedel, J.; Held, C.; Hervet, M.; Plomer, M.; Tschammer, N.; Hübner, H.; Gmeiner, P. Discovery of Highly Potent and Neurotensin Receptor 2 Selective Neurotensin Mimetics. *J. Med. Chem.* **2011**, *54*, 2915–2923.
7. Einsiedel, J.; Hübner, H.; Hervet, M.; Harterich, S.; Koschatzky, S.; Gmeiner, P. Peptide backbone modifications on the C-terminal hexapeptide of neurotensin. *Bioorg. Med. Chem. Lett.* **2008**, *18*, 2013–2018.
8. Härterich, S.; Koschatzky, S.; Einsiedel, J.; Gmeiner, P. Novel insights into GPCR—Peptide interactions: Mutations in extracellular loop 1, ligand backbone methylations and molecular modeling of neurotensin receptor 1. *Bioorgan. Med. Chem.* **2008**, *16*, 9359–9368.
9. Held, C.; Hübner, H.; Kling, R.; Nagel, Y.A.; Wennemers, H.; Gmeiner, P. Impact of the Proline Residue on Ligand Binding of Neurotensin Receptor 2 (NTS2)-Selective Peptide-Peptoid Hybrids. *ChemMedChem* **2013**, *8*, 772–778.
10. Held, C.; Plomer, M.; Hübner, H.; Meltretter, J.; Pischetsrieder, M.; Gmeiner, P. Development of a Metabolically Stable Neurotensin Receptor 2 (NTS2) Ligand. *ChemMedChem* **2013**, *8*, 75–81.
11. Heyl, D.L.; Sefler, A.M.; He, J.X.; Sawyer, T.K.; Wustrow, D.J.; Akunne, H.C.; Davis, M.D.; Pugsley, T.A.; Heffner, T.G.; Corbin, A.E.; *et al.* Structure-Activity and Conformational Studies of a Series of Modified C-Terminal Hexapeptide Neurotensin Analogs. *Int. J. Pept. Prot. Res.* **1994**, *44*, 233–238.
12. Hong, F.; Cusack, B.; Fauq, A.; Richelson, E. Peptidic and non-peptidic neurotensin analogs. *Curr. Med. Chem.* **1997**, *4*, 421–434.
13. Lundquist, J.T.; Bullesbach, E.E.; Golden, P.L.; Dix, T.A. Topography of the neurotensin (NT)(8–9) binding site of human NT receptor-1 probed with NT(8–13) analogs. *J. Pept. Res.* **2002**, *59*, 55–61.
14. Reubi, J.C.; Waser, B.; Friess, H.; Buchler, M.; Laissue, J. Neurotensin receptors: A new marker for human ductal pancreatic adenocarcinoma. *Gut* **1998**, *42*, 546–550.
15. Wu, Z.; Martinez-Fong, D.; Tredaniel, J.; Forgez, P. Neurotensin and its high affinity receptor 1 as a potential pharmacological target in cancer therapy. *Front. Endocrinol.* **2012**, *3*, doi:10.3389/fendo.2012.00184.

16. Dupouy, S.; Mourra, N.; Doan, V.K.; Gompel, A.; Alifano, M.; Forgez, P. The potential use of the neurotensin high affinity receptor 1 as a biomarker for cancer progression and as a component of personalized medicine in selective cancers. *Biochimie* **2011**, *93*, 1369–1378.
17. Myers, R.M.; Shearman, J.W.; Kitching, M.O.; Ramos-Montoya, A.; Neal, D.E.; Ley, S.V. Cancer, Chemistry, and the Cell: Molecules that Interact with the Neurotensin Receptors. *ACS Chem. Biol.* **2009**, *4*, 503–525.
18. Buchegger, F.; Bonvin, F.; Kosinski, M.; Schaffland, A.O.; Prior, J.; Reubi, J.C.; Blauenstein, P.; Tourwé, D.; Garayoa, E.G.; Delaloye, A.B. Radiolabeled neurotensin analog, Tc-99m-NT-XI, evaluated in ductal pancreatic adenocarcinoma patients. *J. Nucl. Med.* **2003**, *44*, 1649–1654.
19. Zhang, K.J.; An, R.; Gao, Z.R.; Zhang, Y.X.; Aruva, M.R. Radionuclide imaging of small-cell lung cancer (SCLC) using Tc-99m-labeled neurotensin peptide 8-13. *Nucl. Med. Biol.* **2006**, *33*, 505–512.
20. Nock, B.A.; Nikolopoulou, A.; Reubi, J.C.; Maes, V.; Conrath, P.; Tourwe, D.; Maina, T. Toward stable N-4-modified neurotensins for NTS1-receptor-targeted tumor imaging with Tc-99m. *J. Med. Chem.* **2006**, *49*, 4767–4776.
21. Maina, T.; Nikolopoulou, A.; Stathopoulou, E.; Galanis, A.S.; Cordopatis, P.; Nock, B.A. [^{99m}Tc]Demotensin 5 and 6 in the NTS1-R-targeted imaging of tumours: Synthesis and preclinical results. *Eur. J. Nucl. Med. Mol. Imaging* **2007**, *34*, 1804–1814.
22. Garcia-Garayoa, E.; Maes, V.; Blauenstein, P.; Blanc, A.; Hohn, A.; Tourwé, D.; Schubiger, P.A. Double-stabilized neurotensin analogues as potential radiopharmaceuticals for NTR-positive tumors. *Nucl. Med. Biol.* **2006**, *33*, 495–503.
23. Orwig, K.S.; Lassetter, M.R.; Hadden, M.K.; Dix, T.A. Comparison of N-Terminal Modifications on Neurotensin(8-13) Analogues Correlates Peptide Stability but Not Binding Affinity with *in Vivo* Efficacy. *J. Med. Chem.* **2009**, *52*, 1803–1813.
24. Garcia-Garayoa, E.; Blauenstein, P.; Blanc, A.; Maes, V.; Tourwé, D.; Schubiger, P.A. A stable neurotensin-based radiopharmaceutical for targeted imaging and therapy of neurotensin receptor-positive tumours. *Eur. J. Nucl. Med. Mol. Imaging* **2009**, *36*, 37–47.
25. Alshoukr, F.; Prignon, A.; Brans, L.; Jallane, A.; Mendes, S.; Talbot, J.N.; Tourwé, D.; Barbet, J.; Gruaz-Guyon, A. Novel DOTA-Neurotensin Analogues for In-111 Scintigraphy and Ga-68 PET Imaging of Neurotensin Receptor-Positive Tumors. *Bioconjugate Chem.* **2011**, *22*, 1374–1385.
26. De Visser, M.; Janssen, P.J.; Srinivasan, A.; Reubi, J.C.; Waser, B.; Erion, J.L.; Schmidt, M.A.; Krenning, E.P.; de Jong, M. Stabilised In-111-labelled DTPA- and DOTA-conjugated neurotensin analogues for imaging and therapy of exocrine pancreatic cancer. *Eur. J. Nucl. Med. Mol. Imaging* **2003**, *30*, 1134–1139.
27. Janssen, P.J.; de Visser, M.; Verwijnen, S.M.; Bernard, B.F.; Srinivasan, A.; Erion, J.L.; Breeman, W.A.; Vulto, A.G.; Krenning, E.P.; de Jong, M. Five stabilized ^{111}In-labeled neurotensin analogs in nude mice bearing HT29 tumors. *Cancer Biother. Radiopharm.* **2007**, *22*, 374–381.
28. Maschauer, S.; Einsiedel, J.; Haubner, R.; Hocke, C.; Ocker, M.; Hübner, H.; Kuwert, T.; Gmeiner, P.; Prante, O. Labeling and Glycosylation of Peptides Using Click Chemistry: A General Approach to ^{18}F-Glycopeptides as Effective Imaging Probes for Positron Emission Tomography. *Angew. Chem. Int. Ed.* **2010**, *49*, 976–979.

29. Maschauer, S.; Einsiedel, J.; Hocke, C.; Hübner, H.; Kuwert, T.; Gmeiner, P.; Prante, O. Synthesis of a ^{68}Ga-Labeled Peptoid-Peptide Hybrid for Imaging of Neurotensin Receptor Expression *in Vivo*. *ACS Med. Chem. Lett.* **2010**, *1*, 224–228.
30. Aumailley, M.; Gurrath, M.; Muller, G.; Calvete, J.; Timpl, R.; Kessler, H. Arg-Gly-Asp constrained within cyclic pentapeptides. Strong and selective inhibitors of cell adhesion to vitronectin and laminin fragment P1. *FEBS Lett.* **1991**, *291*, 50–54.
31. Haubner, R.; Beer, A.J.; Wang, H.; Chen, X. Positron emission tomography tracers for imaging angiogenesis. *Eur. J. Nucl. Med. Mol. Imaging* **2010**, *37*, S86–S103.
32. Haubner, R. PET radiopharmaceuticals in radiation treatment planning—Synthesis and biological characteristics. *Radiother. Oncol.* **2010**, *96*, 280–287.
33. Battle, M.R.; Goggi, J.L.; Allen, L.; Barnett, J.; Morrison, M.S. Monitoring tumor response to antiangiogenic sunitinib therapy with ^{18}F-fluciclatide, an ^{18}F-labeled $\alpha_v\beta_3$-integrin and $\alpha_v\beta_5$-integrin imaging agent. *J. Nucl. Med.* **2011**, *52*, 424–430.
34. Sun, X.; Yan, Y.; Liu, S.; Cao, Q.; Yang, M.; Neamati, N.; Shen, B.; Niu, G.; Chen, X. ^{18}F-FPPRGD2 and ^{18}F-FDG PET of response to Abraxane therapy. *J. Nucl. Med.* **2011**, *52*, 140–146.
35. Decristoforo, C.; Hernandez Gonzalez, I.; Carlsen, J.; Rupprich, M.; Huisman, M.; Virgolini, I.; Wester, H.J.; Haubner, R. ^{68}Ga- and ^{111}In-labelled DOTA-RGD peptides for imaging of $\alpha_v\beta_3$ integrin expression. *Eur. J. Nucl. Med. Mol. Imaging* **2008**, *35*, 1507–1515.
36. Hübner, H.; Haubmann, C.; Utz, W.; Gmeiner, P. Conjugated enynes as nonaromatic catechol bioisosteres: Synthesis, binding experiments, and computational studies of novel dopamine receptor agonists recognizing preferentially the D-3 subtype. *J. Med. Chem.* **2000**, *43*, 756–762.
37. Lowry, O.H.; Rosebrough, N.J.; Farr, A.L.; Randall, R.J. Protein measurement with the Folin phenol reagent. *J. Biol. Chem.* **1951**, *193*, 265–275.
38. Cheng, Y.; Prusoff, W.H. Relationship between the inhibition constant (K1) and the concentration of inhibitor which causes 50 per cent inhibition (I50) of an enzymatic reaction. *Biochem. Pharmacol.* **1973**, *22*, 3099–3108.
39. Kitabgi, P.; Poustis, C.; Granier, C.; Vanrietschoten, J.; Rivier, J.; Morgat, J.L.; Freychet, P. Neurotensin Binding to Extraneural and Neural Receptors—Comparison with Biological-Activity and Structure-Activity-Relationships. *Mol. Pharmacol.* **1980**, *18*, 11–19.
40. Heppeler, A.; Froidevaux, S.; Macke, H.R.; Jermann, E.; Behe, M.; Powell, P.; Hennig, M. Radiometal-labelled macrocyclic chelator-derivatised somatostatin analogue with superb tumour-targeting properties and potential for receptor-mediated internal radiotherapy. *Chem. Eur. J.* **1999**, *5*, 1974–1981.
41. Wouters, B.G.; Skarsgard, L.D. Low-dose radiation sensitivity and induced radioresistance to cell killing in HT-29 cells is distinct from the "adaptive response" and cannot be explained by a subpopulation of sensitive cells. *Radiat. Res.* **1997**, *148*, 435–442.
42. Weber, W.A. Assessing tumor response to therapy. *J. Nucl. Med.* **2009**, *50*, 1S–10S.
43. El Kaffas, A.; Al-Mahrouki, A.; Tran, W.T.; Giles, A.; Czarnota, G.J. Sunitinib effects on the radiation response of endothelial and breast tumor cells. *Microvasc. Res.* **2014**, *92*,1–9.

Figure S1. Radiochemical purity of [^{177}Lu]**NT127** after incubation in human serum in vitro at 37 °C for up to 3.5 h as determined by radio-HPLC.

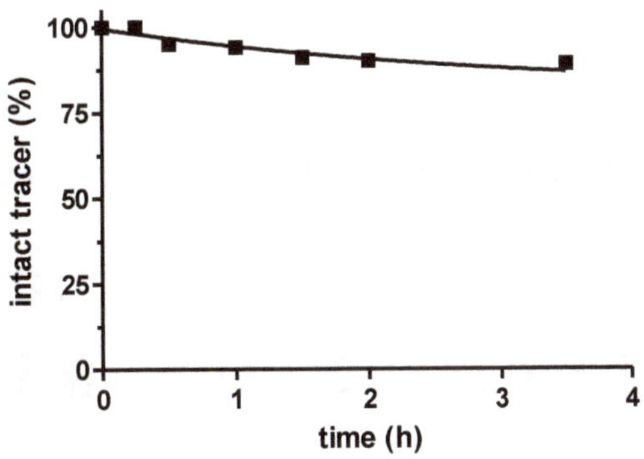

Figure S2. [^{177}Lu]**NT127** after incubation in human serum in vitro at 37 °C for 15 min (**upper HPLC chromatogram**), and for 3.5 h (**lower HPLC chromatogram**).

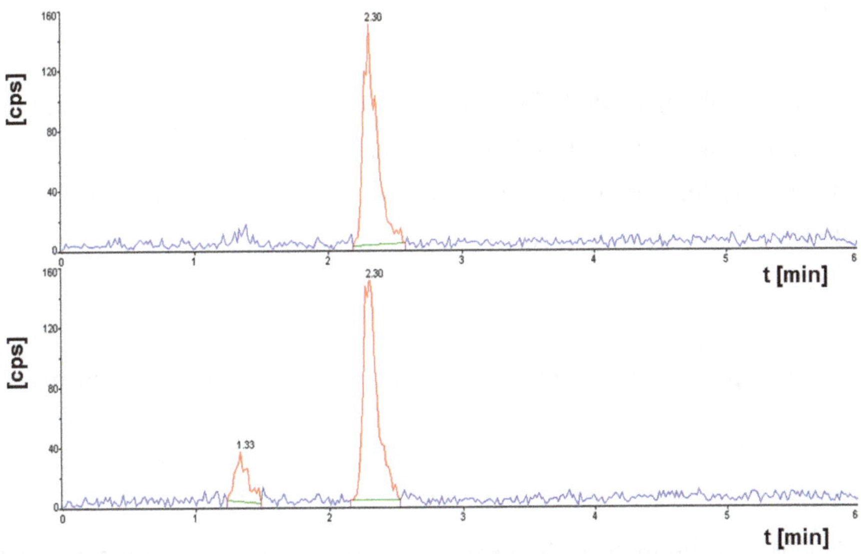

Figure S3. Relative change in body weight of the nude mice after a single high (**right**) dose or a two-time (**left**) or four-time (**middle**) sequential dose of [^{177}Lu]**NT127** in comparison with sham-treated animals (control). Data are expressed as mean ± standard deviation.

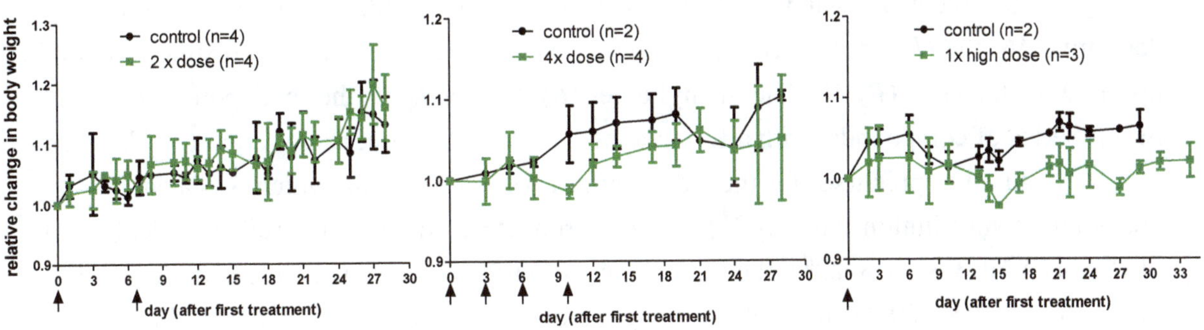

8

Asymmetric Synthesis of Spirocyclic 2-Benzopyrans for Positron Emission Tomography of σ_1 Receptors in the Brain

Katharina Holl [1], Dirk Schepmann [1], Steffen Fischer [2], Friedrich-Alexander Ludwig [2], Achim Hiller [2], Cornelius K. Donat [2], Winnie Deuther-Conrad [2], Peter Brust [2] and Bernhard Wünsch [1,*]

[1] Institut für Pharmazeutische und Medizinische Chemie der Westfälischen Wilhelms-Universität Münster, Corrensstraße 48, Münster D-48149, Germany

[2] Helmholtz-Zentrum Dresden-Rossendorf, Institut für Radiopharmazeutische Krebsforschung, Forschungsstelle Leipzig, Abteilung Neuroradiopharmaka, Permoserstraße 15, Leipzig D-04318, Germany

* Author to whom correspondence should be addressed; E-Mail: wuensch@uni-muenster.de

---

Abstract: *Sharpless* asymmetric dihydroxylation of styrene derivative **6** afforded chiral triols **(*R*)-7** and **(*S*)-7**, which were cyclized with tosyl chloride in the presence of Bu_2SnO to provide 2-benzopyrans **(*R*)-4** and **(*S*)-4** with high regioselectivity. The additional hydroxy moiety in the 4-position was exploited for the introduction of various substituents. Williamson ether synthesis and replacement of the Boc protective group with a benzyl moiety led to potent σ_1 ligands with high σ_1/σ_2-selectivity. With exception of the ethoxy derivative **16**, the (*R*)-configured enantiomers represent eutomers with eudismic ratios of up to 29 for the ester **(*R*)-18**. The methyl ether **(*R*)-15** represents the most potent σ_1 ligand of this series of compounds, with a K_i value of 1.2 nM and an eudismic ratio of 7. Tosylate **(*R*)-21** was used as precursor for the radiosynthesis of $[^{18}F]$-**(*R*)-20**, which was available by nucleophilic substitution with $K[^{18}F]F$ K222 carbonate complex. The radiochemical yield of $[^{18}F]$-**(*R*)-20** was 18%–20%, the radiochemical purity greater than 97% and the specific radioactivity 175–300 GBq/µmol. Although radiometabolites were detected in plasma, urine and liver samples, radiometabolites were not found in brain samples. After 30 min, the uptake of the radiotracer in the brain was 3.4% of injected dose per gram of tissue and could be reduced by coadministration of the σ_1 antagonist haloperidol. $[^{18}F]$-**(*R*)-20** was able to label those regions of the brain, which were reported to have high density of σ_1 receptors.

Keywords: 2-benzopyrans; Sharpless Asymmetric Dihydroxylation; spirocycles; σ affinity; radiochemistry; positron emission tomography; autoradiography; organ distribution

1. Introduction

The σ receptor was firstly described in 1976 by Martin *et al.* It was named after the ligand SKF-10047 and initially regarded as opioid receptor subtype [1]. Further research resulted in the classification of σ receptors as a distinct receptor class. In 1990, the existence of at least two σ receptor subtypes was discovered, which were named σ_1 and σ_2 receptor [2]. The σ_1 receptor has been cloned from different species and tissues including guinea pig liver [3], mouse and rat brain and a human placental tumor cell line. The transmembrane protein consists of 223 amino acids [4] with a molecular weight of 25.3 kDa. A homology with another known mammalian protein was not found, but a 30% homology with the yeast enzyme sterol-Δ^8/Δ^7-ismerase, encoded by the gene ERG2, was detected [3]. The σ_1 receptor has not been crystallized so far, but a structural model was published in 2002 [5] and a 3D homology model was established in 2011 [6]. σ_1 receptors are found in the central nervous system [7], but also in peripheral organs, like liver, kidney [8] and heart [9]. Endogenous ligands have not been clearly identified so far, although some neurosteroids (e.g., progesterone, dehydro-epiandrosterone) and *N,N*-dimethyltryptamine were proposed as endogenous ligands [10,11]. The σ_1 receptor is supposed to have an influence the permeability of ion channels [12,13] and the activity of neurotransmitter systems [14,15]. In 2007, Hayashi and Su postulated the role of the σ_1 receptor as a ligand-operated chaperon [16].

Because of the manifold modulatory effects of the σ_1 receptor, potent and selective σ_1 receptor ligands represent potential therapeutics mainly for neurological and psychiatric diseases such as Alzheimer's Disease [17], neuropathic pain [18], schizophrenia [19,20] and Major Depression [15,21,22]. PET tracers, which are able to label selectively σ_1 receptors, are of high interest not only to gain further insight into the physiological role of the σ_1 receptor, but also for the diagnosis of diseases in which the σ_1 receptor is involved.

A number of PET tracers for the imaging of σ_1 receptors, labeled with [^{11}C] or [^{18}F], have already been developed [23–26]. Very recently, we have reported on the homologous series of fluorinated spirocyclic piperidines **2a–d** (n = 1–4, Figure 1), which were derived from the potent σ_1 receptor antagonist **1**. The use of the 2-benzofuran-based [^{18}F]-labeled spirocyclic σ_1 receptor ligands [^{18}F]**2** was carefully evaluated *in vivo* [27–31]. Moreover, (*R*)- and (*S*)-configured enantiomers of **2a–c** (n = 1–3) were prepared and it was shown that the corresponding enantiomers differ considerably in σ_1 receptor affinity, selectivity over the σ_2 subtype, rate of biotransformation and number and nature of formed metabolites. Additionally, the accumulation of the enantiomeric fluorinated PET tracers in the central nervous system was considerably different [32–34].

Figure 1. Development of fluorinated PET tracers

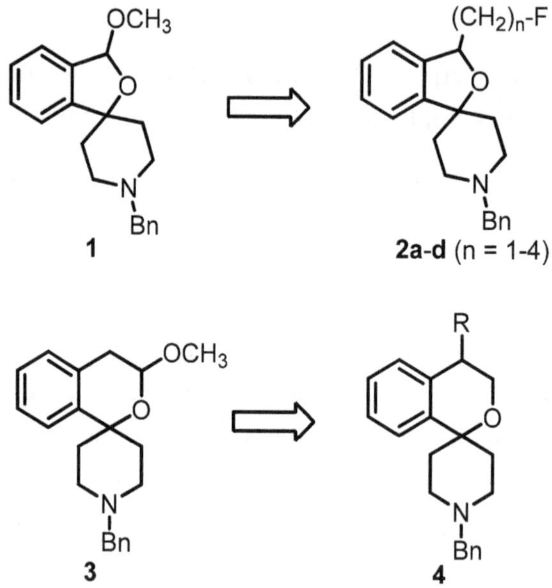

The fluoroalkyl substituted 2-benzofurans **2a–d** (n = 1–4) were derived from the spirocyclic 2-benzofuran **1**; the potent σ_1 antagonist **3** represents the lead for the enantiomerically pure 2-benzopyrans **4**. Although the 2-benzopyran **3** (K_i = 1.3 nM) represents a very potent σ_1 receptor antagonist [35], enantiomers of 2-benzopyran based σ_1 ligands were not yet investigated. Due to their structural similarity to the spirocyclic 3-substituted 2-benzopyrans **3** [36] and 2-benzofurans **1** and **2**, 4-substituted 2-benzopyrans **4** were considered as new type of σ_1 receptor ligands. Moreover, the 2-benzopyran scaffold was not exploited for the development of a fluorinated PET tracer so far. In this communication we report the first enantioselective synthesis of 4-substituted spirocyclic 2-benzopyrans of type **4**, their affinity towards σ receptors and the generation and biological evaluation of a [^{18}F]-labeled PET tracer based on this scaffold.

2. Experimental

2.1. Synthesis

2.1.1. General

Solvents: THF: distilled from sodium/benzophenone; CH_2Cl_2: distilled from calcium hydride. Flash chromatography: silica gel 60 (40–63 μm); parentheses include: diameter of the column (ø), height of the stationary phase (*h*), eluent and fraction size (*V*). Thin layer chromatography: TLC silica gel 60 F_{254} on aluminum sheets. Melting points (mp): uncorrected. Polarimetry: sodium D line (589 nm); length (*l*): 1 dm; temperature +20 °C; unit of specific rotation [deg mL dm^{-1} g^{-1}] is omitted; parentheses include: concentration of the sample [mg/mL] and solvent: ^{1}H-NMR: 400.3 MHz; ^{13}C-NMR: 100.3 MHz; chemical shifts in [ppm] against TMS; in some cases, ^{1}H and ^{13}C-NMR spectroscopy were supported by 2D NMR techniques. IR spectroscopy: ATR technique.

Mass spectrometry: Exact masses (APCI and LC-MS): Deviations of the found exact masses from the calculated exact masses: 5 mDa or less. LC-HRMS: column: Kinetex™, 2.6 μm, C18, 100 Å;

50 mm/2.1 mm, guard column: Security Guard Standard C18 Cartridge, 4 mm/2mm, temperature: 30 °C, solvents: A: acetonitrile-NH_4HCOO (10 mM) = 10:90 + 0.1% (*v/v*) HCO_2H, B: acetonitrile-NH_4HCO_2 (10 mM) = 90:10 + 0.1% (v/v) HCO_2H, gradient elution: (A%): 0–5 min: gradient from 100% to 0%, flow rate: 0.4 mL/min, 5–6.5 min: 0%, flow rate: 0.4 mL/min, 6.5–7 min: gradient from 0% to 100%, flow rate: 0.4 mL/min, 10 min: 100%, flow rate: 0.6 mL/min, injection volume: 0.5–1 μL, sample temperature: 5 °C, UV detection wavelength: 200–350 nm.

HPLC for determination of compound purity (method 1): column: LiChrospher® 60 RP-select B (5 μm), LiChroCART® 250-4 mm cartridge; guard Column: LiChrospher® 60 RP-select B (5 μm), LiCroCART® 4-4 mm cartridge (No.: 1.50963.0001) using manu-CART® NT cartridge holder; solvents: A: water with 0.05% (v/v) trifluoroacetic acid; B: acetonitrile with 0.05% (v/v) trifluoroacetic acid; gradient elution: (A %): 0–4 min: 90%, 4–29 min: gradient from 90% to 0%, 29–31 min: 0%, 31–31.5 min: gradient from 0% to 90%, 31.5–40 min: 90%; flow rate: 1.0 mL/min; injection volume: 5.0 μL; UV detection wavelength: 210 nm; stop time: 30.0 min. Chiral HPLC for determination of enantiomeric purity (method 2): UV detection wavelength: 210 nm; stop time: 30.0 min; parentheses include: column, solvent, flow rate, injection volume.

2.1.2. Synthetic Procedures

tert-Butyl-4-hydroxy-4-(2-vinylphenyl)piperidine-1-carboxylate (**6**)

2-Bromostyrene (**5**, 3.1 g, 16.9 mmol) was dissolved in THF (125 mL). The solution was cooled to −78 °C under N_2 atmosphere. A solution of *n*-butyllithium in hexanes (15 mL, 24 mmol) was added dropwise and the mixture was stirred for 15 min. Then *tert*-butyl 4-oxopiperidine-1-carboxylate (4 m, 4.1 g, 20.6 mmol), dissolved in THF (50 mL), was added and the mixture was stirred at −78 °C for 2.5 h. Then the solution was warmed to ambient temperature. A solution of $LiBH_4$ in THF (5 mL, 20 mmol) was added dropwise and the mixture was stirred for 1 h at ambient temperature. The reaction was stopped by the addition of water and a 1 M aqueous solution of HCl. After separation of the layers, the aqueous layer was extracted with CH_2Cl_2 (3×). The combined organic layers were dried (Na_2SO_4), filtered and the solvent was removed *in vacuo*. The crude product was purified by flash column chromatography (Ø = 8 cm, h = 16 cm, cyclohexane-ethyl acetate = 9:1, V = 100 mL) to give **6** as a colorless solid (R_f = 0.34, cyclohexane-ethyl acetate = 8:2), mp 104 °C, yield 3.83 g (75%). $C_{18}H_{25}NO_3$ (303.4 g/mol). Purity (HPLC method 1): 99.4%, t_R = 20.4 min. Exact mass (APCI): *m/z* = 304.1882 (calcd. 304.1907 for $C_{18}H_{26}NO_3$ $[M+H]^+$). ^{1}H-NMR ($CDCl_3$): δ (ppm) = 1.47 (s, 9H, $CO_2C(CH_3)_3$), 1.64 (s br, 1H, O*H*), 1.93–2.10 (m, 4H, $N(CH_2CH_2)_2$), 3.32–3.36 (m, 2H, $N(CH_2CH_2)_2$), 3.89–4.13 (m, 2H, $N(CH_2CH_2)_2$), 5.28 (dd, *J* = 10.9/1.8 Hz, 1H, HC=C*H*$_2$), 5.51 (dd, *J* = 17.4/1.8 Hz, 1H, HC=C*H*$_2$), 7.24–7.31 (m, 2H, 3-$H_{arom.}$, 4-$H_{arom.}$), 7.34–7.39 (m, 1H, 6-$H_{arom.}$), 7.45–7.50 (m, 1H, 5-$H_{arom.}$), 7.65 (dd, *J* = 17.4/10.9 Hz, 1H, *H*C=CH_2). ^{13}C NMR ($CDCl_3$): δ (ppm) = 28.6 (3C, $CO_2C(CH_3)_3$), 37.4 (br, 2C, $N(CH_2CH_2)_2$), 39.5 (br, 1C, $N(CH_2CH_2)_2$), 40.3 (br, 1C, $N(CH_2CH_2)_2$), 72.5 (1C, Ar*C*OH), 79.6 (1C, $CO_2C(CH_3)_3$), 115.7 (1C, HC=CH_2), 124.9 (1C, C-$6_{arom.}$), 127.7 (1C, C-$4_{arom.}$), 127.8 (1C, C-$3_{arom.}$), 129.1 (1C, C-$5_{arom.}$), 137.9 (1C, C-$2_{arom.}$), 138.0 (1C, *H*C=CH_2), 143.8 (1C, C-$1_{arom.}$), 155.0 (1C, $CO_2C(CH_3)_3$). FT-IR (neat): $\tilde{\nu}$ (cm^{-1}) = 3387 (O-H), 2967, 2932, (C-H), 1655 (C=O), 756 (1,2-disubst. arom.).

tert-Butyl (*R*)-4-[2-(1,2-dihydroxyethyl)phenyl]-4-hydroxypiperidine-1-carboxylate ((***R***)-7)

AD-mix-β (27.1 g) was added to a mixture of *tert*-butyl alcohol (600 mL) and water (600 mL). The mixture was cooled to 0 °C, **6** (5.9 g, 19.5 mmol) was added and the reaction mixture was stirred at 0 °C for 3 d. Then sodium sulfite (29 g) was added and the mixture was allowed to warm to room temperature and stirred for 20 min. Ethyl acetate was added to the reaction mixture, and after separation of the layers, the aqueous layer was extracted with ethyl acetate (3×). The combined organic layers were dried (Na_2SO_4), filtered and the solvent was removed *in vacuo*. The crude product was purified by flash column chromatography (Ø = 8 cm, h = 18 cm, cyclohexane-ethyl acetate = 1:2 → ethyl acetate, V = 100 mL) to give (***R***)-**7** as a colorless solid (R_f = 0.11, cyclohexane-ethyl acetate = 5:5), mp 93 °C, yield 5.4 g (82%). $C_{18}H_{27}NO_5$ (337.4 g/mol). Specific rotation: $[\alpha]_D^{20}$: = –24.5 (3.5; CH_2Cl_2). Purity (HPLC method 1): 99.5%, t_R = 15.3 min.

tert-Butyl (*S*)-4-(2-[1,2-dihydroxyethyl)phenyl]-4-hydroxypiperidine-1-carboxylate ((***S***)-7)

AD-mix-α (15.2 g) was added to a mixture of *tert*-butyl alcohol (325 mL) and water (325 mL). The mixture was cooled to 0 °C, **6** (4.5 g, 14.9 mmol) was added and the reaction mixture was stirred overnight at 0 °C. Then methanesulfonamide (1.0 g, 10.5 mmol) was added and the mixture was stirred overnight at ambient temperature. Then sodium sulfite (16.2 g) was added and the mixture stirred for 30 min. Ethyl acetate was added to the reaction mixture, and after separation of the layers, the aqueous layer was extracted with ethyl acetate (3×). The combined organic layers were washed with a 2 M aqueous solution of NaOH, dried (Na_2SO_4), filtered and the solvent was removed *in vacuo*. The crude product was purified by flash column chromatography (Ø = 8 cm, h = 15 cm, cyclohexane-ethyl acetate = 1:2 → ethyl acetate, V = 100 mL) to give (***S***)-**7** as a colorless solid (R_f = 0.11, cyclohexane:ethyl acetate = 5:5), mp 87 °C, yield 2.7 (74%) $C_{18}H_{27}NO_5$ (337.4 g/mol). Specific rotation: $[\alpha]_D^{20}$: = +25.8 (3.7; CH_2Cl_2). Purity (HPLC method 1): 95.5%, t_R = 15.5 min.

Spectroscopic data for (***R***)-**7** and (***S***)-**7**

LC-HRMS: *m/z* = 360.1800 (calcd. 360.1781 for $C_{18}H_{27}NNaO_5$ $[M+Na]^+$). ^{1}H-NMR ($CDCl_3$): δ (ppm) = 1.47 (s, 9H, $CO_2(CH_3)_3$), 1.82–2.11 (m, 4H, $N(CH_2CH_2)_2$), 3.24 (t, *J* = 12.6 Hz, 2H, $N(CH_2CH_2)_2$), 3.78 (dd, *J* = 10.9/4.2 Hz, 1H, $HOCHCH_2OH$), 3.86 (dd, *J* = 10.9/7.7 Hz, 1H, $HOCHCH_2OH$), 3.95–4.05 (m, 2H, $N(CH_2CH_2)_2$), 5.64 (dd, *J* = 7.7/4.2 Hz, 1H, $HOCHCH_2OH$), 7.23–7.32 (m, 3H, $H_{arom.}$), 7.48–7.52 (m, 1H, $H_{arom.}$). Signals for the OH protons are not visible in the spectrum. ^{13}C-NMR ($CDCl_3$): δ (ppm) = 28.6 (3C, $CO_2C(CH_3)_3$), 38.3 (br, 1C, $N(CH_2CH_2)_2$), 38.6 (br, 1C, $N(CH_2CH_2)_2$), 39.4 (br, 1C, $N(CH_2CH_2)_2$), 40.0 (br, 1C, $N(CH_2CH_2)_2$), 68.0 (1C, $HOCHCH_2OH$), 72.1 (1C, $HOCHCH_2OH$), 72.7 (1C, ArCOH), 79.8 (1C, $CO_2C(CH_3)_3$), 125.6 (1C, $C_{arom.}$), 127.8 (1C, $C_{arom.}$), 127.9 (1C, $C_{arom.}$), 129.1 (1C, $C_{arom.}$), 139.5 (1C, $C_{arom.}$), 145.0 (1C, $C_{arom.}$), 155.1 (1C, $CO_2C(CH_3)_3$). IR (neat): $\tilde{\nu}$ (cm^{-1}) = 3387 (O-H), 2974, 2925, (C-H), 1663 (C=O), 1246, 1161 (C-O-C ester), 756 (1,2-disubst. arom.).

tert-Butyl (*S*)-3-[(tosyloxy)methyl]-3*H*-spiro[[2]benzofuran-1,4′-piperidine]-1′-carboxylate (**(*S*)-8**)

(*R*)-7 (98 mg, 0.29 mmol) was dissolved in CH_2Cl_2 (10 mL). 4-Dimethylaminopyridine (12 mg, 0.10 mmol), triethylamine (210 µL, 1.5 mmol) and 4-toulenesulfonyl chloride (110 mg, 0.58 mmol) were added and the mixture was stirred for 3 h at ambient temperature. Then water was added and after separation of the layers, the aqueous layer was extracted with CH_2Cl_2 (3×). The combined organic layers were dried (Na_2SO_4), filtered and the solvent was removed *in vacuo*. The crude product was purified by flash column chromatography (Ø = 2 cm, h = 16 cm, cyclohexane-ethyl acetate = 9:1, V = 10 mL) to give **(*S*)-8** as a colorless oil (R_f = 0.28, cyclohexane-ethyl acetate = 8:2), mp 124 °C, yield 69 mg (50%). $C_{25}H_{31}NO_6S$ (473.6 g/mol). Specific rotation: $[\alpha]_D^{20}$: = +19.2 (7.6; CH_2Cl_2). Purity (HPLC method 1): 98.8%, t_R = 22.8 min. Exact mass (APCI): *m/z* = 474.1969 (calcd. 474.1945 for $C_{25}H_{32}NO_6S$ $[M+H]^+$). ^{1}H-NMR ($CDCl_3$): δ (ppm) = 1.48 (s, 9H, $CO_2C(CH_3)_3$), 1.51–1.70 (m, 2H, $N(CH_2CH_2)_2$), 1.70 (td, *J* = 13.1/4.8 Hz, 1H, $N(CH_2CH_2)_2$), 1.82 (td, *J* = 13.1/4.8 Hz, 1H, $N(CH_2CH_2)_2$), 2.44 (s, 3H, CH_3), 3.02 (td, *J* = 12.9/2.9 Hz, 1H, $N(CH_2CH_2)_2$), 3.12 (td, *J* = 12.9/2.9 Hz, 1H, $N(CH_2CH_2)_2$), 3.95–4.07 (m, 2H, $N(CH_2CH_2)_2$), 4.15 (dd, *J* = 10.2/5.3 Hz, 1H, CH_2OTos), 4.24 (dd, *J* = 10.2/4.1 Hz, 1H, CH_2OTos), 5.37 (t, *J* = 4.7 Hz 1H, ArC*H*O), 7.04–7.08 (m, 1H, $H_{arom.}$), 7.12–7.17 (m, 1H, $H_{arom.}$), 7.24–7.35 (m, 4H, 3-H_{tosyl}, 5-H_{tosyl}, $H_{arom.}$ (2H)), 7.71–7.75 (m, 2H, 2-H_{tosyl}, 6-H_{tosyl}). ^{13}C-NMR ($CDCl_3$): δ (ppm) = 21.8 (1C, CH_3), 28.6 (3C, $CO_2C(CH_3)_3$), 37.2 (1C, $N(CH_2CH_2)_2$), 37.9 (1C, $N(CH_2CH_2)_2$), 40.4 (1C, $N(CH_2CH_2)_2$), 40.6 (1C, $N(CH_2CH_2)_2$), 72.2 (1C, CH_2OTos), 79.4 (1C, ArCHO), 79.6 (1C, $CO_2C(CH_3)_3$), 85.4 (1C, ArCO), 121.1 (1C, $C_{arom.}$), 122.0 (1C, $C_{arom.}$), 128.1 (2C, C-2_{tosyl}, C-6_{tosyl}), 128.3 (1C, $C_{arom.}$), 128.8 (1C, $C_{arom.}$), 130.0 (2C, C-3_{tosyl}, C-5_{tosyl}), 133.0 (1C, $C_{arom.}$), 136.9 (1C, $C_{arom.}$), 145.1 (1C, $C_{arom.}$), 145.8 (1C, $C_{arom.}$), 155.1 (1C, $CO_2C(CH_3)_3$). IR (neat): $\tilde{\nu}$ (cm^{-1}) = 2978, 2870 (C-H), 1686 (C=O), 1362 (O=S=O), 1234, 1173 (C-O-C, ester), 1069 (C-O-C, ether), 768 (1,2-disubst. arom.).

tert-Butyl (*R*)-4-hydroxy-3,4-dihydrospiro[[2]benzopyran-1,4′-piperidine]-1′-carboxylate (**(*R*)-11**)

(*R*)-7 (908 mg, 2.7 mmol) was dissolved in THF (25 mL). Dibutyltin oxide (75 mg, 0.30 mmol), triethylamine (744 µL, 5.4 mmol) and toluene-4-sulfonyl chloride (1.0 g, 5.3 mmol) were added and the mixture was stirred for 3 h at ambient temperature. Then water and CH_2Cl_2 were added. After separation of the layers, the aqueous layer was extracted with CH_2Cl_2 (3×). The combined organic layers were dried (Na_2SO_4), filtered and the solvent was removed *in vacuo*. The crude product was purified by flash column chromatography (Ø = 5 cm, h = 15 cm, cyclohexane-ethyl acetate = 3:1, V = 30 mL) to give **(*R*)-11** as a colorless solid (R_f = 0.25, cyclohexane-ethyl acetate = 2:1), mp 161 °C, yield 538 mg (62%). $C_{18}H_{25}NO_4$ (319.4 g/mol). Specific rotation: $[\alpha]_D^{20}$: = −4.9 (11.0; CH_2Cl_2). Purity (HPLC method 1): 96.0%, t_R = 18.6 min. Enantiomeric ratio (HPLC method 2, Daicel Chiralpak AD-H, 5 µm, 250 mm/4.6 mm, isohexane:methanol = 95:5, flow rate: 1.0 mL/min, injection volume: 10 µL): (*R*):(*S*) = 92.5:7.5, t_R = 11.4 min.

tert-Butyl (*S*)-4-hydroxy-3,4-dihydrospiro[[2]benzopyran-1,4′-piperidine]-1′-carboxylate (**(*S*)-11**)

(*S*)-7 (996 mg, 3.0 mmol) was dissolved in THF (15 mL). Dibutyltin oxide (86 mg, 0.35 mmol), triethylamine (2.0 mL, 14.8 mmol) and toluene-4-sulfonyl chloride (2.1 g, 6.3 mmol) were added and the mixture was stirred for 3 days at ambient temperature. Then water and CH_2Cl_2 were added. After separation of the layers, the aqueous layer was extracted with CH_2Cl_2 (3×). The combined organic layers were dried (Na_2SO_4), filtered and the solvent was removed *in vacuo*. The crude product was purified by flash column chromatography (Ø = 5 cm, h = 15 cm, cyclohexane-ethyl acetate = 3:1, V = 65 mL) to give **(*S*)-11** as a colorless solid (R_f = 0.25, cyclohexane-ethyl acetate = 2:1), mp 158 °C, yield 447 mg (47%). $C_{18}H_{25}NO_4$ (319.4 g/mol). Specific rotation: $[\alpha]_D^{20}$: = +5.2 (4.4; CH_2Cl_2). Purity (HPLC method 1): 98.3%, t_R = 18.3 min. Enantiomeric ratio (HPLC method 2, Daicel Chiralpak AD-H, 5 µm, 250 mm/4.6 mm, isohexane:methanol = 95:5, flow rate: 1.0 mL/min, injection volume: 10 µL): (*R*):(*S*) = 11.4:88.6, t_R = 20.7 min.

Spectroscopic data for **(*R*)-11** and **(*S*)-11**

Exact mass (APCI): *m/z* = 320.1894 (calcd. 320.1856 for $C_{18}H_{26}NO_4$ $[M+H]^+$). ^{1}H-NMR ($CDCl_3$): δ (ppm) = 1.49 (s, 9H, $CO_2(CH_3)_3$), 1.69–1.83 (m, 2H, $N(CH_2CH_2)_2$), 1.90–2.05 (m, 2H, $N(CH_2CH_2)_2$), 3.11 (t, *J* = 13.0 Hz, 1H, $N(CH_2CH_2)_2$), 3.22 (t, *J* = 13.0 Hz, 1H, $N(CH_2CH_2)_2$), 3.92 (dd, *J* = 12.1/3.3 Hz, 1H, $HOCHCH_2O$), 3.98 (dd, *J* = 12.1/2.7 Hz, 1H, $HOCHCH_2O$), 3.99–4.07 (m, 2H, $N(CH_2CH_2)_2$), 4.54 (t, *J* = 3.0 Hz, 1H, $HOCHCH_2O$), 7.10 (dd, *J* = 7.4/1.6 Hz, 1H, 8-$H_{arom.}$), 7.25–7.34 (m, 2H, 6-$H_{arom.}$, 7-$H_{arom.}$), 7.42 (dd, *J* = 7.2/1.8 Hz, 1H, 5-$H_{arom.}$). A signal for the OH proton is not visible in the spectrum. ^{13}C-NMR ($CDCl_3$): δ (ppm) = 28.6 (3C, $CO_2C(CH_3)_3$), 34.3 (br, 1C, $N(CH_2CH_2)_2$), 37.6 (br, 1C, $N(CH_2CH_2)_2$), 39.5 (br, 1C, $N(CH_2CH_2)_2$), 40.1 (br, 1C, $N(CH_2CH_2)_2$), 64.8 (1C, $HOCHCH_2O$), 66.0 (1C, $HOCHCH_2O$), 73.8 (1C, ArCO), 79.7 (1C, $CO_2C(CH_3)_3$), 125.2 (1C, C-$8_{arom.}$), 127.3 (1C, C-$6_{arom.}$), 128.6 (1C, C-$7_{arom.}$), 129.1 (1C, C-$5_{arom.}$), 135.3 (1C, C-$8a_{arom.}$), 141.2 (1C, C-$4a_{arom.}$), 155.1 (1C, $CO_2C(CH_3)_3$). IR (neat): $\tilde{\nu}$ [cm^{-1}] = 3314 (O-H), 2974, 2928 (C-H), 1686 (C=O), 1169 (C-O-C ether), 768 (1,2-disubst. arom.).

(*R*)-1′-Benzyl-3,4-dihydrospiro[[2]benzopyran-1,4′-piperidin]-4-ol (**(*R*)-12**)

(*R*)-11 (105 mg, 0.33 mmol) was dissolved in CH_2Cl_2 (4 mL). The solution was cooled to 0 °C. Then trifluoroacetic acid (200 µL) was added and the mixture was stirred for 3.5 h at 0 °C. Then a 2 M aqueous solution of sodium hydroxide (4 mL) was added, and after separation of the layers, the aqueous layer was extracted with CH_2Cl_2 (3×). The combined organic layers were dried (Na_2SO_4), filtered and the solvent was removed *in vacuo*. The residue was dissolved in CH_2Cl_2 (5 mL), benzaldehyde (35 µL, 0.35 mmol) and sodium triacetoxyborohydride (85 mg, 0.40 mmol) were added and the mixture was stirred overnight at ambient temperature. The reaction was stopped by the addition of a 2 M aqueous solution of sodium hydroxide, and after separation of the layers, the aqueous layer was extracted with CH_2Cl_2 (4×). The combined organic layers were dried (Na_2SO_4), filtered and the solvent was removed *in vacuo*. The crude product was purified by flash column chromatography (Ø = 1.5 cm, h = 16 cm, cyclohexane-ethyl acetate = 5:1 + 1% *N,N*-dimethylethylamine, V = 5 mL) to give **(*R*)-12** as a colorless solid (R_f = 0.14, cyclohexane-ethyl acetate = 5:5), mp 55 °C), yield 57 mg

(56%). $C_{20}H_{23}NO_2$ (309.4 g/mol). Specific rotation: $[\alpha]_D^{20}$: = −8.4 (2.3; CH_2Cl_2). Purity (HPLC method 1): 95.3%, t_R = 13.5 min. Enantiomeric ratio (HPLC method 2, Daicel Chiralpak AD-H, 5 μm, 250 mm/4.6 mm, isohexane-isopropanol = 95:5, flow rate: 1.0 mL/min, injection volume: 10 μL): (*R*):(*S*) = 96.1:3.9, t_R = 9.7 min).

(*S*)-1′-Benzyl-3,4-dihydrospiro[2-benzopyran-1,4′-piperidin]-4-ol (**(*S*)-12**)

(*R*)-11 (56 mg, 0.18 mmol) was dissolved in CH_2Cl_2 (10 mL). Trifluoroacetic acid (200 μL) was added and the mixture was stirred overnight at ambient temperature. Then water was added, and after separation of the layers, the aqueous layer was extracted with CH_2Cl_2 (3×). The combined organic layers were dried (Na_2SO_4), filtered and the solvent was removed *in vacuo*. The residue was dissolved in CH_2Cl_2 (10 mL), benzaldehyde (50 μL, 0.45 mmol) and sodium triacetoxyborohydride (50 mg, 0.24 mmol) were added and the mixture was stirred for 5.5 h at ambient temperature. Then benzaldehyde (50 μL, 0.35 mmol) and sodium triacetoxyborohydride (60 mg, 0.28 mmol) were added and the mixture was stirred overnight at ambient temperature). The reaction was stopped by the addition of a 2 M aqueous solution of sodium hydroxide, and after separation of the layers, the aqueous layer was extracted with CH_2Cl_2 (3×). The combined organic layers were dried (Na_2SO_4), filtered and the solvent was removed *in vacuo*. The crude product was purified by flash column chromatography (Ø = 1 cm, h = 15 cm, cyclohexane-ethyl acetate = 5:1 + 1% *N,N*-dimethylethylamine, V = 5 mL) to give **(*S*)-12** as a colorless solid (R_f = 0.14, cyclohexane-ethyl acetate = 5:5) mp 53 °C, yield 12 mg (22%). $C_{20}H_{23}NO_2$ (309.4 g/mol). Specific rotation: $[\alpha]_D^{20}$: = +8.8 (2.2; CH_2Cl_2). Purity (HPLC method 1): 98.3%, t_R = 13.4 min. Enantiomeric ratio (HPLC method 2, Daicel Chiralpak AD-H, 5 μm, 250 mm/4.6 mm, isohexane:isopropanol = 95:5, flow rate: 1.0 mL/min, injection volume: 10 μL): (*R*):(*S*) = 11.9:88.1, t_R = 12.9 min.

Spectroscopic data for **(*R*)-12** and **(*S*)-12**

Exact mass (APCI): *m/z* = 310.1802 (calcd. 310.1802 for $C_{20}H_{24}NO_2$ $[M+H]^+$). ^{1}H-NMR ($CDCl_3$): δ (ppm) = 1.78–1.98 (m, 3H, N(CH_2CH_2)$_2$), 2.18 (td, *J* = 13.1/4.6 Hz, 1H, N(CH_2CH_2)$_2$), 2.39 (dd, *J* = 11.9/3.0 Hz, 1H, N(CH_2CH_2)$_2$), 2.46–2.54 (m, 1H, N(CH_2CH_2)$_2$), 2.75 (t, *J* = 13.1/Hz, 2H, N(CH_2CH_2)$_2$), 3.58 (s, 2H, NCH_2Ph), 3.89 (dd, *J* = 12.1/3.3 Hz, 1H, CHCH_2O), 3.97 (dd, *J* = 12.1/2.6 Hz, 1H, CHCH_2O), 4.51 (t, *J* = 2.9 Hz, 1H, C*H*CH$_2$O), 7.20–7.41 (m, 9H, $H_{arom.}$). A signal for the OH proton is not visible in the spectrum. ^{13}C-NMR ($CDCl_3$): δ (ppm) = 34.7 (1C, N(CH_2CH_2)$_2$), 38.0 (1C, N(CH_2CH_2)$_2$), 49.3 (1C, N(CH_2CH_2)$_2$), 49.3 (1C, N(CH_2CH_2)$_2$), 63.5 (1C, NCH_2Ph), 64.5 (1C, CHCH_2O), 66.1 (1C, *C*HCH$_2$O), 73.9 (1C, ArCO), 125.3 (1C, $C_{arom.}$), 127.0 (1C, $C_{arom.}$), 127.1 (1C, $C_{arom.}$), 128.3 (2C, $C_{arom.}$), 128.5 (1C, $C_{arom.}$), 128.9 (1C, $C_{arom.}$), 129.4 (2C, $C_{arom.}$), 135.5 (1C, $C_{arom.}$), 138.6 (1C, $C_{arom.}$), 141.8 (1C, $C_{arom.}$). IR (neat): $\tilde{\nu}$ (cm^{-1}) = 3329 (O-H), 2924, 2817 (C-H), 1072 (C-O-C), 733 (1,2-disubst. arom.), 698 (monosubst. arom.).

tert-Butyl (*R*)-4-methoxy-3,4-dihydrospiro[[2]benzopyran-1,4′-piperidine]-1′-carboxylate (**(*R*)-13**)

(*R*)-10 (450 mg, 1.4 mmol) was dissolved in THF (12 mL). NaH (60% dispersion in paraffin liquid, 112 mg, 2.8 mmol) was added and the mixture was stirred for 1 h at ambient temperature. Then iodomethane (176 µL, 2.8 mmol) was added dropwise and the mixture was stirred for 1 h at ambient temperature. The solvent was removed *in vacuo*. The crude product was purified by flash column chromatography (Ø = 2.5 cm, h = 16.5 cm, cyclohexane-ethyl acetate = 9:1, V = 10 mL) to give ***(R)*-13** as a colorless oil (R_f = 0.28, cyclohexane-ethyl acetate = 8:2), yield 465 mg (99%). $C_{19}H_{27}NO_4$ (333.4 g/mol). Specific rotation: $[\alpha]_D^{20}$ = −8.0 (4.4; CH_2Cl_2). Purity (HPLC method 1): 96.6%, t_R = 20.4 min.

tert-Butyl (*S*)-4-methoxy-3,4-dihydrospiro[2-benzopyran-1,4′-piperidine]-1′-carboxylate (***(S)*-13**)

***(S)*-10** (180 mg, 0.56 mmol) was dissolved in THF (2.5 mL). NaH (60% dispersion in paraffin liquid, 50 mg, 1.3 mmol) was added and the mixture was stirred for 1 h at ambient temperature. Then iodomethane (77 µL, 1.2 mmol) was added dropwise and the mixture was stirred overnight at ambient temperature. The solvent was removed *in vacuo*. The crude product was purified by flash column chromatography (Ø = 2 cm, h = 15 cm, cyclohexane:ethyl acetate = 9:1, V = 10 mL) to give ***(S)*-13** as a pale yellow oil (R_f = 0.28, cyclohexane:ethyl acetate = 8:2), yield 128 mg (69%). $C_{19}H_{27}NO_4$ (333.4 g/mol). Specific rotation: $[\alpha]_D^{20}$: = +7.4 (7.9; CH_2Cl_2). Purity (HPLC method 1): 97.7%, t_R = 20.4 min.

Spectroscopic data for ***(R)*-13** and ***(S)*-13**

Exact mass (APCI): *m/z* = 334.2009 (calcd. 334.2013 for $C_{19}H_{28}NO_4$ $[M+H]^+$). ^{1}H-NMR ($CDCl_3$): δ (ppm) = 1.49 (s, 9H, $CO_2(CH_3)_3$), 1.75 (td, *J* = 13.2/4.9 Hz, 1H, $N(CH_2CH_2)_2$), 1.84–1.99 (m, 3H, $N(CH_2CH_2)_2$), 3.03–3.28 (m, 2H, $N(CH_2CH_2)_2$), 3.50 (s, 3H, OCH_3), 3.93–4.06 (m, 4H, $N(CH_2CH_2)_2$ (2), $CHCH_2O$ (2)), 4.19 (t, *J* = 3.4 Hz, 1H, $CHCH_2O$), 7.11 (dd, *J* = 7.7/1.4 Hz, 1H, $H_{arom.}$), 7.25 (td, *J* = 7.4/1.4 Hz, 1H, $H_{arom.}$), 7.30 (td, *J* = 7.4/1.6 Hz, 1H, $H_{arom.}$), 7.37 (dd, *J* = 7.4/1.6 Hz, 1H, $H_{arom.}$). ^{13}C-NMR ($CDCl_3$): δ (ppm) = 28.6 (3C, $CO_2C(CH_3)_3$), 34.9 (br, 1C, $N(CH_2CH_2)_2$), 37.0 (br, 1C, $N(CH_2CH_2)_2$), 39.4 (br, 1C, $N(CH_2CH_2)_2$), 40.2 (br, 1C, $N(CH_2CH_2)_2$), 56.9 (1C, OCH_3), 61.6 (1C, $CHCH_2O$), 73.5 (1C, ArCO), 74.0 (1C, $CHCH_2O$), 79.5 (1C, $CO_2C(CH_3)_3$), 125.1 (1C, $C_{arom.}$), 126.7 (1C, $C_{arom.}$), 128.4 (1C, $C_{arom.}$), 129.1 (1C, $C_{arom.}$), 132.8 (1C, $C_{arom.}$), 141.8 (1C, $C_{arom.}$), 155.0 (1C, $CO_2C(CH_3)_3$). IR (neat): $\tilde{\nu}$ (cm^{-1}) = 2970, 2928 ($_{C\text{-}H}$), 1686 ($_{C=O}$), 1084 ($_{C\text{-}O\text{-}C\ ether}$), 756 (1,2-disubst. arom.).

tert-Butyl (*R*)-4-ethoxy-3,4-dihyrospiro[[2]benzopyran-1,4′-piperidine]-1′-carboxylate (***(R)*-14**)

***(R)*-10** (210 mg, 0.66 mmol) was dissolved in THF (15 mL). NaH (60% dispersion in paraffin liquid, 80 mg, 2.0 mmol) was added and the mixture was stirred for 1 h at ambient temperature. Then iodoethane (0.53 mL, 6.6 mmol) was added dropwise and the mixture was stirred for 2.5 h at ambient temperature. A 1 m solution of lithium bis(trimethylsilyl)amide (4.5 mL) was added and the mixture was heated to reflux overnight. The mixture was allowed to cool to ambient temperature and stirred overnight. Then water and CH_2Cl_2 were added. After separation of the layers, the aqueous layer was extracted with CH_2Cl_2 (3×). The combined organic layers were dried (Na_2SO_4), filtered and the solvent removed *in vacuo*. The crude product was purified by flash column chromatography (Ø = 2 cm, h = 15 cm, cyclohexane-ethyl acetate = 9:1, V = 10 mL) to give ***(R)*-14** as a pale yellow oil (R_f = 0.15, cyclo-hexane-ethyl acetate = 9:1), yield 66 mg (29%). $C_{20}H_{29}NO_4$ (347.4 g/mol). Specific rotation: $[\alpha]_D^{20}$: = −2.2 (3.2; CH_2Cl_2). Purity (HPLC method 1): 96.3%, t_R = 21.3 min.

tert-Butyl (*S*)-4-ethoxy-3,4-dihydrospiro[[2]benzopyran-1,4′-piperidine]-1′-carboxylate (***(S)*-14**)

***(S)*-10** (200 mg, 0.63 mmol) was dissolved in THF (5 mL). A 1 m solution of lithium bis(trimethylsilyl)amide (6.3 mL) was added and the mixture was stirred for 1 h at ambient temperature. Then iodoethane (500 µL, 6.3 mmol) was added dropwise and the mixture was stirred for 16 h at ambient temperature. NaH (60% dispersion in paraffin liquid, 250 mg, 6.3 mmol) and iodoethane (500 µL, 6.3 mmol) were added and the mixture was heated to reflux overnight. The mixture was allowed to cool to ambient temperature and stirred for 3 days. Then water was added. After separation of the layers, the aqueous layer was extracted with ethyl acetate (3×). The combined organic layers were dried (Na_2SO_4), filtered and the solvent was removed *in vacuo*. The crude product was purified by flash column chromatography three times (1. Ø = 2 cm, h = 15 cm, cyclohexane-ethyl acetate = 9:1, V = 10 mL; 2. Ø = 1.5 cm, h = 15 cm, cyclohexane-ethyl acetate = 9:1, V = 5 mL; 3. Ø = 1.5 cm, h = 15 cm, cyclohexane-ethyl acetate = 95:5, V = 5 mL) to give ***(S)*-14** as a pale yellow oil (R_f = 0.15, cyclohexane-ethyl acetate = 9:1), yield 110 mg (50%). $C_{20}H_{29}NO_4$ (347.4 g/mol). Specific rotation: $[\alpha]_D^{20}$: = +2.4 (3.9; CH_2Cl_2). Purity (HPLC method 1): 98.4%, t_R = 21.5 min.

Spectroscopic data for ***(R)*-14** and ***(S)*-14**

Exact mass (APCI): *m/z* = 348.2199 (calcd. 348.2169 for $C_{20}H_{30}NO_4$ $[M+H]^+$). ^{1}H-NMR ($CDCl_3$): δ (ppm) = 1.28 (t, *J* = 7.0 Hz, 3H, OCH_2CH_3), 1.49 (s, 9H, $CO_2(CH_3)_3$), 1.76–1.86 (m, 2H, $N(CH_2CH_2)_2$), 1.86–1.96 (m, 2H, $N(CH_2CH_2)_2$), 3.04–3.26 (m, 2H, $N(CH_2CH_2)_2$), 3.64–3.78 (m, 2H, OCH_2CH_3), 3.86–4.08 (m, 2H, $N(CH_2CH_2)_2$), 3.89 (dd, *J* = 12.0/5.4 Hz, 1H, $CHCH_2O$), 4.00 (dd, *J* = 12.0/3.7 Hz, 1H, $CHCH_2O$), 4.35 (t, *J* = 4.5 Hz, 1H, $CHCH_2O$), 7.08 (dd, *J* = 7.2/2.0 Hz, 1H, $H_{arom.}$), 7.20–7.32 (m, 2H, $H_{arom.}$), 7.42 (dd, *J* = 6.9/2.3 Hz, 1H, $H_{arom.}$). ^{13}C-NMR ($CDCl_3$): δ (ppm) = 15.9 (1C, OCH_2CH_3), 28.7 (3C, $CO_2C(CH_3)_3$), 35.8 (br, 1C, $N(CH_2CH_2)_2$), 36.4 (br, 1C, $N(CH_2CH_2)_2$), 39.5 (br, 1C, $N(CH_2CH_2)_2$), 40.3 (br, 1C, $N(CH_2CH_2)_2$), 62.1 (1C, $CHCH_2O$), 64.9 (1C, OCH_2CH_3), 72.4 (1C, $CHCH_2O$), 73.7 (1C, $CO_2C(CH_3)_3$), 79.6 (1C, ArCO), 125.1 (1C, $C_{arom.}$), 126.8 (1C, $C_{arom.}$), 128.1 (1C, $C_{arom.}$), 128.5 (1C, $C_{arom.}$), 134.0 (1C, $C_{arom.}$), 141.8 (1C, $C_{arom.}$), 155.1 (1C, $CO_2C(CH_3)_3$). IR (neat): $\tilde{\nu}$ (cm^{-1}) = 2970, 2928 (C-H), 1690 (C=O), 1092 (C-O-C ether), 756 (1,2-disubst. arom.).

(*R*)-1′-Benzyl-4-methoxy-3,4-dihydrospiro[[2]benzopyran-1,4′-piperidine] (***(R)*-15**)

(*R*)-**13** (360 mg, 1.1 mmol) was dissolved in CH_2Cl_2 (5 mL). The solution was cooled to 0 °C. Trifluoroacetic acid (0.7 mL) was added and the mixture was stirred for 2 h at 0 °C. Then a 2 M aqueous solution of NaOH was added. After separation of the layers, the aqueous layer was extracted with CH_2Cl_2 (3×). The combined organic layers were dried (Na_2SO_4), filtered and the solvent was removed *in vacuo*. The residue was dissolved in CH_2Cl_2 (5 mL). Benzaldehyde (30 µL, 0.30 mmol) and sodium triacetoxyborohydride (76 mg, 0.36 mmol) were added and the mixture was stirred for 26 h at ambient temperature. Then a 2 M aqueous solution of NaOH (3 mL) and water (3 mL) were added. After separation of the layers, the aqueous layer was extracted with CH_2Cl_2 (3×). The combined organic layers were dried (Na_2SO_4), filtered and the solvent was removed *in vacuo*. The crude product was purified by flash column chromatography (Ø = 0.75 cm, h = 15 cm, cyclohexane-ethyl acetate = 4:1, V = 5 mL) to give ***(R)*-15** as a colorless oil (R_f = 0.27, cyclohexane-ethyl acetate = 5:5), yield 31 mg (9%). $C_{21}H_{25}NO_2$ (323.4 G/mol). Specific rotation: $[\alpha]_D^{20}$: = −8.6 (2.8; CH_2Cl_2). Purity (HPLC method 1): 98.2%, t_R = 15.8 min. Enantiomeric ratio (HPLC method 2, Daicel Chiralpak IB, 5 μm, 250 mm/4.6 mm, isohexane-methanol = 97:3, flow rate: 1.0 mL/min, injection volume: 5 μL): (*R*):(*S*) = 94.8:5.2, t_R = 7.2 min.

(*S*)-1′-Benzyl-4-methoxy-3,4-dihydrospiro[[2]benzopyran-1,4′-piperidine] (***(S)*-15**)

***(S)*-13** (50 mg, 0.15 mmol) was dissolved in CH_2Cl_2 (5 mL). Trifluoroacetic acid (200 μL) was added and the mixture was stirred for 4.5 h at ambient temperature. Then a 2 M aqueous solution of NaOH was added. After separation of the layers, the aqueous layer was extracted with CH_2Cl_2 (3×). The combined organic layers were dried (Na_2SO_4), filtered and the solvent was removed *in vacuo*. The residue was dissolved in CH_2Cl_2 (10 mL). Benzaldehyde (70 μL, 0.69 mmol) and sodium triacetoxyborohydride (96 mg, 0.45 mmol) were added and the mixture was stirred overnight at ambient temperature. The reaction was stopped by the addition of a 2 M aqueous solution of NaOH. After separation of the layers, the aqueous layer was extracted with CH_2Cl_2 (3×). The combined organic layers were dried (Na_2SO_4), filtered and the solvent was removed *in vacuo*. The crude product was purified by flash column chromatography twice (1. Ø = 1.5 cm, h = 16 cm, cyclohexane-ethyl acetate = 4:1, V = 5 mL; 2. Ø = 1.5 cm, h = 15 cm, cyclohexane-ethyl acetate = 6:1, V = 5 mL) to give ***(S)*-15** as a yellowish oil (R_f = 0.27, cyclohexane-ethyl acetate = 5:5), yield 39 mg (80%). $C_{21}H_{25}NO_2$ (323.4 g/mol). Specific rotation: $[\alpha]_D^{20}$: = +7.7 (8.3; CH_2Cl_2). Purity (HPLC method 1): 97.3%, t_R = 15.6 min. Enantiomeric ratio (HPLC method 2, Daicel Chiralpak IB, 5 μm, 250 mm/4.6 mm, isohexane:methanol = 97:3, flow rate: 1.0 mL/min, injection volume: 5 μL): (*R*):(*S*) = 9.0:91.0, t_R = 8.6 min.

Spectroscopic data for ***(R)*-15** and ***(S)*-15**

Exact mass (APCI): *m/z* = 324.1950 (calcd. 324.1958 for $C_{21}H_{26}NO_2$ $[M+H]^+$). ^{1}H-NMR ($CDCl_3$): δ (ppm) = 1.87–1.95 (m, 3H, N(CH_2CH_2)$_2$), 2.13 (td, *J* = 13.0/4.6 Hz, 1H, N(CH_2CH_2)$_2$), 2.36–2.44 (m, 1H, N(CH_2CH_2)$_2$), 2.51 (td, *J* = 13.0/2.5 Hz, 1H, N(CH_2CH_2)$_2$), 2.70–2.79 (m, 2H, N(CH_2CH_2)$_2$), 3.50 (s, 3H, OCH_3), 3.56 (d, *J* = 13.0 Hz, 1H, NCH_2Ph), 3.60 (d, *J* = 13.0 Hz, 1H, NCH_2Ph), 3.93–4.06 (d, *J* = 3.6 Hz, 2H, CHCH_2O), 4.19 (t, *J* = 3.6 Hz, 1H, *C*HCH$_2$O), 7.21–7.39 (m, 9H, $H_{arom.}$). ^{13}C-NMR ($CDCl_3$): δ (ppm) = 35.5 (1C, N(CH_2CH_2)$_2$), 37.3 (1C, N(CH_2CH_2)$_2$), 49.4 (1C, N(CH_2CH_2)$_2$), 49.4 (1C, N(CH_2CH_2)$_2$), 56.9 (1C, OCH_3), 61.3 (1C, CHCH_2O), 63.5 (1C, NCH_2Ph), 73.5 (1C, Ar*C*O), 74.1 (1C, *C*HCH$_2$O), 125.3 (1C, $C_{arom.}$), 126.5 (1C, $C_{arom.}$), 127.1 (1C, $C_{arom.}$), 128.3 (1C, $C_{arom.}$), 128.3 (2C, 3-C_{benzyl}, 5-C_{benzyl}), 129.0 (1C, 6-$C_{arom.}$), 129.4 (2C, 2-C_{benzyl}, 6-C_{benzyl}), 133.1 (1C, 2-$C_{arom.}$), 138.7 (1C, 1-Cbenzyl), 142.5 (1C, 1-Carom.). IR (neat): $\tilde{\nu}$ (cm^{-1}) = 2924, 2816 (C-H), 1088 (C-O-C), 737 (1,2-disubst. arom.), 737 (monosubst. arom.).

(*R*)-1′-Benzyl-4-ethoxy-3,4-dihydrospiro[[2]benzopyran-1,4′-piperidine] (**(*R*)-16**)

(*R*)-14 (49 mg, 0.14 mmol) was dissolved in CH_2Cl_2 (10 mL). Trifluoroacetic acid (200 µL) was added and the mixture was stirred for 3 h at ambient temperature. Then a 2 M aqueous solution of NaOH (10 mL) was added. After separation of the layers, the aqueous layer was extracted with CH_2Cl_2 (3×). The combined organic layers were dried (Na_2SO_4), filtered and the solvent was removed *in vacuo*. The residue was dissolved in CH_2Cl_2 (10 mL). Benzaldehyde (60 µL, 0.59 mmol) and (after 45 min) sodium triacetoxyborohydride (181 mg, 0.85 mmol) were added and the mixture was stirred overnight at ambient temperature. The reaction was stopped by the addition of a 2 M aqueous solution of NaOH. After separation of the layers, the aqueous layer was extracted with CH_2Cl_2 (2×) and ethyl acetate (1×). The combined organic layers were dried (Na_2SO_4), filtered and the solvent was removed *in vacuo*. The crude product was purified by flash column chromatography twice (1. Ø = 1.5 cm, h = 17 cm, cyclohexane-ethyl acetate = 4:1, V = 5 mL; 2. Ø = 1.5 cm, h = 17 cm, cyclohexane-ethyl acetate = 6:1, V = 5 mL) to give **(*R*)-16** as a pale yellow oil (R_f = 0.31, cyclohexane-ethyl acetate = 5:5), yield 33 mg (70%). $C_{22}H_{27}NO_2$ (337.5 g/mol). Specific rotation: $[\alpha]_D^{20}$: = −3.3 (7.7; CH_2Cl_2). Purity (HPLC method 1): 99.1%, t_R = 17.0 min.

(*S*)-1′-Benzyl-4-ethoxy-3,4-dihydrospiro[[2]benzopyran-1,4′-piperidine] (**(*S*)-16**)

(*S*)-14 (63 mg, 0.18 mmol) was dissolved in CH_2Cl_2 (5 mL). Trifluoroacetic acid (300 µL) was added and the mixture was stirred for 2 h at ambient temperature. Then a 2 M aqueous solution of NaOH was added. After separation of the layers, the aqueous layer was extracted with ethyl acetate (3×). The combined organic layers were dried (Na_2SO_4), filtered and the solvent was removed *in vacuo*. The residue was dissolved in CH_2Cl_2 (5 mL). Benzaldehyde (40 µL, 0.39 mmol) and after 15 min, sodium triacetoxyborohydride (120 mg, 0.57 mmol) were added and the mixture was stirred at ambient temperature for 8 h. The reaction was stopped by the addition of a 2 M aqueous solution of NaOH. After separation of the layers, the aqueous layer was extracted with CH_2Cl_2 (3×). The combined organic layers were dried (Na_2SO_4), filtered and the solvent was removed *in vacuo*. The crude product was purified by flash column chromatography (Ø = 1.25 cm, h = 15 cm, cyclohexane-ethyl acetate = 6:1, V = 5 mL) to give (*S*)-16 as a pale yellow oil (R_f = 0.31, cyclohexane-ethyl acetate = 5:5), yield 28 mg (46%). $C_{22}H_{27}NO_2$ (337.5 g/mol). Specific rotation: $[\alpha]_D^{20}$: = +2.6 (11.7; CH_2Cl_2). Purity (HPLC method 1): 96.6%, t_R = 17.0 min.

Spectroscopic data for **(*R*)-16** and **(*S*)-16**

Exact mass (APCI): *m/z* = 338.2130 (calcd. 338.2115 for $C_{22}H_{28}NO_2$ $[M+H]^+$) ^{1}H-NMR ($CDCl_3$): δ (ppm) = 1.20 (t, *J* = 6.9 Hz, 3H, OCH_2CH_3), 1.74–2.04 (m, 4H, $N(CH_2CH_2)_2$), 2.28–2.24 (m, 2H, $N(CH_2CH_2)_2$), 2.62–2.70 (m, 2H, $N(CH_2CH_2)_2$), 3.50 (s, 2H, NCH_2Ph), 3.58–3.68 (m, 2H, OCH_2CH_3), 3.79 (dd, *J* = 11.9/5.4 Hz, 1H, $CHCH_2O$), 3.93 (dd, *J* = 11.9/3.9 Hz, 1H, $CHCH_2O$), 4.28 (t, *J* = 4.6 Hz, 1H, $CHCH_2O$), 7.11–7.35 (m, 9H, $H_{arom.}$). ^{13}C-NMR ($CDCl_3$): δ (ppm) = 15.9 (1C, OCH_2CH_3), 36.3 (1C, $N(CH_2CH_2)_2$), 36.7 (1C, $N(CH_2CH_2)_2$), 49.3 (1C, $N(CH_2CH_2)_2$), 49.5 (1C, $N(CH_2CH_2)_2$), 61.8 (1C, $CHCH_2O$), 63.6 (1C, NCH_2Ph), 64.8 (1C, OCH_2CH_3), 72.5 (1C, $CHCH_2O$), 73.7 (1C, ArCO), 125.2 (1C, $C_{arom.}$), 126.6 (1C, $C_{arom.}$), 127.1 (1C, $C_{arom.}$), 128.0 (1C, $C_{arom.}$), 128.2 (1C, $C_{arom.}$),

128.3 (2C, $C_{arom.}$), 129.4 (2C, $C_{arom.}$), 134.2 (1C, $C_{arom.}$), 138.7 (1C, $C_{arom.}$), 142.4 (1C, $C_{arom.}$). IR (neat): $\tilde{\nu}$ (cm^{-1}) = 2928, 2812 (C-H), 1092 (C-O-C ether), 737 (1,2-disubst. arom.), 698 (monosubst. arom.).

tert-Butyl (*R*)-4-(2-ethoxy-2-oxoethoxy)-3,4-dihydrospiro[[2]benzopyran-1,4′-piperidine]-1′-carboxylate (**(R)-17**)

***(R)*-11** (1.6 g, 5.0 mmol) was dissolved in THF (60 mL). A 1 M solution of lithium bis(trimethyl-silyl)amide (41 mL, 41 mmol) was added and the mixture was stirred for 1 h at ambient temperature. Then ethyl 2-bromoacetate (4.6 mL, 41.5 mmol) and tetrabutylammonium iodide (191 mg, 0.52 mmol) were added and the mixture was heated to reflux overnight. The solvent was removed *in vacuo*. The crude product was purified by flash column chromatography (Ø = 5.5 cm, h = 15 cm, cyclohexane-ethyl acetate = 9:1, V = 65 mL) to give ***(R)*-17** as a pale yellow oil (R_f = 0.17, cyclohexane-ethyl acetate = 5:1), yield 1.2 g (59%). $C_{22}H_{31}NO_6$ (405.5 g/mol). Specific rotation: $[\alpha]_D^{20}$: = −14.7 (5.5; CH_2Cl_2). Purity (HPLC method 1): 97.3%, t_R = 21.3 min.

tert-Butyl (*S*)-4-(2-ethoxy-2-oxoethoxy)-3,4-dihydrospiro[2-benzopyran-1,4′-piperidine]-1′-carboxylate (**(*S*)-17**)

***(S)*-11** (2.0 g, 6.3 mmol) was dissolved in THF (50 mL). A 1 M solution of lithium bis(trimethyl-silyl)amide (50 mL, 50 mmol) was added and the mixture was stirred for 45 min at ambient temperature. Then ethyl 2-bromoacetate (50 mL, 50.5 mmol) and tetrabutylammonium iodide (247 mg, 0.67 mmol) were added and the mixture was heated to reflux overnight. The solvent was removed *in vacuo*. The crude product was purified by flash column chromatography (Ø = 5 cm, h = 17 cm, cyclohexane-ethyl acetate = 9:1, V = 30 mL) to give ***(S)*-17** as a pale yellow oil (R_f = 0.17, cyclo-hexane-ethyl acetate = 5:1), yield 1.4 g (55%). $C_{22}H_{31}NO_6$ (405.5 g/mol). Specific rotation: $[\alpha]_D^{20}$: = +14.3 (3.6; CH_2Cl_2). Purity (HPLC method 1): 96.0%, t_R = 20.9 min.

Spectroscopic data for ***(R)*-17** and ***(S)*-17**

Exact mass (APCI): *m/z* = 406.2224 (calcd. 406.2224 for $C_{22}H_{32}NO_6$ $[M+H]^+$). ^{1}H-NMR ($CDCl_3$): δ (ppm) = 1.29 (t, *J* = 7.1 Hz, 3H, CH_2CH_3), 1.49 (s, 9H, $CO_2C(CH_3)_3$), 1.68–1.79 (m, 1H, $N(CH_2CH_2)_2$), 1.83–2.02 (m, 3H, $N(CH_2CH_2)_2$), 3.01–3.29 (m, 2H, $N(CH_2CH_2)_2$), 3.93–4.11 (m, 4H, $N(CH_2CH_2)_2$ (2H), $CHCH_2O$ (2H)), 4.17–4.28 (m, 4H, CH_2CH_3 (2), OCH_2CO_2 (2)), 4.52 (t, *J* = 3.4 Hz, 1H, $CHCH_2O$), 7.11 (dd, *J* = 7.6/1.5 Hz, 1H, $H_{arom.}$), 7.25–7.35 (m, 2H, $H_{arom.}$), 7.55 (dd, *J* = 7.5/1.7 Hz, 1H, H_{arom}). ^{13}C-NMR ($CDCl_3$): δ (ppm) = 14.4 (1C, CH_2CH_3), 28.7 (3C, $CO_2C(CH_3)_3$), 34.7 (br, 1C, $N(CH_2CH_2)_2$), 37.1 (br, 1C, $N(CH_2CH_2)_2$), 39.5 (br, 1C, $N(CH_2CH_2)_2$), 40.1 (br, 1C, $N(CH_2CH_2)_2$), 61.0 (1C, CH_2CH_3), 62.0 (1C, $CHCH_2O$), 65.7 (1C, OCH_2CO_2), 72.6 (1C, $CHCH_2O$), 73.6 (1C, $CO_2C(CH_3)_3$), 79.6 (1C, ArCO), 125.0 (1C, $C_{arom.}$), 127.0 (1C, $C_{arom.}$), 128.8 (1C, $C_{arom.}$), 129.5 (1C, $C_{arom.}$), 131.8 (1C, $C_{arom.}$), 142.1 (1C, $C_{arom.}$), 155.0 (1C, $CO_2C(CH_3)_3$), 170.9 (1C, OCH2CO2). IR (neat): $\tilde{\nu}$ (cm^{-1}) = 2974, 2928 (C-H), 1751, 1690 (C=O), 1165, 1099 (C-O-C ether), 759 (1,2-disubst. arom.).

Ethyl (*R*)-2-[(1′-benzyl-3,4-dihydrospiro[[2]benzopyran-1,4′-piperidin]-4-yl)oxy]acetate (**(*R*)-18**)

(*R*)-17 (86 mg, 0.21 mmol) was dissolved in CH_2Cl_2 (4 mL). Trifluoroacetic acid (200 μL) was added and the mixture was stirred overnight at ambient temperature. Then water was added. After separation of the layers, the aqueous layer was extracted with ethyl acetate (3×). The combined organic layers were dried (Na_2SO_4), filtered and the solvent was removed *in vacuo*. The residue was dissolved in CH_2Cl_2 (2 mL). Benzaldehyde (103 μL, 1.0 mmol) and sodium triacetoxyborohydride (161 mg, 0.76 mmol) were added and the mixture was stirred at ambient temperature for 4 days. The reaction was stopped by the addition of a 2 M aqueous solution of NaOH. After separation of the layers, the aqueous layer was extracted with CH_2Cl_2 (3×). The combined organic layers were dried (Na_2SO_4), filtered and the solvent was removed *in vacuo*. The crude product was purified by flash column chromatography (Ø = 1.5 cm, h = 14 cm, cyclohexane-ethyl acetate = 3:1, V = 5 mL) to give **(*R*)-18** as a yellowish oil (R_f = 0.16, cyclohexane-ethyl acetate = 5:5), yield 36 mg (43%). $C_{24}H_{29}NO_4$ (395.5 g/mol). Specific rotation: $[\alpha]_D^{20}$: = −16.0 (3.3; CH_2Cl_2). Purity (HPLC method 1): 95.4%, t_R = 17.7 min.

Ethyl (*S*)-2-[(1′-benzyl-3,4-dihydro-3,4-dihydrospiro[2-benzopyran-1,4′-piperidin]-4-yl)oxy]acetate (**(*S*)-18**)

(*S*)-17 (1.3 mg, 3.2 mmol) was dissolved in CH_2Cl_2 (60 mL). Trifluoroacetic acid (3.5 mL) was added and the mixture was stirred for 7 h at ambient temperature. Then a 2 M aqueous solution of NaOH was added. After separation of the layers, the aqueous layer was extracted with CH_2Cl_2 (3×). The combined organic layers were dried (Na_2SO_4), filtered and the solvent was removed *in vacuo*. The residue was dissolved in CH_2Cl_2 (50 mL). Benzaldehyde (1.0 mL, 9.9 mmol) and, after 15 min, sodium triacetoxyborohydride (2.0 g, 9.4 mmol) were added and the mixture was stirred overnight at ambient temperature. The reaction was stopped by the addition of a 2 M aqueous solution of NaOH and worked up as described for **(*R*)-18**. The crude product was purified by flash column chromatography (Ø = 5 cm, h = 15 cm, cyclohexane-ethyl acetate = 3:1, V = 30 mL) to give **(*S*)-18** as a yellowish oil (R_f = 0.16, cyclohexane-ethyl acetate = 5:5), yield 36 mg (43%). $C_{24}H_{29}NO_4$ (395.5 g/mol). Specific rotation: $[\alpha]_D^{20}$: = +15.3 (3.4; CH_2Cl_2). Purity (HPLC method 1): 93.1%, t_R = 17.3 min.

Spectroscopic data for **(*R*)-18** and **(*S*)-18**

Exact mass (APCI): m/z = 396.2177 (calcd. 396.2169 for $C_{24}H_{30}NO_4$ $[M+H]^+$). ^{1}H-NMR ($CDCl_3$): δ (ppm) = 1.30 (t, J = 7.1 Hz, 3H, CH_2CH_3), 1.87–1.95 (m, 3H, $N(CH_2CH_2)_2$), 2.16 (td, J = 13.1/4.6 Hz, 1H, $N(CH_2CH_2)_2$), 2.34–2.45 (m, 1H, $N(CH_2CH_2)_2$), 2.47–2.55 (m, 1H, $N(CH_2CH_2)_2$), 2.70–2.81 (m, 2H, $N(CH_2CH_2)_2$), 3.57 (d, J = 13.1 Hz, 1H, NCH_2Ph), 3.61 (d, J = 13.1 Hz, 1H, NCH_2Ph), 3.98 (dd, J = 12.4/3.3 Hz, 1H, $CHCH_2O$), 4.05 (dd, J = 12.4/3.8 Hz, 1H, $CHCH_2O$), 4.16–4.29 (m, 4H, CH_2CH_3 (2H), OCH_2CO_2 (2H)), 4.53 (t, J = 3.5 Hz, $CHCH_2O$), 7.22–7.41 (m, 8H, $H_{arom.}$), 7.53–7.57 (m, 1H, $H_{arom.}$). ^{13}C-NMR ($CDCl_3$): δ (ppm) = 14.4 (1C, CH_2CH_3), 35.1 (1C, $N(CH_2CH_2)_2$), 37.4 (1C, $N(CH_2CH_2)_2$), 49.3 (1C, $N(CH_2CH_2)_2$), 49.4 (1C, $N(CH_2CH_2)_2$), 61.0 (1C, CH_2CH_3), 61.7 (1C, $CHCH_2O$), 63.5 (1C, NCH_2Ph), 65.6 (1C, OCH_2CO_2), 72.7 (1C, $CHCH_2O$), 73.6 (1C, ArCO), 125.2

(1C, $C_{arom.}$), 126.8 (1C, $C_{arom.}$), 127.1 (1C, $C_{arom.}$), 128.3 (2C, $C_{arom.}$), 128.6 (1C, $C_{arom.}$), 129.4 (1C, $C_{arom.}$), 129.4 (2C, $C_{arom.}$), 132.0 (1C, 4a-$C_{arom.}$), 138.6 (1C, 1-C_{benzyl}), 142.8 (1C, 8a-$C_{arom.}$), 170.9 (1C, OCH2*C*O2). IR (neat): $\tilde{\nu}$ (cm^{-1}) = 2920, 2866 (C-H), 1748 (C=O), 1099, 1053 (C-O-C ether), 737 (1,2-disubst. arom.), 698 (monosubst. arom.).

(*R*)-2-[(1′-Benzyl-3,4-dihydrospiro[[2]benzopyran-1,4′-piperidin]-4-yl)oxy]ethanol (**(*R*)-19**)

(*R*)-18 (480 mg, 1.21 mmol) was dissolved in THF (5 mL). A 1 m solution of $LiAlH_4$ in THF (6 mL, 6 mmol) was added and the mixture was stirred overnight at ambient temperature. Then water was added. After separation of the layers, the aqueous layer was extracted with CH_2Cl_2 (3×). The combined organic layers were washed with water (2×) and brine (1×), dried (Na_2SO_4), filtered and the solvent was removed *in vacuo*. The crude product was purified by flash column chromatography (Ø = 3 cm, h = 15 cm, cyclohexane-ethyl acetate = 5:5, V = 20 mL) to give **(*R*)-19** as a yellowish oil (R_f = 0.06, ethyl acetate), yield 254 mg (59%). $C_{22}H_{27}NO_3$ (353.5 g/mol). Specific rotation: $[\alpha]_D^{20}$: = −2.2 (1.7; CH_2Cl_2). Purity (HPLC method 1): 95.1%, t_R = 13.8 min.

(*S*)-2-[(1′-Benzyl-3,4-dihydrospiro[[2]benzopyran-1,4′-piperidin]-4-yl)oxy]ethanol (**(*S*)-19**)

(*S*)-18 (451 mg, 1.14 mmol) was dissolved in THF (10 mL). A 1 M solution of $LiAlH_4$ in THF (2.5 mL, 2.5 mmol) was added and the mixture was stirred overnight at ambient temperature. Then water and CH_2Cl_2 were added. The reaction was worked up as described for **(*R*)-19**. The crude product was purified by flash column chromatography (Ø = 2 cm, h = 15 cm, cyclohexane-ethyl acetate = 5:5, V = 10 mL) to give **(*S*)-19** as a pale yellow oil (R_f = 0.06, ethyl acetate), yield 302 mg (75%). $C_{22}H_{27}NO_3$ (353.5 g/mol). Specific rotation: $[\alpha]_D^{20}$: = +2.1 (1.8; CH_2Cl_2). Purity (HPLC method 1): 94.3%, t_R = 13.9 min.

Spectroscopic data for **(*R*)-19** and **(*S*)-19**

Exact mass (APCI): *m/z* = 354.2039 (calcd. 354.2064 for $C_{22}H_{28}NO_3$ $[M+H]^+$). ^{1}H-NMR ($CDCl_3$): δ (ppm) = 1.85–1.99 (m, 3H, N(CH_2CH_2)$_2$), 2.13 (td, *J* = 13.3/4.6 Hz, 1H, N(CH_2*C*H_2)$_2$), 2.30–2.44 (s br, 1H, O*H*), 2.40 (td, *J* = 10.9/4.6 Hz, 1H, N(*C*H_2CH_2)$_2$), 2.45–2.53 (m, 1H, N(*C*H_2CH_2)$_2$), 2.70–2.79 (m, 2H, N(*C*H_2CH_2)$_2$), 3.58 (s, 2H, NC*H*$_2$Ph), 3.72–3.81 (m, 4H, OC*H*$_2$C*H*$_2$OH), 3.94 (dd, *J* = 12.3/3.3 Hz, 1H, CHC*H*$_2$O), 4.01 (dd, *J* = 12.3/3.9 Hz, 1H, CHC*H*$_2$O), 4.36 (t, *J* = 3.6 Hz, 1H, C*H*CH$_2$O), 7.22–7.39 (m, 9H, $H_{arom.}$). ^{13}C-NMR ($CDCl_3$): δ (ppm) = 35.4 (1C, N(CH_2*C*H_2)$_2$), 37.4 (1C, N(CH_2*C*H_2)$_2$), 49.3 (1C, N(*C*H_2CH_2)$_2$), 49.4 (1C, N(*C*H_2CH_2)$_2$), 61.6 (1C, CH*C*H_2O), 62.2 (1C, OCH_2*C*H_2OH), 63.5 (1C, N*C*H_2Ph), 70.1 (1C, O*C*H_2CH_2OH), 73.1 (1C, *C*HCH_2O), 73.7 (1C, Ar*C*O), 125.4 (1C, $C_{arom.}$), 126.7 (1C, $C_{arom.}$), 127.1 (1C, $C_{arom.}$), 128.3 (2C, $C_{arom.}$), 128.5 (1C, $C_{arom.}$), 128.9 (1C, $C_{arom.}$), 129.4 (2C, $C_{arom.}$), 133.1 (1C, $C_{arom.}$), 138.7 (1C, $C_{arom.}$), 142.5 (1C, $C_{arom.}$). IR (neat): $\tilde{\nu}$ (cm^{-1}) = 3399 (O-H), 2924, 2816 (C-H), 1092, 1076 (C-O-C, ether), 741 (1,2-disubst. arom.), 698 (monosubst. arom.).

(*R*)-1′-Benzyl-4-(2-fluoroethoxy)-3,4-dihydrospiro[[2]benzopyran-1,4′-piperidine] ((***R***)-**20**)

(Diethylamino)difluorosulfonium tetrafluoroborate (Xtal-Fluor E®, 46 mg, 0.20 mmol) and triethylamine trihydrofluoride (45 μL, 0.28 mmol) were dissolved in CH_2Cl_2 (1 mL). The solution was cooled to −78 °C. (***R***)**-19** (48 mg, 0.14 mmol) was added and the mixture was stirred at –78 °C for 1 h, then at 0 °C for 1 h and at ambient temperature for 1 h. A 5% aqueous solution of $NaHCO_3$ (3 mL) was added and the mixture was stirred for 15 min. The aqueous layer was extracted with CH_2Cl_2 (2×). The combined organic layers were dried (Na_2SO_4), filtered and the solvent was removed *in vacuo*. The crude product was purified by flash column chromatography (Ø = 0.75 cm, h = 16 cm, cyclohexane-ethyl acetate = 2:1, V = 5 mL) to give (***R***)**-20** as a pale yellow oil (R_f = 0.34, cyclohexane-ethyl acetate = 5:5), yield 27 mg (54%). $C_{22}H_{26}FNO_2$ (355.4 g/mol). Specific rotation: $[\alpha]_D^{20}$: = −6.4 (5.8; CH_2Cl_2). Purity (HPLC method 1): 97.0%, t_R = 16.4 min.

(*S*)-1′-Benzyl-4-(2-fluoroethoxy)-3,4-dohydrospiro[[2]benzopyran-1,4′-piperidine] ((***S***)-**20**)

(Diethylamino)difluorosulfonium tetrafluoroborate (Xtal-Fluor E®, 120 mg, 0.52 mmol) and triethylamine trihydrofluoride (305 μL, 1.87 mmol) were dissolved in CH_2Cl_2 (2 mL). The solution was cooled to −78 °C. (***S***)**-19** (120 mg, 0.34 mmol) dissolved in CH_2Cl_2 (2 mL), was added and the mixture was stirred at -78 °C for 1 h, then at 0 °C for 1 h and at ambient temperature overnight. A 20% aqueous solution of $NaHCO_3$ (4 mL) was added and the mixture was stirred for 15 min. The aqueous layer was extracted with CH_2Cl_2 (2×). The combined organic layers were dried (Na_2SO_4), filtered and the solvent was removed *in vacuo*. The crude product was purified by flash column chromatography (Ø = 1.5 cm, h = 18 cm, cyclohexane-ethyl acetate = 3:1, V = 5 mL) to give (***S***)**-20** as a pale yellow oil (R_f = 0.34, cyclohexane-ethyl acetate = 5:5), yield 86 mg (71%). $C_{22}H_{26}FNO_2$ (355.4 g/mol). Specific rotation: $[\alpha]_D^{20}$: = +5.9 (4.4; CH_2Cl_2). Purity (HPLC method 1): 95.1%, t_R = 16.1 min.

Spectroscopic data for (***R***)**-20** and (***S***)**-20**

Exact mass (APCI): *m/z* = 356.2032 (calcd. 356.2020 for $C_{22}H_{27}FNO_2$ $[M+H]^+$). ^{1}H-NMR ($CDCl_3$): δ (ppm) = 1.85–2.00 (m, 3H, $N(CH_2CH_2)_2$), 2.10 (td, *J* = 13.3/4.6 Hz, 1H, $N(CH_2CH_2)_2$), 2.39 (td, *J* = 11.6/3.1 Hz, 1H, $N(CH_2CH_2)_2$), 2.48 (td, *J* = 11.6/2.5 Hz, 1H, $N(CH_2CH_2)_2$), 2.69–2.78 (m, 2H, $N(CH_2CH_2)_2$), 3.57 (s, 2H, NCH_2Ph), 3.78–3.87 (m, 1H, OCH_2CH_2F), 3.87–3.94 (m, 1H, OCH_2CH_2F), 3.94 (dd, *J* = 12.1/4.7 Hz, 1H, $CHCH_2O$), 4.01 (dd, *J* = 12.1/3.7 Hz, 1H, $CHCH_2O$), 4.45 (t, *J* = 4.2 Hz, 1H, $CHCH_2O$), 4.59 (dt, *J* = 47.7/4.2 Hz, 2H, OCH_2CH_2F), 7.21–7.38 (m, 8H, $H_{arom.}$), 7.41–7.44 (m, 1H, $H_{arom.}$). ^{13}C-NMR ($CDCl_3$): δ (ppm) = 35.7 (1C, $N(CH_2CH_2)_2$), 37.0 (1C, $N(CH_2CH_2)_2$), 49.3 (1C, $N(CH_2CH_2)_2$), 49.4 (1C, $N(CH_2CH_2)_2$), 61.8 (1C, $CHCH_2O$), 63.5 (1C, NCH_2Ph), 68.0 (d, *J* = 20.3 Hz, 1C, OCH_2CH_2F), 73.1 (1C, $CHCH_2O$), 73.6 (1C, ArCO), 83.5 (d, *J* = 179.1 Hz, 1C, OCH_2CH_2F), 125.3 (1C, $C_{arom.}$), 126.7 (1C, $C_{arom.}$), 127.2 (1C, $C_{arom.}$), 128.4 (2C, $C_{arom.}$), 128.7 (1C, $C_{arom.}$), 129.5 (2C, $C_{arom.}$), 129.6 (1C, $C_{arom.}$), 133.0 (1C, $C_{arom.}$), 138.4 (1C, $C_{arom.}$), 142.5 (1C, Carom.). IR (neat): $\tilde{\boldsymbol{\nu}}$ (cm^{-1}) = 2934, 2812 (C-H), 1096 (C-O-C, ether), 737 (1,2-disubst. arom.), 698 (monosubst. arom.).

{(*R*)-2-[(1′-Benzyl-3,4-dihydrospiro[[2]benzopyran-1,4′-piperidin]-4-yl)oxy]ethyl} 4-methylbenzene-sulfonate ((***R***)-**21**)

(***R***)-**19** (90 mg, 0.25 mmol) was dissolved in CH_2Cl_2 (13 mL). 4-Dimethylaminopyridine (8 mg, 0.07 mmol), triethylamine (176 µL, 1.3 mmol) and 4-toulenesulfonyl chloride (108 mg, 0.57 mmol) were added and the mixture was stirred overnight at ambient temperature. Then a 2 M aqueous solution of NaOH was added. After separation of the layers, the aqueous layer was extracted with CH_2Cl_2 (3×). The combined organic layers were dried (Na_2SO_4), filtered and the solvent was removed *in vacuo*. The crude product was purified by flash column chromatography (Ø = 1.5 cm, h = 16 cm, cyclohexane-ethyl acetate = 7:3, V = 5 mL) to give (***R***)-**21** as a colorless oil (R_f = 0.13, cyclohexane-ethyl acetate = 5:5), yield 59 mg (46%). $C_{29}H_{33}NO_5S$ (507.6 g/mol). Specific rotation: $[\alpha]_D^{20}$: = −5.9 (21.8; CH_2Cl_2). Purity (HPLC method 1): 94.5%, t_R = 20.3 min.

{(*S*)-2-[(1′-Benzyl-3,4-dihydrospiro[[2]benzopyran-1,4′-piperidin]-4-yl)oxy]ethyl} 4-methylbenzene-sulfonate ((***S***)-**21**)

(***S***)-**19** (140 mg, 0.40 mmol) was dissolved in CH_2Cl_2 (20 mL). Triethylamine (274 µL, 2.0 mmol), 4-dimethylaminopyridine (16 mg, 0.13 mmol) and 4-toulenesulfonyl chloride (152 mg, 0.80 mmol) were added and the mixture was stirred overnight at ambient temperature. Then reaction was worked up as described for (***R***)-**21**. The crude product was purified by flash column chromatography (Ø = 2 cm, h = 15 cm, cyclohexane-ethyl acetate = 7:3, V = 10 mL) to give (***S***)-**21** as a yellow oil (R_f = 0.13, cyclohexane-ethyl acetate = 5:5), yield 66 mg (32%). $C_{29}H_{33}NO_5S$ (507.6 g/mol). Specific rotation: $[\alpha]_D^{20}$: = +7.5 (23.8; CH_2Cl_2). Purity (HPLC method 1): 95.1%, t_R = 19.6 min.

Spectroscopic data for (***R***)-**21** and (***S***)-**21**

Exact mass (APCI): *m/z* = 508.2151 (calcd. 508.2152 for $C_{29}H_{35}NO_5S$ $[M+H]^+$). ^{1}H-NMR ($CDCl_3$): δ (ppm) = 1.78–1.90 (m, 2H, $N(CH_2CH_2)_2$), 1.91–2.03 (m, 1H, $N(CH_2CH_2)_2$), 2.14 (br t, *J* = 12.9 Hz, 1H, $N(CH_2CH_2)_2$), 2.41 (s, 3H, CH_3), 2.45–2.62 (m, 2H, $N(CH_2CH_2)_2$), 2.77–2.82 (m, 2H, $N(CH_2CH_2)_2$), 3.62 (s, 2H, NCH_2Ph), 3.70–3.87 (m, 3H, OCH_2CH_2OTos (2H), $CHCH_2O$ (1H)), 3.91 (dd, *J* = 12.2/3.4 Hz, 1H, $CHCH_2O$), 4.09–4.25 (m, 2H, OCH_2CH_2OTos), 4.33 (t, *J* = 3.8 Hz, $CHCH_2O$), 7.08–7.57 (m, 11H, $H_{arom.}$), 7.71–7.83 (m, 2H, H-2_{tosyl}, H-6_{tosyl}). ^{13}C-NMR ($CDCl_3$): δ (ppm) = 21.8 (1C, CH_3), 35.2 (1C, $N(CH_2CH_2)_2$), 36.8 (1C, $N(CH_2CH_2)_2$), 49.2 (1C, $N(CH_2CH_2)_2$), 49.3 (1C, $N(CH_2CH_2)_2$), 61.7 (1C, $CHCH_2O$), 63.3 (1C, NCH_2Ph), 66.1 (1C, OCH_2CH_2OTos), 69.7 (1C, OCH_2CH_2OTos), 73.0 (1C, $CHCH_2O$), 73.4 (1C, ArCO), 125.2 (1C, $C_{arom.}$), 126.1 (1C, $C_{arom.}$), 126.7 (1C, $C_{arom.}$), 128.1 (2C, $C_{arom.}$), 128.4 (2C, $C_{arom.}$), 128.7 (1C, $C_{arom.}$), 128.8 (2C, $C_{arom.}$), 129.6 (1C, $C_{arom.}$), 129,9 (2C, $C_{arom.}$), 132.2 (1C, $C_{arom.}$), 133.0 (1C, $C_{arom.}$), 133.9 (1C, $C_{arom.}$), 144.9 (1C, $C_{arom.}$), 146.0 (1C, Carom.). IR (neat): $\tilde{\nu}$ [cm^{-1}] = 2924, 2812 (C-H), 1358(m), 1177 (O=S=O), 1096 (C-O-C), 741 (1,2-disubst. arom.), 698 (monosubst. arom.).

2.2. Receptor Bindings Studies

2.2.1. Materials

The guinea pig brain and rat liver for the σ_1 and σ_2 receptor binding assays were commercially available (Harlan-Winkelmann, Borchen, Germany). Homogenizer: Elvehjem Potter (B. Braun Biotech International, Melsungen, Germany). Cooling centrifuge model Rotina 35R (Hettich, Tuttlingen, Germany) and High-speed cooling centrifuge model Sorvall RC-5C plus (Thermo Fisher Scientific, Langenselbold, Germany). Multiplates: standard 96-well multiplates (Diagonal, Muenster, Germany). Shaker: self-made device with adjustable temperature and tumbling speed (scientific workshop of the institute). Vortexer: Vortex Genie 2 (Thermo Fisher Scientific, Langenselbold, Germany). Harvester: MicroBeta FilterMate-96 Harvester. Filter: Printed Filtermat Typ A and B. Scintillator: Meltilex (Typ A or B) solid state scintillator. Scintillation analyzer: MicroBeta Trilux (all Perkin Elmer LAS, Rodgau-Jügesheim, Germany). Chemicals and reagents were purchased from different commercial sources and of analytical grade.

2.2.2. Preparation of Membrane Homogenates from Guinea Pig Brain

According to [35–37]: five guinea pig brains were homogenized with the Potter (500–800 rpm, 10 up-and-down strokes) in 6 volumes of cold 0.32 M sucrose. The suspension was centrifuged at 1,200 × *g* for 10 min at 4 °C. The supernatant was separated and centrifuged at 23,500 × *g* for 20 min at 4 °C. The pellet was resuspended in 5-6 volumes of buffer (50 mM TRIS, pH 7.4) and centrifuged again at 23,500 × *g* (20 min, 4 °C). This procedure was repeated twice. The final pellet was resuspended in 5-6 volumes of buffer and frozen (−80 °C) in 1.5 mL portions containing about 1.5 mg protein/mL.

2.2.3. Preparation of Membrane Homogenates from Rat Liver

According to [35–37]: two rat livers were cut into small pieces and homogenized with the Potter (500–800 rpm, 10 up-and-down strokes) in 6 volumes of cold 0.32 M sucrose. The suspension was centrifuged at 1,200 × *g* for 10 min at 4 °C. The supernatant was separated and centrifuged at 31,000 × *g* for 20 min at 4 °C. The pellet was resuspended in 5–6 volumes of buffer (50 mM TRIS, pH 8.0) and incubated at room temperature for 30 min. After the incubation, the suspension was centrifuged again at 31,000 × *g* for 20 min at 4 °C. The final pellet was resuspended in 5–6 volumes of buffer and stored at −80 °C in 1.5 mL portions containing about 2 mg protein/mL.

2.2.4. Protein Determination

The protein concentration was determined by the method of Bradford [38], modified by Stoscheck [39]. The Bradford solution was prepared by dissolving 5 mg of Coomassie Brilliant Blue G 250 in 2.5 mL of EtOH (95%, v/v). 10 mL deionized H_2O and 5 mL phosphoric acid (85%, m/v) were added to this solution, the mixture was stirred and filled to a total volume of 50.0 mL with deionized water. The calibration was carried out using bovine serum albumin as a standard in 9 concentrations (0.1, 0.2, 0.4, 0.6, 0.8, 1.0, 1.5, 2.0 and 4.0 mg/mL). In a 96-well standard multiplate, 10 μL of the calibration solution or 10 μL of the membrane receptor preparation were mixed with 190 μL of the Bradford solution, respectively. After 5 min, the UV absorption of the protein-dye complex at $\lambda = 595$ nm was measured with a platereader (Tecan Genios, Tecan, Crailsheim, Germany).

2.2.5. General Protocol for the Binding Assays

According to [35–37]: the test compound solutions were prepared by dissolving approximately 10 μmol (usually 2–4 mg) of test compound in DMSO so that a 10 mM stock solution was obtained. To obtain the required test solutions for the assay, the DMSO stock solution was diluted with the respective assay buffer. The filtermats were presoaked in 0.5% aqueous polyethylenimine solution for 2 h at room temperature before use. All binding experiments were carried out in duplicates in 96-well multiplates. The concentrations given are the final concentrations in the assay. Generally, the assays were performed by addition of 50 μL of the respective assay buffer, 50 μL test compound solution in various concentrations (10^{-5}, 10^{-6}, 10^{-7}, 10^{-8}, 10^{-9} and 10^{-10} mol/L), 50 μL of corresponding radioligand solution and 50 μL of the respective receptor preparation into each well of the multiplate (total volume 200 μL). The receptor preparation was always added last. During the incubation, the multiplates were shaken at a speed of 500–600 rpm at the specified temperature. Unless otherwise noted, the assays were terminated after 120 min by rapid filtration using the harvester. During the filtration each well was washed five times with 300 μL of water. Subsequently, the filtermats were dried at 95 °C. The solid scintillator was melted on the dried filtermats at a temperature of 95 °C for 5 min. After solidifying of the scintillator at room temperature, the trapped radioactivity in the filtermats was measured with the scintillation analyzer. Each position on the filtermat corresponding to one well of the multiplate was measured for 5 min with the [^{3}H]-counting protocol. The overall counting efficiency was 20%. The IC_{50}-values were calculated with the program GraphPad Prism® 3.0 (GraphPad Software, San Diego, CA, USA) by non-linear regression analysis. Subsequently, the IC_{50} values were transformed into K_i-values using the equation of Cheng and Prusoff [40]. The K_i-values are given as mean value ± SEM from three independent experiments.

2.2.6. Protocol of the σ_1 Receptor Binding Assay

According to [35–37]: the assay was performed with the radioligand [^{3}H]-(+)-pentazocine (22.0 Ci/mmol; Perkin Elmer). The thawed membrane preparation of guinea pig brain cortex (about 100 μg of protein) was incubated with various concentrations of test compounds, 2 nM [^{3}H]-(+)-pentazocine, and TRIS buffer (50 mM, pH 7.4) at 37 °C. The non-specific binding was determined with 10 μM unlabeled (+)-pentazocine. The K_d-value of (+)-pentazocine is 2.9 nM [41].

2.2.7. Protocol of the σ_2 Receptor Binding Assay

According to [35–37]: the assays were performed with the radioligand [^{3}H]DTG (specific activity 50 Ci/mmol; ARC, St. Louis, MO, USA). The thawed membrane preparation of rat liver (about 100 μg of protein) was incubated with various concentrations of the test compound, 3 nM [^{3}H]DTG and buffer containing (+)-pentazocine (500 nM (+)-pentazocine in 50 mM TRIS, pH 8.0) at room temperature.

The non-specific binding was determined with 10 μM non-labeled DTG. The K_d value of [^{3}H]DTG is 17.9 nM [42].

2.3. Radiochemistry

2.3.1. General

For Solid Phase Extraction (SPE), Sep-Pak® C18 cartridges Plus, Plus short and Plus light (Waters, Eschborn, Germany) as well as Chromabond HR-X® cartridges (Machery-Nagel, Düren, Germany) were tried and C18 cartridges Plus were applied routinely.

Analytical radio-HPLC was performed using an Jasco device series 2000 consisting of autosampler, quaternary pump, degasser, UV-Vis detector, and NaI(Tl)-scintillation detector (bte, Braunschweig, Germany) for gamma detection. A Multospher 120 RP18-AQ column (250x4.6 mm, particle size 5 μm p.s.; CS Chromatographie Service, , Langerwehe, Germany) was applied in gradient mode (0–10 min: 5% MeCN+ 20 mM NH_4OAc aq.; 10–55 min: 10%–80% MeCN + 20 mM NH_4OAc aq.) at a flow rate of 1.0 mL/min.

Separation of the crude ^{18}F-labeled product was conducted via semi-preparative radio-HPLC in isocratic mode using a Multospher 120 RP18-AQ column (150×10 mm, 5 μm) with 50% acetonitrile + 20 mM NH_4OAc aq. as eluent at a flow rate of 2 mL/min. The device consisted of an S1021 pump (SYKAM Chromatographie, Fürstenfeldbruck, Germany), UV detector (Well-ChromK-2001, KNAUER, Berlin, Germany), and NaI(Tl)-counter and data acquisition was performed by NINA software version 4.8 rev. 4 (Nuclear Interface, München, Germany).

Radioluminescence thin-layer chromatography (radio-TLC) was performed on alumina coated platelets (Alugram® ALOX N/UV_{254}) with petroleum ether/ethyl acetate 7:3 (v/v) as solvent. Radioactive spots were visualised by radioluminescence using a BAS-1800 II system (Bioimaging Analyzer, Fuji Film, Düsseldorf, Germany). Images were evaluated with AIDA 2.31 software (raytest, Straubenhardt, Germany) using the non-radioactive reference compounds after visualization under UV (254 nm).

2.3.2. Synthesis of [^{18}F]fluoride Labeled Radiotracer [^{18}F]-***(R)*-20**

Aqueous [^{18}F]fluoride was added to a solution of K222 (11.2 mg, 29.7 μmol) and aqueous K_2CO_3 (1.78 mg, 12.9 μmol) in acetonitrile (0.5 mL). The solvent was removed azeotropically in an Ar atmosphere under reduced pressure to produce anhydrous reactive K[^{18}F]F-K222-carbonate complex. To this mixture a solution of tosylate precursor ***(R)*-21** (2.0–2.5 mg) in acetonitrile (0.5 mL) was added and the reaction mixture was heated to 82 °C for 20 min (total reaction volume 1.0 mL). These optimized reaction conditions led to reproducible labelling yields of 25%–32% (n = 8) as determined by radio-TLC (petroleum ether-ethyl acetate 7: 3 (v/v). TLC retention values: [^{18}F]-***(R)*-20**: R_f = 0.83; (*R*)-**21**: R_f = 0.27.

2.4. In vitro *stability and lipophilicity of* [^{18}F]-**(*R*)-20**

For pharmacological characterization of the radiotracer [^{18}F]-***(R)*-20**, chemical stability was investigated *in vitro* in different buffer systems over 2 h at 40 °C: 50 mM phosphate buffer (pH 7.2), phosphate-saline-solution (Dulbecco; pH 7.2) and 0.01 M TRIS-HCl (pH 7.4). *In-vitro* stability in native mouse plasma was investigated by incubation of 200 μL plasma plus 5 μL [^{18}F]-***(R)*-20** (~50 MBq) in isotonic NaCl (containing 10% ethanol) for 30 min at 37 °C.

To get information about the blood-brain barrier permeability of [^{18}F]-***(R)*-20**, the distribution coefficient logD was determined by conventional shake-flask experiments using *n*-octanol/phosphate buffer pH 7.2, *n*-octanol/phosphate-saline-solution pH 7.2 and *n*-octanol/TRIS-HCl pH 7.4 extraction systems. The amount of the radiotracer [^{18}F]-***(R)*-20** in the respective layer was determined using a calibrated γ-counter (Wallac WIZARD, Perkin Elmer, Rodgau-Jügesheim, Germany). The determination of the $logD_{7.4}$ value by HPLC (RP-HPLC; column: ReproSil-Pur AQ, 5 μm, 250 × 4 mm, Dr. Maisch HPLC GmbH, Ammerbruch, Germany; solvent A: NH_4OAc 20 mM aq., solvent B: acetonitrile using a gradient for B: 0–10 min 10%, 10–40 min 10%–90%; flow: 1 ml/min; detection: 254 nm) was achieved after calibration using reference compounds following the EU guideline 67/548/EWG based on OECD guidelines 2004 [43]. The following reference compounds have been used for calibration (reference compound (*logD*)): phenol (*1.5*), benzene (*2.1*), toluene (*2.7*), benzyl alcohol (*1.1*), *o*-nitrophenol (*1.8*), benzyl chloride (*2.3*), 1,4-dibromobenzene (*3.8*), nitrobenzene (*1.9*), benzophenone (*3.2*), diphenyl ether (*4.2*), fluoranthene (*5.1*), *p*-nitrophenol (*1.9*), chlorobenzene (*2.8*), naphthalene (*3.6*), trichloroethylene (*2.4*), biphenyl (*4.0*), phenanthrene (*4.5*), dibenzyl (*4.8*), thiourea (for determination of t_0). For the reference compounds as well as **(*R*)-20**, multiple measurements were conducted (n = 3–6). The following regression equation was obtained: log k = 0.07189 × logD + 0.84472 (R^2 = 0.7988). The $logD_{7.4}$ value of [^{18}F]-*(S)*-**20** was recorded six times. Furthermore, the logD value was calculated via ACD ChemSketch2012 software.

2.5. Biological Evaluation

2.5.1. General

The experimental protocols were approved by the local ethics committee and conducted according to the national and EU regulations for animal research. Female CD1 mice (10–12 weeks old, 33.8 ± 6.2 g) were obtained from the Medizinisch-Experimentelles Zentrum, Universität Leipzig and housed under a 12 h/12 h light/dark cycle with free access to food and water for at least 24 h before experiments. Animals were sacrificed by CO_2 asphyxiation after anaesthesia with O_2/CO_2 mixture.

2.5.2. *In Vivo* Metabolism of [^{18}F]-**(*R*)-20**

The metabolism of [^{18}F]-***(R)*-20** was investigated at 30 min after injection of the radiotracer (166.4 ± 65.4 MBq, dissolved in *ca.* 150 μL saline) into the left or right vena caudalis lateralis. Metabolites were investigated in plasma, urine, brain and liver samples. Urine samples were analyzed directly. Plasma samples were obtained by centrifugation of EDTA blood (12,000 rpm, 4 °C, 10 min) obtained by heart puncture. Brain and liver samples were acquired by homogenization of the organs in ice-cold 50 mM TRIS-HCl buffer (pH 7.4) using a PotterS® Homogeizer (B. Braun). The tissues were treated in a borosilicate glass cylinder by 10 strokes of a PTFE plunge at a speed of 800–1000 min^{-1}.

The precipitation of proteins in plasma, brain, and liver samples was performed using twofold extraction of aliquots with ice-cold MeCN (1:4 v/v; for plasma 1:7 v/v), centrifugation of precipitates, and gentle concentration of the combined supernatants (~60°C, argon flow). In addition, precipitation experiments were supplemented by an alternative precipitation method using aqueous MeOH ($MeOH/H_2O$ 9:1). The percentages of the parent radiotracer and radiometabolites were analysed by radio-HPLC and radio-TLC. The extraction efficiency was controlled using a calibrated γ-counter (Wallac WIZARD, Perkin Elmer).

2.5.3. *Ex Vivo* Autoradiography Studies

The tracer distribution in the brain under control and blocking conditions was determined by *ex vivo* autoradiography studies. [^{18}F]-(*R*)-**20** was administered via right vena caudalis lateralis without (31.0 MBq) or with (31.7 MBq) co-application 1 mg/kg haloperidol (Tocris, Bristol, UK) [44]. Animals were sacrificed at 30 min p.i. Blood was collected by heart puncture, the brain quickly removed and transferred on ice, and all samples were weighed. Radioactivity in brain and plasma samples was counted using an automated γ-counter and expressed as percentage of injected dose per gram (%ID/g). For autoradiography, the brain hemispheres were frozen immediately after isolation in 2-methylbutane (Carl Roth, Karlsruhe, Germany) at −30 °C (>2 min). Serial sagittal slices of 12 µm thickness were cut on a cryostat (Microm, Walldorf, Germany) from approx. midline, +500 µm, +1,000 µm and +1,500 µm. Slices were exposed overnight on an imaging plate (SR 2025, Fuji, Tokyo, Japan), scanned afterwards with a high-resolution phosphorimager (HD-CR 35 Bio, raytest). 2D densitometry of the whole brain was performed with AIDA software (raytest).

3. Results and Discussion

3.1. Synthesis

The synthesis of enantiomerically pure 2-benzopyrans of type **4** started with 2-bromostyrene (**5**). Bromine lithium exchange with *n*-BuLi at −78 °C led to an aryllithium intermediate, which was treated with 1-Boc-piperidin-4-one to yield the styrene derivative **6**. The Boc-protected piperidone was chosen because the handling (work-up, purification, isolation) of the resulting carbamate was much easier than the handling of alternative benzyl substituted tertiary amines (e.g., **12**). Removal of the excess of 1-Boc-piperidin-4-one was performed by $LiBH_4$ reduction of the keto group after complete reaction of the ketone with the lithiated vinylbenzene derivative. Flash chromatographic separation of the resulting 1-Boc-piperidin-4-ol resulted in 75% yield of the tertiary alcohol **6**.

The Sharpless Asymmetric Dihydroxylation of terminal alkene **6** with AD-mix-β employing the standard protocol [45–47], led only to low yields of diol ***(R)*-7** (Scheme 1). Increasing of the amount of chiral ligand $(DHQD)_2PHAL$, oxidant (K_2OsO_4) and cooxidant ($Na_3[Fe(CN)_6]$ and a longer reaction time did not lead to reproducible high yields of diol **(*R*)-7**. It was assumed that the reason for the low yields of **(*R*)-7** was the low solubility of alkene **6** in a 1:1 *tert*-butanol-water solvent mixture. Despite the addition of different cosolvents (e.g., *tert*-butyl methyl ether, THF) to the solvent mixture, the yields were not improved. However, the yield was considerably raised when increasing the amount of solvent mixture from 10 mL to 60 mL/mmol alkene. The (*R*)-configured triol **(*R*)-7** was obtained in a reproducible yield of 82%. Analogously the (*S*)-configured enantiomer **(*S*)-7** was accessible in 74% yield, when using AD-mix-α for the dihydroxylation step.

Reaction of triol **(*R*)-7** with tosyl chloride, NEt_3 and DMAP provided the 2-benzofuran **(*S*)-8** in 50% yield. It is assumed that tosyl chloride reacts predominantly with the primary OH-moiety of triol **(*R*)-7**. In the presence of base the resulting primary tosylate forms an oxirane, which is opened by the tertiary alcohol giving the five-membered 2-benzofuran. Finally the primary alcohol reacts with a second equivalent tosyl chloride to form the tosylate **(*S*)-8**. Reaction of 2-(2-bromophenyl)oxirane **(*R*)-9** with n-BuLi and subsequently with 1-Boc-piperidin-4-one led to an analogous 2-benzofuran (**(*S*)-10**) upon regioselective opening of the oxirane ring by the intermediate lithium alcoholate [35].

Scheme 1. Regioselective synthesis of 2-benzopyrans and 2-benzofurans.

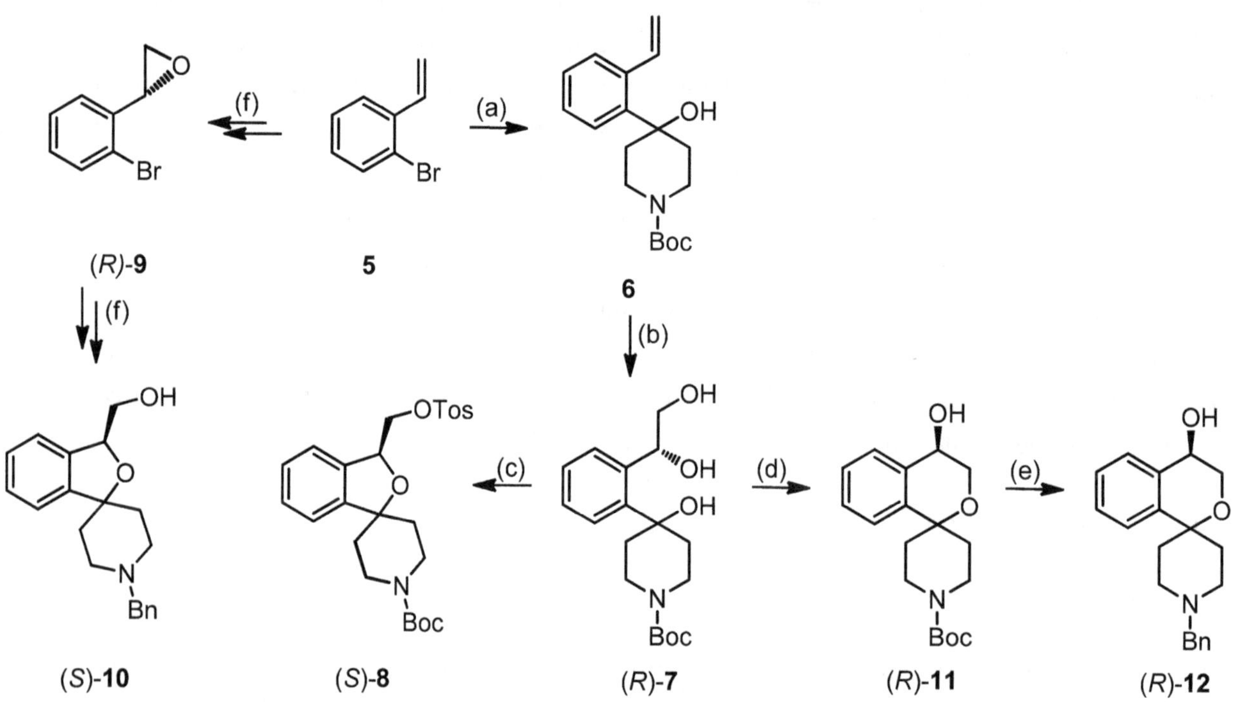

Reagents and conditions: (a) *n*-BuLi, THF, then 1-Bocpiperidin-4-one, then $LiBH_4$, 75%. (b) AD-mix-β, *t*-BuOH/H_2O = 1:1, 82%. (c) *p*-TosCl, NEt_3, 4-DMAP, CH_2Cl_2, 50%. (d) *p*-TosCl, NEt_3, Bu_2SnO, THF, 62%. (e) TFA, CH_2Cl_2, then PhCH=O, $NaBH(OAc)_3$, CH_2Cl_2, 56%. (f) see ref. [33]. Bromostyrene **5** was transformed in the same manner into the corresponding (*S*)-configured enantiomers by using AD-mix-α. (*S*)-7: 74%. (S)-**11**: 47%. (S)-**12**: 22%.

However, addition of catalytic amounts of Bu_2SnO during the tosylation of triol **(*R*)-7** afforded selectively the 2-benzopyran **(*R*)-11**, which was isolated in 62% yield. The addition of Bu_2SnO was crucial for the synthesis of the 2-benzopyran scaffold. Bu_2SnO is described as additive for the selective tosylation of the primary OH-moiety of diols by shielding the other OH-moiety [48]. In case of triol **(*R*)-7**, shielding of the secondary OH-moiety by Bu_2SnO leads to selective activation (*i.e.*, tosylation) of the primary OH-moiety for the nucleophilic substitution.

The enantiomeric purity of **(*R*)-11** and **(*S*)-11**, which was prepared analogously, was analyzed by chiral HPLC using Daicel Chiralpak IB column, resulting in 85% ee for **(*R*)-11** and 77.2% ee for **(*S*)-11**. The moderate enantiomeric excess is explained by the high solvent amount used for the Sharpless Asymmetric Dihydroxylation leading to a lower concentration of the chiral alkaloid ligand due to dilution effect. The lower concentration of the chiral catalyst may lead to an increased amount of uncatalyzed dihydroxylation of alkene **6**. This effect has already been described in the literature [33].

For the introduction of the desired benzyl group at the piperidine ring the Boc protective group of **(*R*)-11** was cleaved off with trifluoroacetic acid (TFA). Without further purification, the resulting secondary amine was reductively alkylated with benzaldehyde and $NaBH(OAc)_3$ to afford the benzyl-substituted alcohol **(*R*)-12**. After synthesis of the enantiomer **(*S*)-12**, the enantiomeric purity of both enantiomers was determined by chiral HPLC using a Daicel Chiralpak AD-H column, which resulted in 92.2% ee for **(*R*)-12** and 76.2% ee for **(*S*)-12**.

The structure of the 2-benzopyran **(*R*)-12** was unambiguously identified by comparison of its NMR spectra with those of the hydroxymethyl substituted 2-benzofuran **(*S*)-10**, which was obtained from the oxirane **(*R*)-9** as reported previously by halogen/metal exchange, addition to piperidinone and exchange of the Boc-protective group with a benzyl group [33]. The ^{1}H-NMR spectra of the 2-benzopyran **(*R*)-12** and the 2-benzofuran **(*S*)-10** show three doublets of doublets for the $ArCH(OR)CH_2OR$ substructure. However the chemical shift of the dd for the methine proton of the 2-benzopyran **(*R*)-12** is around 0.8 ppm high-field shifted (4.51 ppm) compared to the dd for the methine proton of the five-membered 2-benzofuran **(*S*)-10** (5.29 ppm). After assigning the ^{13}C-NMR signals on the basis of the gHSQC (= gradient heteronuclear single quantum coherence) NMR spectrum, the identity of the 2-benzopyran substructure was proved by 2D gHMBC (= gradient heteronuclear multiple bond correlation) NMR spectroscopy. In this NMR experiment, couplings between protons and carbon atoms over 2–3 bonds are detected. In the 2D gHMBC NMR spectrum of the 2-benzopyran **(*R*)-12** (Figure 2) a coupling between the OCH_2 signals and the quaternary spiro-C-atom is observed indicating a distance of 2–3 bonds. On the contrary a corresponding crosspeak for the 2-benzofuran **(*S*)-10** is not seen, since four bonds separate the corresponding protons and C-atom.

Figure 2. Part of the gHMBC NMR spectrum of 2-benzopyran **(*R*)-12**. The crosspeak between the OCH_2 protons and the spiro-C-atom is marked.

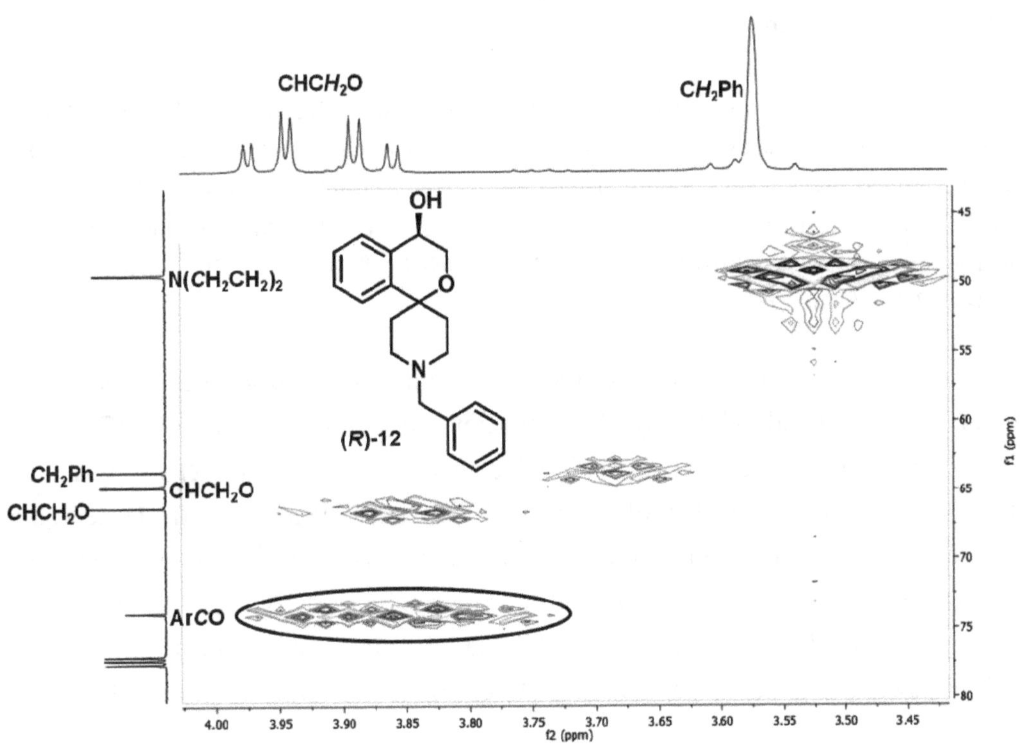

Methyl and ethyl ethers ***(R)*-15** and ***(S)*-16** were synthesized by alkylation of the alcohol ***(R)*-11** with methyl iodide and ethyl iodide, respectively, cleavage of the Boc-protective group with trifluoroacetic acid and subsequent reductive alkylation with benzaldehyde and $NaBH(OAc)_3$. (Scheme 2) The enantiomeric purity of the methyl ethers was determined via chiral HPLC, resulting in ee-values of 89.6% for ***(R)*-15**, 82% for ***(S)*-15**.

Scheme 2. Synthesis of ethers ***(R)*-15**, ***(R)*-16**, and ***(R)*-20**.

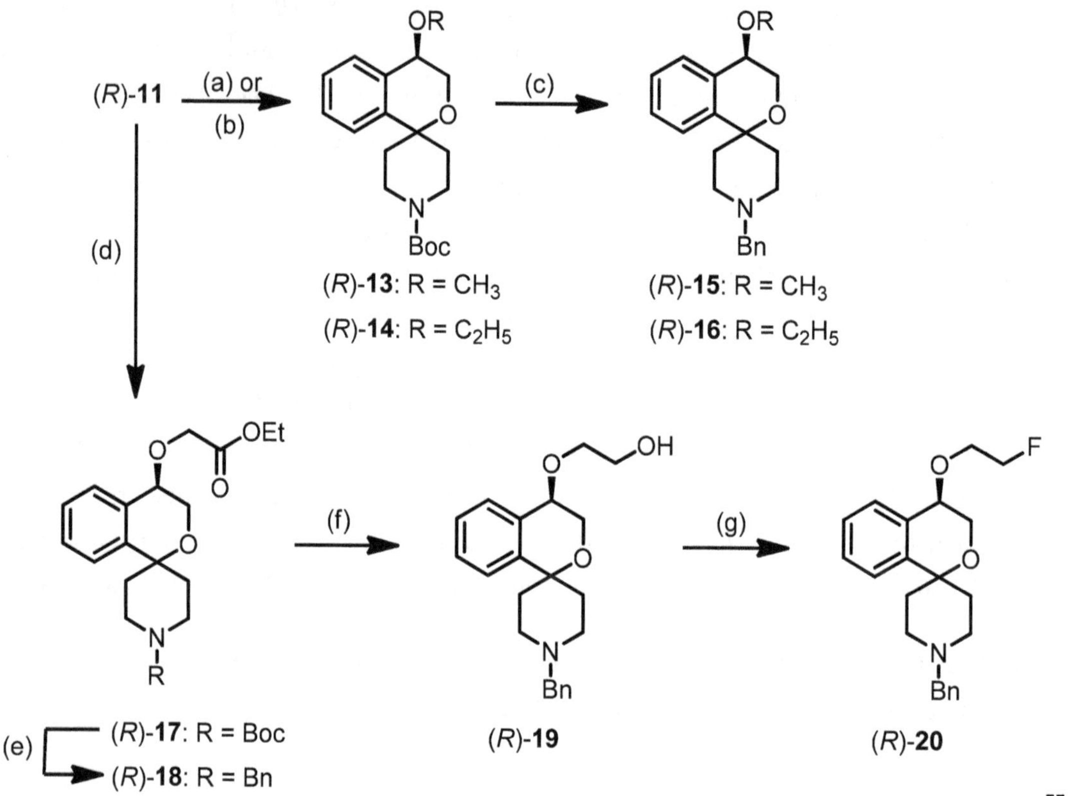

Reagents and conditions: (**a**) NaH, THF, then CH_3I, 99%. (**b**) NaH, THF, then C_2H_5I, then LiHMDS, 29%. (**c**) TFA, CH_2Cl_2, then benzaldehyde, $NaBH(OAc)_3$, CH_2Cl_2, 9% (R)-**15**, 70% (R)-**16**. (**d**) LiHMDS, THF, then ethyl 2-bromoacetate, TBAI, 59%. (**e**) TFA, CH_2Cl_2, then benzaldehyde, $NaBH(OAc)_3$, CH_2Cl_2, 43%. (**f**) $LiALH_4$, THF, 59%. (**g**) Xtal-Fluor E®, $NEt_3 \times 3HF$, CH_2Cl_2, 54%. The (*S*)-configured enantiomers were prepared in the same manner: **(*S*)-13**: 69%. **(*S*)-14**: 50%. **(*S*)-15**: 80%. **(*S*)-16**: 46%. **(*S*)-17**: 55%. **(*S*)-18**: 43%. **(*S*)-19**: 75%. **(*S*)-20**: 71%.

In order to introduce a fluorine atom into the substituent in 4-position of the 2-benzopyran ring the alcohol ***(S)*-11** was alkylated with ethyl bromoacetate to yield the ester ***(R)*-17**. Removal of the Boc-protective group and reductive benzylation led to the benzylamine ***(R)*-18**, which was reduced with $LiAlH_4$ to afford the primary alcohol ***(R)*-19** in 59% yield. The alcohol ***(R)*-19** served as precursor for the introduction of [^{19}F]fluorine as well as the radioactive isotope [^{18}F]fluorine into the side chain. Reaction of ***(R)*-19** with XtalFluor-E® provided the fluoroethoxy derivative ***(R)*-20** in 54% yield. For the radiosynthesis the alcohol ***(R)*-11** had to be activated for nucleophilic substitution (see Scheme 3 in the section Radiosynthesis). The corresponding (*S*)-configured enantiomers ***(S)*-17–20** were prepared in the same manner.

3.2. Receptor Binding Studies

σ_1 and σ_2 receptor affinities were measured in competition experiments with radioligands. The σ_1 receptor binding assay was carried out using a receptor preparation from guinea pig brain and [^{3}H]-(+)-pentazocine as a high-affinity and selective radioligand. The σ_2 receptor affinity was conducted with a receptor preparation from rat liver and [^{3}H]di-*o*-toylguanidine ([^{3}H]DTG) was used as radioligand. Since DTG is not selective for the σ_2 subtype over the σ_1 subtype, σ_1 receptors binding sites were masked by addition of non-labeled (+)-pentazocine [35–37].

The σ_1 and σ_2 affinities of the spirocyclic 2-benzopyrans are listed in Table 1. Most of the representatives of this new class of compounds show high σ_1 affinity with K_i-values in the low nanomolar range. All 2-benzopyrans are selective towards the σ_2 receptor subtype with high selectivity factors. With exception of the ethyl ether **16** (eudismic ratio 1), the (*R*) enantiomers represent the eutomers. The eudismic ratio varies from 1.2 (compounds **19**, **20**) indicating low enantioselective receptor binding up to 29 (esters **18**) revealing very high enantioselective receptor interaction.

Table 1. σ_1 and σ_2 receptor affinities of (*R*)- and (*S*)-configured spirocyclic 2-benzopyrans.

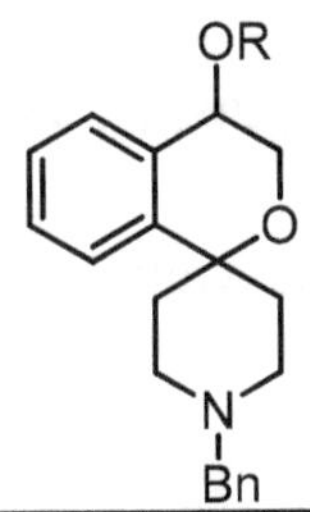

Entry	Compound	R	Configuration	$K_i \pm$ SEM [nM]		Selectivity
				σ_1	σ_2	σ_1/σ_2
1	**(*R*)-11**	H	*R*	5.2 ± 0.3	2150	413
2	**(*S*)-11**	H	*S*	18 ± 5	24% *	>55
3	**(*R*)-15**	Me	*R*	1.2 ± 0.3	1150	958
4	**(*S*)-15**	Me	*S*	8.8 ± 1.1	676	77
5	**(*R*)-16**	Et	*R*	5.0 ± 1.2	954	191
6	**(*S*)-16**	Et	*S*	4.2 ± 0.8	31% *	>235
7	**(*R*)-18**	CH_2CO_2Et	*R*	4.0 ± 0.8	552	138
8	**(*S*)-18**	CH_2CO_2Et	*S*	114	12% *	>5
9	**(*R*)-19**	CH_2CH_2OH	*R*	55 ± 1.0	0% *	>15
10	**(*S*)-19**	CH_2CH_2OH	*S*	64 ± 0.9	0% *	>15
11	**(*R*)-20**	CH_2CH_2F	*R*	4.7 ± 0.7	14% *	>210
12	**(*S*)-20**	CH_2CH_2F	*S*	5.9 ± 2.9	10% *	>170
13		(+)-Pentazocine		5.7 ± 2.2	--	--
14		Haloperidol		6.3 ± 1.6	78 ± 2.3	12

* Inhibition of radioligand binding at a concentration of 1 μM.

As previously reported for other spirocyclic σ_1 receptor ligands [28], the hydroxy moiety of **(*R*)-11** acting as H-bond donor is unfavorable in terms of high σ_1 receptor affinity (K_i = 5.2 nM). Methylation of the OH group led to increased σ_1 affinity. The methyl ether **(*R*)-15** (K_i = 1.2 nM) represents the most potent σ_1 receptor ligand of this series of spirocyclic 2-benzopyrans. Larger substituents like an ethyl ((***R***)-**16**) or an ethoxycarbonylethyl group ((***R***)-**18**) reduced the σ_1 affinity slightly, whereas a substituent with a polar OH group in the side chain resulted in 10-fold reduced σ_1 affinity ((***R***)-**19**: $K_i = 55$ nM).

The fluoroethyl derivatives **20** were synthesized having in mind fluorinated PET tracers for labeling of σ_1 receptors in the brain. Due to its similar size the fluorine atom is considered as bioisosteric replacement of a proton, but due its high electronegativity it is also regarded as a bioisostere of an OH moiety. As summarized in Table 1 the ethyl derivative (***R***)**-16** and the fluoroethyl derivative (***R***)**-20** show very similar σ_1 receptor affinity proving the H/F bioisosterism. On the contrary the fluoroethyl derivative (R)-**20** is 10-fold more active than the hydroxyethyl derivative (***R***)**-19** indicating that in this compound class the hydroxy moiety and the fluorine atom cannot be exchanged bioisosterically by each other. The very high σ_1 affinity of the (*R*)-configured fluoroethyl derivative (***R***)**-20** ($K_i = 4.7$ nM), which is slightly higher than the σ_1 affinity of the (*S*)-configured enantiomer (***S***)**-20**, rendered this compound a promising candidate for molecular imaging of σ_1 receptors after labeling with [^{18}F]fluorine.

3.3. Radiosynthesis

For the radiosynthesis of [^{18}F]-(***R***)**-20** (K_i = 4.7 nM) the alcohol (***R***)**-19** was converted into the tosylate precursor (***R***)**-21** upon treatment with *p*-TosCl. (Scheme 3)

Scheme 3. Radiosynthesis of [^{18}F]-(***R***)**-20**.

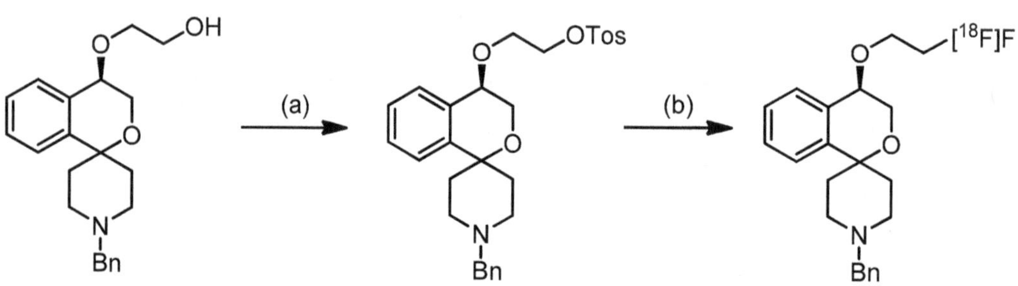

(*R*)-**19** (*R*)-**21** [^{18}F](*R*)-**20**

Reagents and Conditions: **(a)** p-TosCl, NEt_3, 4-DMAP, CH_2Cl_2, RT, overnight, 46%; (***S***)**-21** was obtained in 32% yield starting with (***S***)**-19**. **(b)** K[^{18}F]F, Kryptofix K222, acetonitrile, 82 °C, 20 min.

The one-step introduction of ^{18}F was performed by a S_N2 substitution of the precursor (***R***)**-21** with [^{18}F]fluoride using the K[^{18}F]F-K222-carbonate complex, prepared from a 1:1 mixture of K_2CO_3 and Kryptofix K222. Using this complex, the precursor (***R***)**-21** was readily transformed into the ^{18}F-labeled radiotracer by heating in acetonitrile at 82 °C for 20 min. According to radio-TLC and radio-HPLC analyses, only a few radioactive by-products were formed. Thus, the crude reaction mixture was diluted with water to 4 mL and directly applied to semi-preparative HPLC. The radiotracer eluted at ca. 32 min and was completely free from radioactive and non-radioactive impurities. (Figure 3) Interestingly, a considerable part of ^{18}F activity, mainly from highly polar components remained in the stainless steel loop. Using a PEEK loop in the HPLC device resulted in about 80%–90% elution of [^{18}F]-(***R***)**-20**. Combined isolated fractions were diluted with water (50 mL), adsorbed on a Sep-Pak C18 Plus cartridge and desorbed with pure MeOH in small portions. Adsorption of the total activity

(≥95%) and elution with MeOH (≥95%) were achieved resulting in a total volume of 1.25 to 1.5 mL. The solvent was carefully evaporated at 60 °C, and the final product was dissolved in 0.9% NaCl solution containing 5% EtOH.

Figure 3. Semi-preparative HPLC separation of the crude labelling mixture of [^{18}F]-***(R)*-20**. HPLC chromatogram with radioactivity detection (above) and UV detection (below). The identity of the final radioactive product, [^{18}F]-***(R)*-20**, was validated with stable [^{19}F]-***(R)*-20** as reference.

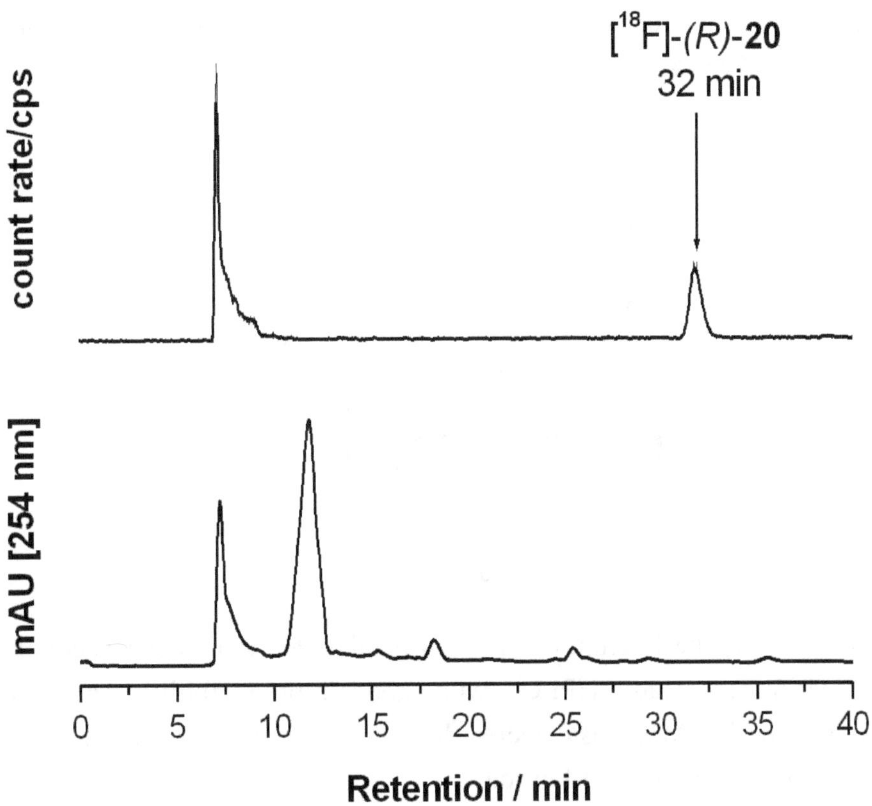

[^{18}F]-***(R)*-20** was obtained with radiochemical yields of 18%–20%, radiochemical purity of ≥97%, and specific activities of about 175–300 GBq/μmol within a total synthesis time of about 2 h.

3.4. In Vitro *Stability and Lipophilicity of* [^{18}F]-***(R)*-20**

According to radio-TLC the radiotracer [^{18}F]-***(R)*-20** proved to be chemically stable in phosphate buffer, Dulbecco buffer and in native mouse plasma over 30 min at 37 °C. No defluorination was observed.

Determination of the distribution coefficient by the shake flask method provided a $\log D_{7.4}$ value of 1.78 ± 0.8. This value is in good accordance with the calculated $\log D_{7.4}$ value of 1.68 (ACD ChemSketch 2012). The $\log D_{7.4}$ value obtained by HPLC method, however, differed by one order of magnitude (2.97±0.32) from these values. The range of the experimentally determined $\log D_{7.4}$ values is very similar to the corresponding $\log D_{7.4}$ values of fluspidine (**2b**, 1.5–1.8), which has been shown to have excellent brain uptake properties.

3.5. Biological Evaluation

3.5.1. Metabolic Stability of [^{18}F]-**(*R*)-20** in Mice

The existence of radiometabolites after injection of the radiotracer [^{18}F]-**(*R*)-20** in mice was analyzed by radio-HPLC and radio-TLC analyses. In Figure 4 HPLC chromatograms of brain, plasma, liver and urine samples are presented in a combined manner.

Figure 4. Stacked analytical radio-HPLC profiles of brain, plasma, liver and urine samples; samples were collected 30 min after injection of the radiotracer [^{18}F]-**(*R*)-20**; t_R of the parent compound *ca.* 42 min.

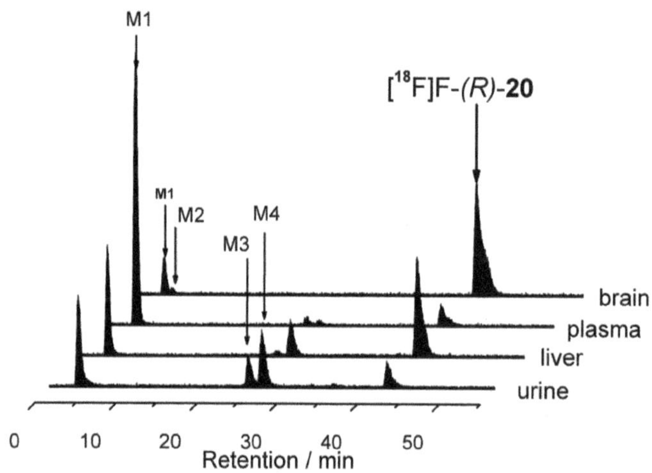

In brain samples (n = 4) the fraction of the non-metabolized radiotracer accounted for 91%–95% (radio-TLC) and 89%–92% (radio-HPLC) with good reproducibility. Only one highly polar (hydrophilic) radiometabolite (M1) was detected. Its retention time (t_R 3.6 min) was similar to but not identical with the retention time of [^{18}F]fluoride.

Analysis of the plasma samples (n = 3) at 30 min p.i. revealed fast biotransformation (15% and 12% of [^{18}F]-**(*R*)-20** remained unchanged as determined by acetonitrile and methanol extraction). Results from radio-HPLC and radio-TLC agreed well. The recovery of total radioactivity was 75% for acetonitrile extraction and up to 90% for methanol extraction. The main radiometabolite in plasma samples was the very polar metabolite M1 (80%–90% of total radioactivity at 30 min p.i.). Additionally, two small peaks for metabolites M2 (t_R ~24.7 min) and M3 t_R ~26.0 min) were detected with an intensity of lower than 3%.

In urine samples (n = 3), a large amount of radiometabolites and a very low amount of the parent radiotracer [^{18}F]-**(*R*)-20** (non-metabolized radiotracer accounting for 2%–20% of total radioactivity) was observed.

The results obtained by analysis of liver homogenates are based on a single experiment and should be treated with caution. About 50% to 56% of the parent radiotracer [^{18}F]-**(*R*)-20** (determined after acetonitrile and methanol extraction, respectively) remained unchanged after 30 min. The recovery of radioactivity was 45% for acetonitrile and 89% for methanol extraction. The same radiometabolite profile as in plasma and urine samples was found.

3.5.2. Comparison of Biotransformation of [^{18}F]-***(R)*-20** with Established PET Tracers [^{18}F]**2b** and [^{18}F]**2c**

With respect to biotransformation the new 2-benzopyran based radiotracer [^{18}F]-***(R)*-20** behaved quite different, when compared with the ^{18}F labelled radiotracers [^{18}F]**2b** and [^{18}F]**2c** with a 2-fluoroethyl or 3-fluoropropyl side chain. After application of all three fluorinated radiotracers radioactive metabolites were not found in the brain. However, in the plasma only 15% of the unchanged tracer [^{18}F]-***(R)*-20** was detected, whereas 89% and 86% of the unchanged parent compounds [^{18}F]**2b** and [^{18}F]**2c** were found in the plasma. Also the amount of parent compound [^{18}F]-***(R)*-20** in liver samples was lower (50%) compared with those of [^{18}F]**2b** (69%) and [^{18}F]**2c** (65%) in liver samples. These results indicate that the 2-benzopyran based radiotracer [^{18}F]-***(R)*-20** with a 2-fluoroethoxy side chain underwent faster biotransformation than the analogous 2-benzofuran based tracers [^{18}F]**2b** and [^{18}F]**2c** with a fluoroethyl or fluoropropyl side chain. The faster metabolic degradation of [^{18}F]-***(R)*-20** could be due to the additional ether in the side chain [49,50]. Nevertheless, as no brain-permeable radiometabolites of the 2-benzopyran-based [^{18}F]-***(R)*-20** were detected, this radiotracer is applicable for brain imaging studies by PET.

3.5.3. *Ex Vivo* Autoradiography Studies

In order to investigate the spatial distribution of [^{18}F]-***(R)*-20** and the specificity of its uptake in the mouse brain, *ex vivo* autoradiography studies were performed under control and blocking conditions. Haloperidol co-application reduced the uptake of radioactivity in the brain at 30 min p.i. by 34% (3.40% ID/g *vs.* 2.24% ID/g under control and blocking conditions, respectively). Although this result indicates target specific binding of [^{18}F]-***(R)*-20**, the corresponding total-to-nonspecific binding ratio of [^{18}F]-***(R)*-20** of 1.5 at 30 min p.i. is lower than previously reported ratios of approx. 3 at 30 min after injection of [^{18}F]fluspidine (**2b**) [29] or the corresponding ^{18}F-labeled fluorobutyl-radiotracer **2d** [29]. This may be attributed to the lower σ_1 affinity of [^{18}F]-***(R)*-20** (K_i = 4.7 nM) compared to fluspidine (**2b**) (K_i = 0.59 nM) and the fluorobutyl derivative **2d** (K_i = 1.2 nM).

Binding of the radiotracer [^{18}F]-***(R)*-20** in the mouse brain, shown in Figure 5A, corresponds to binding of [^{18}F]fluspidine [29] and [^{3}H]1,3-di(2-tolyl)guanidine [7]. Under control conditions, the highest uptake of [^{18}F]-***(R)*-20** was detected in the whole brainstem (most prominent in the facial nucleus) and the pons (pontine reticular nucleus). High to moderate uptake was noted in midbrain, cortex, hippocampus, cerebellum and layers of the olfactory bulb. Low uptake was found in parts of the olfactory bulb, striatum and basal forebrain. 2D densitometric evaluation of whole brain sections confirmed the general blocking effect of haloperidol with a mean decrease of radiotracer uptake in the slices of the whole brain hemisphere of about 40%. (Figure 5B) This effect corresponds to the 34% decrease of uptake reflected by the %ID/g values reported above.

Brain autoradiographs also revealed that regions with high radioligand binding (e.g., pontine nuclei, facial nucleus) showed residual binding (Figure 5B) after co-administration of haloperidol.

Figure 5. *Ex vivo* brain autoradiographs under control (**A**) and blockade (**B**) conditions. Anatomical reference (Mouse Atlas, Paxinos & Franklin) is shown in C. Numbers indicate the following major brain regions: 1, Cerebral cortex; 2, Olfactory bulb; 3, Cerebellum; 4, Basal forebrain; 5, Midbrain; 6, Hypothalamus; 7, Pons; 8, Brainstem.

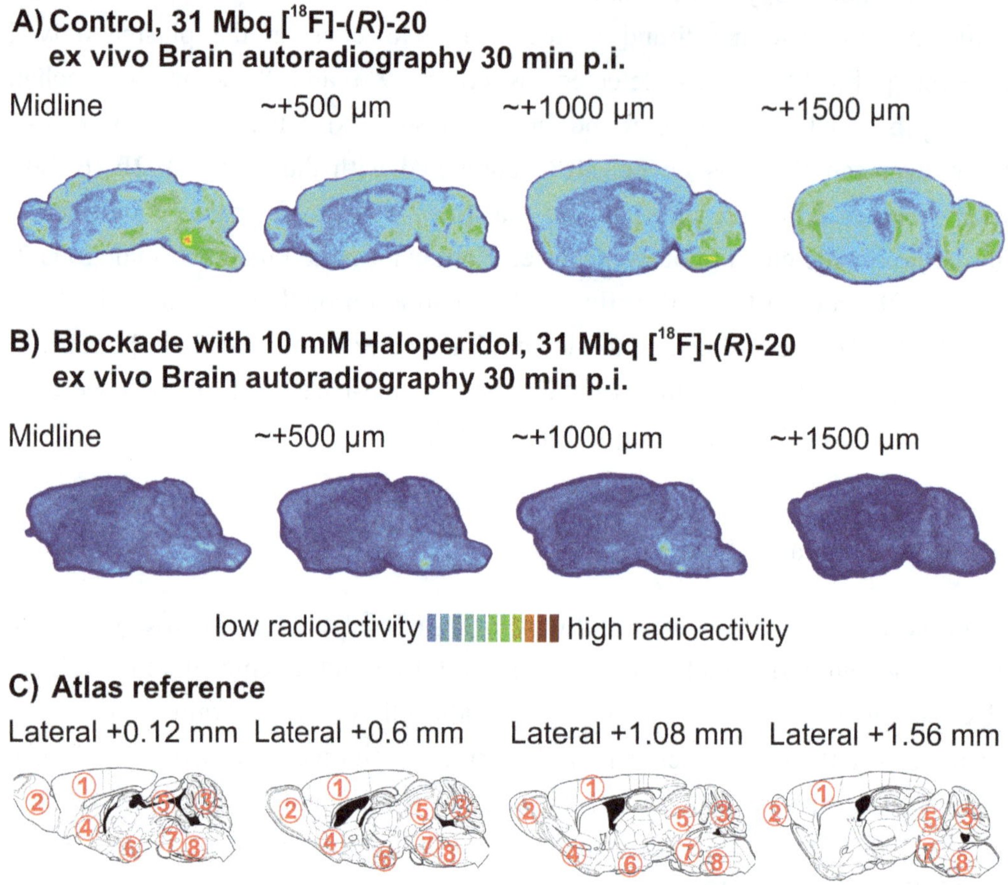

4. Conclusions

In this manuscript the asymmetric synthesis of spirocyclic 2-benzopyrans in enantiomerically pure form is described for the first time. The key step of the synthesis is the asymmetric dihydroxylation according to Sharpless, which allows the preparation of 4-substituted spirocyclic 2-benzopyrans. These compounds represent a new type of potent and subtype selective σ_1 receptor ligands. Some of the compounds show an eudismic ratio up to 29 (ester 18), indicating an enantioselective interaction of the σ_1 receptor with these ligands. The very potent fluorinated fluoroethoxy derivative **(*R*)-20** was developed as fluorinated PET-tracer. The radiosynthesis based on a one-step nucleophilic substitution of tosylate **(*R*)-21** provided the PET tracer $[^{18}F]$-**(*R*)-20** in 18%–20% radiochemical yield. Whereas radiometabolites of $[^{18}F]$-**(*R*)-20** were not found in the brain, plasma, liver and urine samples showed a large amount of radiometabolites. Obviously the 2-benzopyran derivative $[^{18}F]$-**(*R*)-20** with a fluoroethoxy side chain is faster metabolized than the corresponding benzofuran-based radiotracers $[^{18}F]$**2b** and $[^{18}F]$**2c** with fluoroethyl or fluoropropyl side chains. In *ex vivo* autoradiography experiments brain regions with high σ_1 receptor expression are labeled selectively. Altogether, $[^{18}F]$-**(*R*)-20** represents a very good alternative fluorinated PET tracer for imaging of σ_1 receptors in the brain.

Acknowledgments

This work was funded by the *Deutsche Forschungsgemeinschaft*, which is gratefully acknowledged.

References

1. Martin, W.R.; Eades, C.G.; Thompson, J.A.; Huppler, R.E.; Gilbert, P.E. The effects of morphine- and nalorphine-likedrugs in the nondependent and morphine-dependent chronic spinal dog. *J. Pharmacol. Exp. Ther.* **1976**, *197*, 517–532.
2. Hellewell, S.B.; Bowen, W.D. A sigma-like binding site in rat pheochromocytoma (PC12) cells: Decreased affinity for (+)-benzomorphans and lower molecular weight suggest a different sigma receptor form from that of guinea pig brain. *Brain Res.* **1990**, *527*, 244–253.
3. Hanner, M.; Moebius, F.F.; Flandorfer, A.; Knaus, H.; Striessnig, J.; Kempner, E.; Glossman, H. Purification, molecular cloning, and expression of the mammalian sigma1-binding site. *PNAS* **1996**, *93*, 8072–8077.
4. Kekuda, R.; Prasad, P.D.; Fei, Y.; Leibach, F.H.; Ganapathy, V. Cloning and functional expression of the human type 1 sigma receptor (hSigmaR1). *Biochem. Biophys. Res. Commun.* **1996**, *229*, 553–558.
5. Aydar, E.; Palmer, C.P.; Klyachko, V.A.; Jackson, M.B. The sigma receptor as a ligand-regulated auxiliary potassium channel subunit. *Neuron* **2002**, *34*, 399–410.
6. Laurini, E.; Dal, C.; Mamolo, M.G.; Zampieri, D.; Posocco, P.; Fermeglia, M.; Vio, L.; Pricl, S. Homology model and docking-based virtual screening for ligands of the sigma1 receptor. *ACS Med. Chem. Lett.* **2011**, *2*, 834–839.
7. Bouchard, P.; Quirion, R. [^{3}H]1,3-Di(2-tolyl)guanidine and [^{3}H](+)pentazocine binding sites in the rat brain: Autoradiographic visualization of the putative sigma1, and sigma2 receptor subtypes. *Neuroscience* **1997**, *76*, 467–477.
8. Hellewell, S.B.; Bruce, A.; Feinstein, G.; Orringer, J.; Williams, W.; Bowen, W.D. Rat liver and kidney contain high densities of sigma 1 and sigma 2 receptors: Characterization by ligand binding and photoaffinity labeling. *Eur. J. Pharmacol.* **1994**, *268*, 9–18.
9. Ela, C.; Barg, J.; Vogel, Z.; Hasin, Y.; Eilam, Y. Sigma receptor ligands modulate contractility, Ca^{2+} influx and beating rate in cultured cardiac myocytes. *J. Pharmacol. Exp. Ther.* **1994**, *269*, 1300–1309.
10. Su, T.P.; London, E.D.; Jaffe, J.H. Steroid binding at sigma receptors suggests a link between endocrine, nervous, and immune systems. *Science* **1988**, *240*, 219–221.
11. Monnet, F.P.; Mahe, V.; Robel, P.; Baulieu, E. Neurosteroids, via sigma receptors, modulate the [^{3}H]norepinephrine release evoked by N-methyl-D-aspartate in the rat hippocampus. *Proc. Natl. Acad. Sci. USA* **1995**, *92*, 3774–3778.

12. Martina, M.; Turcotte, M.B.; Halman, S.; Bergeron, R. The sigma-1 receptor modulates NMDA receptor synaptic transmission and plasticity via SK channels in rat hippocampus. *J. Physiol.* **2007**, *578*, 143–157.
13. Hayashi, T.; Maurice, T.; Su, T. Ca^{2+} signaling via sigma1-receptors: novel regulatory mechanism affecting intracellular Ca^{2+} concentration. *J. Pharmacol. Exp. Ther.* **2000**, *293*, 788–798.
14. Bergeron, R.; Debonnel, G.; de Montigny, C. Modification of the N-methyl-D-aspartate response by antidepressant sigma receptor ligands. *Eur. J. Pharmacol.* **1993**, *240*, 319–323.
15. Bermack, J.E.; Debonnel, G. Modulation of serotonergic neurotransmission by short- and long-term treatments with sigma ligands. *Br. J. Pharmacol.* **2001**, *134*, 691–699.
16. Hayashi, T.; Su, T. Sigma-1 receptor chaperones at the ER-mitochondrion interface regulate Ca^{2+} signaling and cell survival. *Cell* **2007**, *131*, 596–610.
17. Maurice, T.; Su, T.P.; Privat, A. Sigma1 (sigma 1) receptor agonists and neurosteroids attenuate B25–35-amyloid peptide-induced amnesia in mice through a common mechanism. *Neuroscience* **1998**, *83*, 413–428.
18. De la Puente, B.; Nadal, X.; Portillo-Salido, E.; Sanchez-Arroyos, R.; Ovalle, S.; Palacios, G.; Muro, A.; Romero, L.; Entrena, J.M.; Baeyens, J.M.; *et al.* Sigma-1 receptors regulate activity-induced spinal sensitization and neuropathic pain after peripheral nerve injury. *Pain* **2009**, *145*, 294–303.
19. Weissman, A.D.; Casanova, M.F.; Kleinman, J.E.; London, E.D.; de Souza, E.B. Selective loss of cerebral cortical sigma, but not PCP binding sites in schizophrenia. *Biol. Psychiatry* **1991**, *29*, 41–54.
20. Hayashi, T.; Su, T. Sigma-1 receptor ligands: Potential in the treatment of neuropsychiatric disorders. *CNS Drugs* **2004**, *18*, 269–284.
21. Matsuno, K.; Kobayashi, T.; Tanaka, M.K.; Mita, S. Sigma1 receptor subtype is involved in the relief of behavioral despair in the mouse forced swimming test. *Eur. J. Pharmacol.* **1996**, *312*, 267–271.
22. Bermack, J.E.; Debonnel, G. The role of sigma receptors in depression. *J. Pharmacol. Sci.* **2005**, *97*, 317–336.
23. Waterhouse, R.N.; Lee Collier, T. *In vivo* Evaluation of [^{18}F]1-(3-fluoropropyl)-4-(4-cyanophenoxymethyl)piperidine: A selective sigma-1 receptor radioligand for PET. *Nucl. Med. Biol.* **1997**, *24*, 127–134.
24. Ishiwata, K.; Ishii, K.; Kimura, Y.; Kawamura, K.; Oda, K.; Sasaki, T.; Sakata, M.; Senda, M. Successive positron emission tomography measurement of cerebral blood flow and neuroreceptors in the human brain: An 11C-SA4503 Study. *Ann. Nucl. Med.* **2008**, *22*, 411–416.
25. Elsinga, P.H.; Kawamura, K.; Kobayashi, T.; Tsukada, H.; Senda, M.; Vaalburg, W.; Ishiwata, K. Synthesis and evaluation of [^{18}F]fluoroethyl SA4503 as a PET ligand for the sigma receptor. *Synapse* **2002**, *43*, 259–267.
26. Brust, P.; Deuther-Conrad, W.; Lehmkuhl, K.; Jia, H.; Wünsch, B. Molecular imaging of σ_1 receptors *in vivo*: Current status and perspectives. *Curr. Med. Chem.* **2014**, *21*, 35–69.
27. Maisonial, A.; Große Maestrup, E.; Wiese, C.; Hiller, A.; Schepmann, D.; Fischer, S.; Deuther-Conrad, W.; Steinbach, J.; Brust, P.; Wünsch, B. Synthesis, radiofluorination and pharmacological evaluation of a fluoromethyl spirocyclic PET tracer for central sigma 1 receptors and comparison with fluoroalkyl homologs. *Bioorg. Med. Chem.* **2012**, *20*, 257–269.

28. Große Maestrup, E.; Wiese, C.; Schepmann, D.; Brust, P.; Wünsch, B. Synthesis, pharmacological activity and structure affinity relationships of spirocyclic sigma 1 receptor ligands with a (2-fluoroethyl) residue in 3-position. *Bioorg. Med. Chem.* **2011**, *19*, 393–405.
29. Fischer, S.; Wiese, C.; Große Maestrup, E.; Hiller, A.; Deuther-Conrad, W.; Scheunemann, M.; Schepmann, D.; Steinbach, J.; Wünsch, B.; Brust, P. Molecular imaging of sigma receptors: Synthesis and evaluation of the potent sigma 1 selective radioligand [^{18}F]fluspidine. *Eur. J. Nucl. Med. Mol. Imaging* **2011**, *38*, 540–551.
30. Große Maestrup, E.; Fischer, S.; Wiese, C.; Schepmann, D.; Hiller, A.; Deuther-Conrad, W.; Steinbach, J.; Wünsch, B.; Brust, P. Evaluation of spirocyclic 3-(3-fluoropropyl)-2-benzofurans as sigma 1 receptor ligands for neuroimaging with positron emission tomography. *J. Med. Chem.* **2009**, *52*, 6062–6072.
31. Maisonial, A.; Maestrup, E.G.; Fischer, S.; Hiller, A.; Scheunemann, M.; Wiese, C.; Schepmann, D.; Steinbach, J.; Deuther-Conrad, W.; Wünsch, B.; *et al.* A ^{18}F-labeled fluorobutyl-substituted spirocyclic piperidine derivative as a selective radioligand for PET imaging of sigma receptors. *Chem. Med. Chem.* **2011**, *6*, 1401–1410.
32. Wiese, C.; Große Maestrup, E.G.; Schepmann, D.; Grimme, S.; Humpf, H.; Brust, P.; Wünsch, B. Enantioselective sigma 1 receptor binding and biotransformation of the spirocyclic PET tracer 1′-benzyl-3-(3-fluoropropyl)-3H-spiro[[2]benzofuran-1,4′-piperidine]. *Chirality* **2011**, *23*, 148–154.
33. Holl, K.; Schepmann, D.; Daniliuc, C.G.; Wünsch, B. Sharpless asymmetric dihydroxylation as key step in the enantioselective synthesis of spirocyclic σ_1 receptor ligands. *Tetrahedron Asymmetry* **2014**, in press.
34. Holl, K.; Falck, E.; Köhler, J.; Schepmann, D.; Humpf, H.-U.; Brust, P.; Wünsch, B. Synthesis, characterization and metabolism studies of fluspidine enantiomers. *Chem. Med. Chem.* **2013**, *8*, 2047–2056.
35. Maier, C.A.; Wünsch, B. Novel spiropiperidines as highly potent and subtype selective sigma-receptor ligands. Part 1. *J. Med. Chem.* **2002**, *45*, 438–448.
36. Maier, C.A.; Wünsch, B. Novel sigma receptor ligands. Part 2. SAR of spiro[[2]benzopyran-1,4′-piperidines] and spiro[[2]benzofuran-1,4′-piperidines] with carbon substituents in position 3. *J. Med. Chem.* **2002**, *45*, 4923–4930.
37. Meyer, C.; Neue, B.; Schepmann, D.; Yanagisawa, S.; Yamaguchi, J.; Würthwein, E.-U.; Itami, K.; Wünsch, B. Improvement of σ_1 receptor affinity by late-stage C-H-bond arylation of spirocyclic lactones. *Bioorg. Med. Chem.* **2013**, *21*, 1844–1856.
38. Bradford, M.M. A rapid and sensitive method for the quantitation of microgram quantities of protein utilizing the principle of protein-dye binding. *Anal. Biochem.* **1976**, *72*, 248–254.
39. Stoscheck, C.M. Quantitation of protein. *Methods Enzymol.* **1990**, *182*, 50–68.
40. Cheng, Y.C.; Prusoff, W.H. Relationship between the inhibition constant (K_i) and the concentration of inhibitor which causes 50 per cent inhibition (IC_{50}) of an enzymatic reaction. *Biochem. Pharmacol.* **1973**, *22*, 3099–3108.
41. De-Haven-Hudkins, D.L.; Fleissner, L.C.; Ford-Rice, F.Y. Characterization of the binding of [^{3}H]-(+)-pentazocine to σ recognition sites in guinea pig brain. *Eur. J. Pharmacol. Mol. Pharmacol. Sect.* **1992**, *227*, 371–378.

42. Mach, H.; Smith, C.R.; Childers, S.R. Ibogaine possesses a selective affinity for σ_2 receptors. *Life Sci.* **1995**, *57*, 57–62.
43. OECD (2004). Test No. 117: Partition coefficient (n-octanol/water), HPLC method, OECD Guidelines for the Testing of Chemicals. Available online: http://www.oecd-ilibrary.org/environment/test-no-117-partition-coefficient-n-octanol-water-hplc-method_9789264069824-en;jsessionid=161rftmwk152z.x-oecd-live-01 (accessed on 21 January 2014).
44. Musachio, J.L; Scheffel, U.; Stathis, M.; Ravert, H.T.; Mathews, W.B.; Dannals, R.F. (+)-[C-11]-cis-N-benzyl-normetazocine: A selective ligand for sigma receptors *in vivo*. *Life Sci.* **1994**, *55*, 225–232.
45. Jacobsen, E.N.; Marko, I.; Mungall, W.S.; Schroeder, G.; Sharpless, K.B. Asymmetric dihydroxylation via ligand-accelerated catalysis. *J. Am. Chem. Soc.* **1988**, *110*, 1968–1970.
46. Kolb, H.C.; VanNieuwenhze, M.S.; Sharpless, K.B. Catalytic asymmetric dihydroxylation. *Chem. Rev.* **1994**, *94*, 2483–2547.
47. Katsuki, T. *Asymmetric Oxidation Reactions*; Oxford University Press: Oxford, UK, 2001.
48. Martinelli, M.J.; Vaidyanathan, R.; Pawlak, J.M.; Nayyar, N.K.; Dhokte, U.P.; Doecke, C.W.; Zollars, L.M.H.; Moher, E.D.; van Khau, V.; Kosmrlj, B. Catalytic regioselective sulfonylation of alpha-chelatable alcohols: Scope and mechanistic insight. *J. Am. Chem. Soc.* **2002**, *124*, 3578–3585.
49. Damont, A.; Sik-chung, A.C.; Medrán-Navarette, V.; Kuhnast, B.; Gaudy, H.; Dollé, F. Synthesis and fluorine-18 labelling of a novel pyrazolo[1,5*a*]pyrimidineacetamide, CfO-DPA-714, a compound devoid of the metabolically unstable fluoroalkoxy moiety. *J. Labelled Compd. Radiopharm.* **2011**, *54*, S461.
50. Peyronneau, M.; Damont, A.; Valette, H.; Saba, W.; Delforge, J.; Goutal, S.; Bougeois, S.; Hinnen, F.; Dollé, F.; Bottlaender, M. Metabolism of DPA-714, a new peripheral benzodiazepine receptor PET ligand. *J. Labelled Compd. Radiopharm.* **2009**, *52*, S385.

9

Novel Preclinical and Radiopharmaceutical Aspects of [^{68}Ga]Ga-PSMA-HBED-CC: A New PET Tracer for Imaging of Prostate Cancer

Matthias Eder [1,2,†,*], Oliver Neels [1,2,†], Miriam Müller [1], Ulrike Bauder-Wüst [1], Yvonne Remde [1], Martin Schäfer [1], Ute Hennrich [1,2], Michael Eisenhut [1], Ali Afshar-Oromieh [3], Uwe Haberkorn [3] and Klaus Kopka [1,2]

1 German Cancer Research Center (dkfz), Division of Radiopharmaceutical Chemistry, Im Neuenheimer Feld 280, Heidelberg 69120, Germany; E-Mails: o.neels@dkfz.de (O.N.); miriam.mueller@wak-gmbh.de (M.M.); u.bauder-wuest@dkfz.de (U.B.-W.); y.remde@dkfz.de (Y.R.); martin.schaefer@dkfz.de (M.S.); u.hennrich@dkfz.de (U.He.); m.eisenhut@dkfz.de (M.E.); k.kopka@dkfz.de (K.K.)

2 German Cancer Consortium (DKTK), Im Neuenheimer Feld 280, Heidelberg 69120, Germany

3 Department of Nuclear Medicine, University of Heidelberg, Im Neuenheimer Feld 400, Heidelberg 69120, Germany; E-Mails: Ali.Afshar@med.uni-heidelberg.de (A.A.-O.); Uwe.Haberkorn@med.uni-heidelberg.de (U.Ha.)

† The authors contributed equally to this work.

* Author to whom correspondence should be addressed; E-Mail: m.eder@dkfz.de

---

Abstract: The detection of prostate cancer lesions by PET imaging of the prostate-specific membrane antigen (PSMA) has gained highest clinical impact during the last years. ^{68}Ga-labelled Glu-urea-Lys(Ahx)-HBED-CC ([^{68}Ga]Ga-PSMA-HBED-CC) represents a successful novel PSMA inhibitor radiotracer which has recently demonstrated its suitability in individual first-in-man studies. The radiometal chelator HBED-CC used in this molecule represents a rather rarely used acyclic complexing agent with chemical characteristics favourably influencing the biological functionality of the PSMA inhibitor. The simple replacement of HBED-CC by the prominent radiometal chelator DOTA was shown to dramatically reduce the *in vivo* imaging quality of the respective ^{68}Ga-labelled PSMA-targeted tracer proving that HBED-CC contributes intrinsically to the PSMA binding of the

Glu-urea-Lys(Ahx) pharmacophore. Owing to the obvious growing clinical impact, this work aims to reflect the properties of HBED-CC as acyclic radiometal chelator and presents novel preclinical data and relevant aspects of the radiopharmaceutical production process of [^{68}Ga]Ga-PSMA-HBED-CC.

Keywords: ^{68}Ga-PET imaging; PSMA; HBED-CC; prostate cancer; radiopharmaceutical production; good manufacturing practice; GMP

---

1. Introduction

Early detection of metastases or recurrent prostate cancer (PC) lesions is of utmost clinical relevance in terms of clinical staging, prognosis and therapy management [1,2]. The high clinical impact of targeting the prostate-specific membrane antigen (PSMA) was recently demonstrated in a series of first-in-man examinations with either ^{68}Ga- [3–5] or ^{123}I-labelled [6] PSMA inhibitors. PSMA is a membrane-type zinc protease, also called glutamate carboxypeptidase II (GCPII), which is expressed by nearly all prostate cancers. Enhanced expression levels were found in poorly differentiated, metastatic and hormone-refractory carcinomas [7,8]. Since urea-based inhibitors of PSMA clear rapidly from the circulation and since only low levels of physiological PSMA expression were detected in a few organs like the brain, kidney, salivary gland and small intestine [7,9–11] PSMA represents an ideal biological target for high quality PET imaging of prostate cancer [12–17].

Initial clinical experiences with the ^{68}Ga-labelled PET tracer Glu-NH-CO-NH-Lys-(Ahx)-[[^{68}Ga]Ga(HBED-CC)] ([^{68}Ga]Ga-PSMA-HBED-CC) suggest that this novel tracer detects PC relapses and metastases with higher contrast as compared to ^{18}F-choline. In a retrospective study, the images of 37 patients who received both ^{18}F-choline PET/CT and ^{68}Ga-PSMA PET/CT were analyzed [3]. Especially at low PSA values, PET/CT images obtained with [^{68}Ga]Ga-PSMA-HBED-CC showed more PC lesions as compared to ^{18}F-choline. It was concluded that [^{68}Ga]Ga-PSMA-HBED-CC represents an attractive new imaging agent for the detection of recurrent prostate cancer and metastatic spread.

The chelator HBED-CC (*N,N'*-bis-[2-hydroxy-5-(carboxyethyl)benzyl]ethylenediamine-*N,N'*-diacetic acid), represents a hitherto rarely used acyclic complexing agent especially allowing efficient radiolabelling with ^{68}Ga even at ambient temperature [18,19]. By combining HBED-CC with the PSMA inhibitor Glu-urea-Lys, a favourable aromatic part is introduced into the radiotracer which was found to be a necessary requirement for a sustainable interaction with the PSMA receptor, putatively with the accessory hydrophobic pocket of the PSMA S1 binding site [15,20,21]. We have indeed shown in a preclinical study that the replacement of HBED-CC by DOTA (1,4,7,10-tetraazacyclododecane-*N,N',N'',N'''*-tetraacetic acid) resulted in a molecule not able to image the tumour at all [20]. Moreover, besides these biological advantages, HBED-CC represents a highly effective chelator. Extraordinary high thermodynamic stability constants of $>10^{39}$ were determined for the complexation of Ga with HBED [22]. As mentioned before the structure is acyclic and demands rather low energy for complex formation which allows fast labelling at ambient temperature [19,20]. Moreover, a high kinetic stability of the Ga-HBED-CC complex at physiological pH was reported [23] resulting in a stable complex *in vivo* [24] and in human serum for at least 72 h [25]. Thus, HBED-CC represents a highly attractive radiogallium chelator for high-stability labelling of radiopharmaceuticals. However, in contrast to other clinically well-established radiometal chelators, HBED-CC forms three NMR-distinguishable diastereomers (RR, RS and SS configurations at the amine nitrogens) during gallium complexation, whereas presumably the RR configuration is thermodynamically favoured [24]. Besides the influence of the temperature the formation of the diastereomers was reported to be pH- and concentration-dependent as well [23]. In a standard labelling protocol, [^{68}Ga]Ga-PSMA-HBED-CC is incubated at a pH of ~4 and heated at 95 °C. The thermodynamically favoured diastereomer is formed; however, a small fraction of one of the other two diastereomers is still present in the labelling reaction and would be part of the final formulation prepared for the patient. Thus, it is of utmost importance to analyze the two major diastereomers according to their biological activity in cell-based assays. The aim of this study is to summarize hitherto existing radiochemical experiences with HBED-CC conjugated low-molecular weight compounds and to confirm that the configuration of Ga-HBED-CC does not influence the cell binding properties of the resulting PSMA-targeted radioligand [^{68}Ga]Ga-PSMA-HBED-CC, especially since the chelator has high impact on the interaction with the aforementioned accessory hydrophobic pocket of PSMA. Owing to the high and growing clinical impact, this work aims to present novel important preclinical data of [^{68}Ga]Ga-PSMA-HBED-CC and relevant aspects of its radiopharmaceutical production. The fully automated radiosynthesis as well as the essential quality control parameters according to current EU-GMP regulations for radiopharmaceuticals are given.

2. Experimental Section

2.1. Reagents and Chemical Syntheses

The chemicals were of analytical grade and were used without further purification. Analysis of the synthesised molecules was performed using reversed-phase high performance liquid chromatography (RP-HPLC; Chromolith RP-18e, 100 mm × 4.6 mm; Merck, Darmstadt, Germany) with a linear A–B gradient (0% B to 100% B in 6 min) at a flow rate of 4 mL/min (analysis) or 6 mL/min (purification). Solvent A consisted of 0.1% aqueous trifluoroacetic acid (TFA) and solvent B was 0.1% TFA in acetonitrile. The HPLC system (L6200 A; Merck-Hitachi, Darmstadt, Germany) was equipped with a UV and a gamma detector (Bioscan, Washington, DC, USA). UV absorbance was measured at 214 nm and 254 nm. Mass spectrometry was performed with a MALDI-MS Daltonics Microflex system (Bruker Daltonics, Bremen, Germany). The ^{nat}Ga-labelled reference Glu-urea-Lys(Ahx)-[Ga(HBED-CC)] (DKFZ-GaPSMA-11) was purchased from ABX Advanced Biochemical Compounds (Radeberg, Germany) and dissolved in 40 µL CH_3CN/H_2O (1:1). 2.6 µg were characterised at RT by mass spectrometry using an Agilent 1200 HPLC-MS system connected to an Orbitrap Mass Spectrometer (Exactive, Thermo Fisher Scientific) on a Hypersil Gold C18 column (2.1 mm × 200 mm, 1.9 µm; Thermo Scientific, Bremen, Germany) eluted with a linear gradient (eluent A: 0.05% TFA in water; eluent B: 0.05% TFA in acetonitrile; 0%–30% B in 30 min at RT, flow rate: 0.2 mL/min, absorbance: λ = 214 nm). Full scan single mass spectra (positive mode) were obtained by scanning from m/z = 200–4000.

The peptide c(RGDyK) was synthesised as described previously [26]. HBED-CC was conjugated by reacting with 1.2 equivalents of HBED-CC-TFP-ester which was synthesised as previously described [19]. The reaction mixture was supplemented with two equivalents of DIPEA in *N,N*-dimethylformamide (DMF). After HPLC purification (vide supra) the product was treated with TFA at room temperature for one hour resulting in the final compound. NOTA (1,4,7-triazacyclononane-1,4,7-triacetic acid) conjugation was carried out by reacting the peptide with 3 equivalents of SCN-Bn-NOTA (purchased from Macrocyclics, Dallas, TX, USA) in 0.1 M sodium carbonate buffer (pH 9.5) for 20 h at room temperature. The reaction mixture was purified by semipreparative HPLC. Mass spectrometry was used to confirm the identity of the synthesised compounds (m/z (NOTA-c(RGDyK) = 1071.3 (calc. for $[M+H]^+$ = 1071.2); m/z (HBED-CC-c(RGDyK) = 1035.2 (calc. for $[M+H]^+$ = 1035.2)).

2.2. Preclinical Radiolabelling and Radiochemical Stability

2.2.1. ^{68}Ga-Radiolabelling

^{68}Ga (half-life 68 min; β^+ 89%; $E_{\beta+}$ max. 1.9 MeV) was obtained from a ^{68}Ge/^{68}Ga-generator based on a pyrogallol resin support [27]. For radiolabelling, the conjugates (0.1–1 nmol in 0.1 M HEPES buffer, pH = 7.5, 100 µL) were added to a mixture of 10 µL HEPES (2.1 M in H_2O) and 40 µL [^{68}Ga]Ga^{3+} eluate. The pH of the labelling solution was adjusted using NaOH. The reaction mixture was incubated at room temperature or 95 °C, respectively. The radiochemical yield (RCY) was determined via analytical RP-HPLC and thin layer chromatography (ITLC, Pall, Crailsheim, Germany) with a mixture of 0.9% NaCl and methanol (5:1) as solvent. Free activity was complexed by supplementing with 10 µL 0.1 M EDTA. In case of non-conjugated chelators, 0.9% NaCl was used as solvent.

2.2.2. *^{nat}Ga-Complexes*

A 10 times molar excess of Ga(III)-nitrate (Sigma Aldrich, Munich, Germany) in 10 µL 0.1 N HCl was reacted with the conjugates (1 mM in 0.1 M HEPES buffer pH 7.5, 40 µL) in a mixture of 10 µL 2.1 M HEPES solution and 2 µL 1 N HCl for 2 min at room temperature or 95 °C, respectively.

2.2.3. Radiochemical Stability

The radiochemical stability of the ^{68}Ga-labelled compounds was determined by incubating in both phosphate buffered saline (PBS) and human serum at 37 °C. An equal volume of acetonitrile was added to the samples to precipitate serum proteins. Subsequently, the samples were centrifuged for 5 min at 13,000 rpm (Heraeus Picofuge fresco, Thermo Fisher Scientific Germany, Schwerte, Germany). An aliquot of the supernatant and the PBS sample was analysed by RP-HPLC. In addition, serum samples were run on a Superdex 75 5/150 GL gel filtration column (GE Healthcare, Munich, Germany) in order to analyse protein binding. To investigate the complex stability against human transferrin, a 400 µL aliquot of the ^{68}Ga-labelled peptide was added to 250 µg apo-transferrin and incubated at 37 °C in PBS at pH 7. The complex stability was determined using a Superdex 75 GL 5/150 short column with PBS (pH 7) as eluent.

2.3. In Vitro Testing

2.3.1. Cell Culture

LNCaP cells (metastatic lesion of human prostatic adenocarcinoma, ATCC CRL-1740) were cultured in RPMI medium supplemented with 10% fetal calf serum and Glutamax (PAA, Pasching, Austria). The cells were grown at 37 °C in an incubator with humidified air equilibrated with 5 % CO_2. The cells were harvested using trypsin-ethylenediaminetetraacetic acid (trypsin-EDTA; 0.25% trypsin, 0.02% EDTA, all from PAA, Austria) and washed with PBS.

2.3.2. Cell Binding and Internalisation

The competitive cell binding assay and internalisation experiments were performed as described previously [20]. Briefly, LNCaP cells (10^5 per well) were incubated with the radioligand [^{68}Ga]Ga-PSMA-HBED-CC in the presence of 12 different concentrations of analyte (0–5000 nM, 100 µL/well, ^{nat}Ga-labelled Glu-urea-Lys(Ahx)-HBED-CC prepared either by reaction at room temperature (RT) or by reaction at 95 °C). After incubation, washing was performed using a multiscreen vacuum manifold from Millipore (Billerica, MA, USA). Cell-bound radioactivity was determined using a gamma counter (Packard Cobra II, GMI, Ramsey, MN, USA). The 50% inhibitory concentration (IC_{50}) was calculated using a nonlinear regression algorithm (GraphPad Software, version 5.01, La Jolla, CA, USA). Experiments were performed in triplicate.

The specific cell uptake and internalisation was determined in another cell-based assay. Briefly, 10^5 cells per well were seeded in poly-L-lysine coated 24-well cell culture plates 24 h before incubation. After washing, the cells were incubated with 25 nM of the radiolabelled compounds (either labelled at RT or 95 °C) for 45 min at 37 °C and at 4°C, respectively. Specific cellular uptake was determined by competitive blocking with the PSMA inhibitor 2-(phosphonomethyl)pentanedioic acid (500 µM final concentration, 2-PMPA, Axxora, Loerrach, Germany). Cellular uptake was terminated by washing 4 times with 1 mL of ice-cold PBS. Cells were subsequently incubated twice with 0.5 mL glycine-HCl in PBS (50 mM, pH = 2.8) for 5 min to remove the surface-bound fraction. The cells were washed with 1 mL of ice-cold PBS and lysed using 0.5 mL 0.3 N NaOH. The radioactivity of the probes was measured in a gamma counter. The cell uptake was calculated as per cent of the initially added radioactivity bound to 10^6 cells [%IA/10^6 cells].

2.4. Automated Synthesis

A fully automated synthesis module (Scintomics GRP, Fürstenfeldbruck, Germany) and its ControlCenter and GRP-Interface software were used to transfer the radiosynthesis of [^{68}Ga]Ga-PSMA-HBED-CC into an environment suitable for clinical application. The ^{68}Ge/^{68}Ga-generator used for radiopharmaceutical production was purchased from IDB-Holland BV (Baarle-Nassau, The Netherlands). Disposable cassette kits and chemicals including the precursor PSMA-HBED-CC (DKFZ-PSMA-11) in GMP-compliant grade used for the radiosynthesis were obtained from ABX advanced biochemical compounds. A Dionex Ultimate 3000 HPLC system (Thermo Fisher Scientific, Dreieich, Germany) equipped with a Chromolith Performance RP-18e column (100 mm × 4.6 mm,

Merck) and a NaI radiodetector (Raytest, Straubenhardt, Germany) was used to determine the radiochemical purity. The mobile phase consisted of gradient mixtures of acetonitrile (A) and 0.1% aqueous TFA (B); 0–0.5 min: 95% B; 0.5 to 10 min linear gradient to 80% A; flow rate 2 mL/min. Residual solvents were determined using a 6850 Series gas chromatograph (Agilent Technologies, Böblingen, Germany). Bacterial endotoxin testing was performed using the LAL test with an Endosafe®-PTS device (Charles River Laboratories, Wilmington, DE, USA). The radionuclide was identified by determination of the half-life (67.9 min) using a CRC-15R dose calibrator (Capintec, Ramsey, NJ, USA). Radionuclidic purity of the final product solution and separation cartridges was analysed using gamma spectrometry (HPGe Canberra GC 5020, Meriden, CT, USA). Sterility testing was realised at the Department for Infectiology of the Heidelberg University Hospital. 1.9 µg (2 nmol) of PSMA-HBED-CC were dissolved in a mixture of 1.5 M acetate buffer pH 4.5 (1 mL) and 1 M ascorbic acid (10 µL) and the mixture was transferred into the reaction vessel. The ^{68}Ge/^{68}Ga-generator was eluted with 10 mL of 0.6 M HCl and the eluate diluted with 9 mL of ultrapure water. The mixture was then transferred to a cation exchange cartridge (Macherey-Nagel PS-H+, Size M, Düren, Germany) and eluted with 5 M NaCl solution (1.2 mL) into the preheated reaction vessel (100 °C). The reaction mixture was heated for 10 min. The crude reaction mixture was then removed from the reaction vessel and transferred to a pre-conditioned (1. 10 mL EtOH/ 2. 10 mL ultrapure water) C18 cartridge (Waters Sep-Pak light, Eschborn, Germany). 9 mL ultrapure water was used to rinse the reaction vessel and passed over the C18 cartridge. The C18 cartridge was washed with another 5 mL of ultrapure water. The final product was eluted from the C18 cartridge with 2 mL of EtOH/H_2O (1:1 v:v), sterile filtered (Millipore Cathivex-GV, 0.22 µm) and diluted with 8 mL of PBS solution (according to Ph. Eur. 8.0 (4005000)). All quality control tests except those for sterility and radionuclidic purity were determined prior release of the final product.

3. Results and Discussion

3.1. HBED-CC as Chelator for Highly Efficient Radiolabelling of Peptides

The acyclic radiometal chelator HBED-CC was reported to represent a highly effective ^{68}Ga complexing agent mainly suitable for gentle room temperature-radiolabelling of antibodies and proteins [18,19,24]. However, less is known about labelling kinetics and stability issues of ^{68}Ga-labelled HBED-CC-conjugated peptides. First insights in the quality of HBED-CC as labelling moiety of low-molecular weight compounds were given in the context of HBED-CC-conjugated PSMA inhibitors. We have recently reported that Glu-urea-Lys(Ahx)-HBED-CC can be labelled in less than 2 min with 99% radiochemical yield (RCY) at room temperature [20,28]. Here we summarise our PSMA-independent radiochemical experiences with the HBED-CC-conjugated peptide c(RGDyK) compared to the NOTA-labelled counterpart.

Figure 1A shows a typical dependency of the radiochemical yield (RCY) over time demonstrating the fast labelling kinetics of the examined HBED-CC-conjugated peptides at room temperature. A direct comparison of the labelling kinetics of a NOTA-conjugate and a HBED-CC-conjugate on the basis of proteins was already published previously [18] and is in good agreement with the herein presented data. In comparison to NOTA, HBED-CC complexes [^{68}Ga]Ga^{3+} more efficiently at low concentrations and low temperatures. A concentration of 1.7 μM was found to be sufficient to form the ^{68}Ga-labelled peptide with high radiochemical yields in less than one minute at room temperature. Clear differences were still observed after 20 min incubation of the reaction mixtures (Figure 1B).

Figure 1. The radiochemical yields (RCY) of the HBED-CC- and NOTA-conjugated model-peptide c(RGDyK) as a function of (**A**) peptide concentration (2 min reaction time); and (**B**) reaction time (1.7 μM peptide concentration), respectively. The compounds were incubated with the generator eluate at room temperature in HEPES buffer (pH 4.2). The reaction was stopped by adding 10 μL of a 0.1 M EDTA solution and the reaction mixture was subsequently analysed via radio-HPLC ($n = 6$).

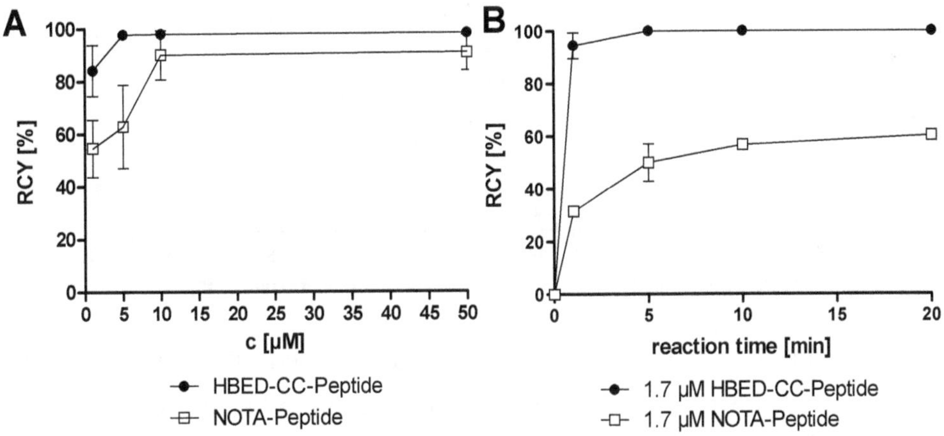

The different labelling kinetics of HBED-CC and NOTA observed in these experiments were also confirmed in a *competition-for-chelation* assay performed with the HBED-CC- and NOTA-conjugated RGD-peptides. Equal concentrations of HBED-CC-c(RGDyK) and NOTA-c(RGDyK) were incubated with [^{68}Ga]Ga^{3+} at room temperature. Also under these conditions, HBED-CC turned out to be the more potent chelator in direct challenging with NOTA, as 16% of the activity was complexed by NOTA-c(RGDyK) whereas 84% of the activity was incorporated in HBED-CC-c(RGDyK).

Labelling the free acid of HBED-CC was effective at pH values between 3.5 and 5 with no significant reduction of RCY between pH 4 and 5 (Figure 2). This fact ensures a high reproducibility and highly reliable radiopharmaceutical production process as a broad range of pH and an efficient radiolabelling at low concentrations of precursor enhance the robustness of the synthesis.

Another aspect which determines the quality and the clinical impact of a radiometal chelator is its serum stability. As metal complexes of open chain ligands generally show a lower degree of kinetic stability compared to cyclic chelators it is of importance to prove the long term stability of Ga-HBED-CC as active pharmaceutical ingredient of a radiopharmaceutical before its clinical use. The long term stability of radiogallium labelled HBED-CC-c(RGDyK) and NOTA-c(RGDyK) in human serum was investigated using the longer living radionuclide ^{67}Ga. Neither the NOTA-conjugate nor the HBED-CC-conjugate showed non-complexed ^{67}Ga in ionic form after 48 h-incubation in human serum at 37 °C. Remarkably, ~3% of the radioactivity was released from the NOTA-conjugate after 1 week in PBS at room temperature while the HBED-CC conjugate remained unchanged (>99% radiochemical purity (RCP)). This might be explained by a slight instability of the NOTA complex which was also demonstrated by analysing the serum samples on gel filtration (Figure 3). About 13% of the original peptide-bound radioactivity was eluted at about the same time as the serum proteins. In order to specify the transfer of ^{67}Ga to the serum proteins, the stability was further investigated by incubating the ^{68}Ga-labelled peptides in the presence of an excess of apo-transferrin for 2 h at 37 °C. However, no radiogallium was transchelated to apo-transferrin in both cases.

Figure 2. The pH dependence of the complexation reaction was determined by incubating the free acid of (**A**) HBED-CC (10 μM) and (**B**) NOTA (10 μM), respectively, at RT for 10 min. The radiochemical yield was determined by ITLC at the indicated time points (n = 6).

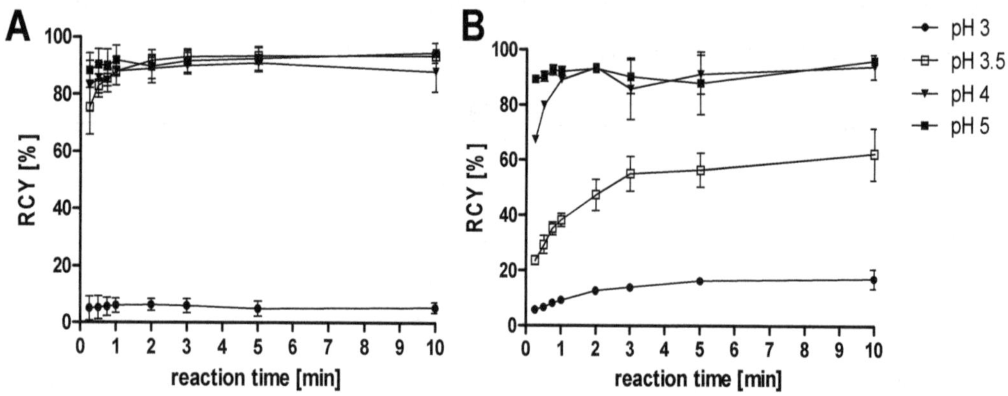

Figure 3. Superdex 75 5/150 GL runs of (**A**) ^{67}Ga-labelled HBED-CC-c(RGDyK); and (**B**) ^{67}Ga-labelled NOTA-c(RGDyK) after 48 h incubation in human serum at 37 °C. Only the radiometric signal is shown. The UV trace showed a major peak at ~3.9 min p.i.; (**C**) which corresponds with the elution time of serum proteins.

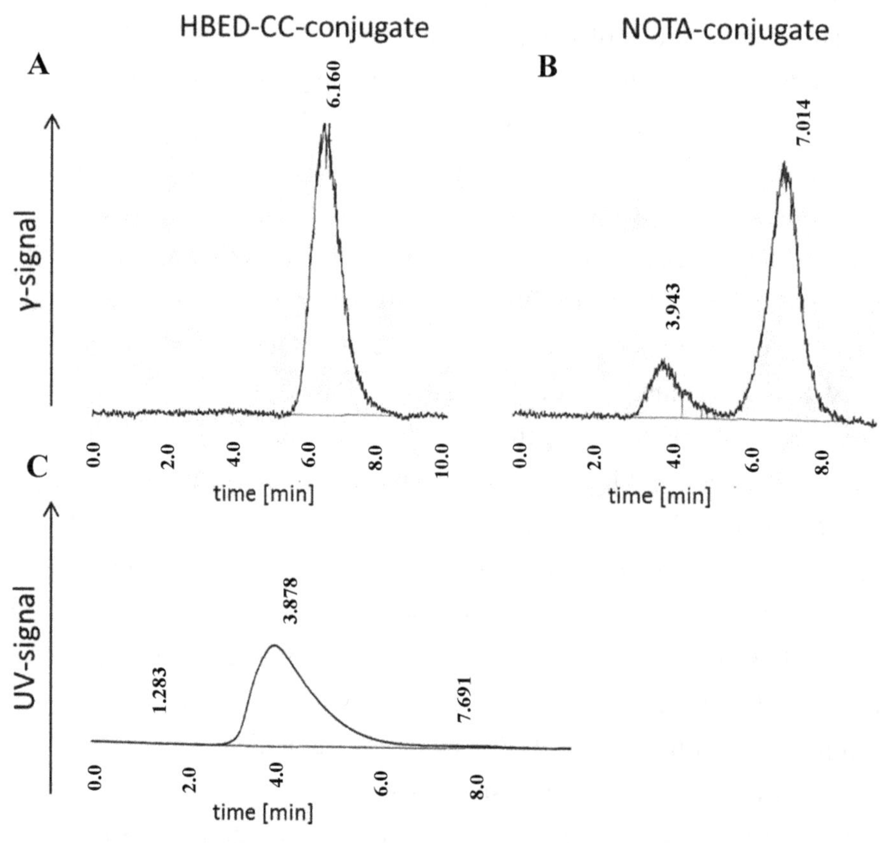

Taken together, HBED-CC represents an attractive acyclic alternative chelator for room temperature radiolabelling of proteins and peptides. Due to its different chemical characteristics compared to NOTA or DOTA such as the higher lipophilicity and the presence of aromatic residues, HBED-CC might have a positive impact on the pharmacokinetics or binding properties of a molecule. For [^{68}Ga]Ga-PSMA-HBED-CC these chemical characteristics, obviously being a part of the pharmacophore, were shown to be advantageous for the PSMA binding behaviour of the molecule, presumably by interacting with the known accessory hydrophobic pocket of the PSMA S1 site [20].

3.2. The Influence of Diastereomers of HBED-CC on the Binding Properties

The active site of a PSMA inhibitor consists of two independent main binding sites, a zinc-containing rigid site and an efferent tunnel with rather lipophilic characteristics [29,30]. The classical binding motif of urea-based PSMA inhibitors typically interacts with its carboxylic groups and the carbonylic oxygen. For efficient internalisation of a PSMA-directed radiotracer, however, the interaction of the linker region of the molecule with the aforementioned rather hydrophobic tunnel region seems of crucial importance. HBED-CC turned out to presumably interact with this region as the replacement of DOTA by HBED-CC has shown a significant influence on the internalisation efficiency of [^{68}Ga]Ga-PSMA-HBED-CC [20]. Due to this specific interaction with the hydrophobic binding pocket, slight chemical differences caused by the known formation of different diastereomers of HBED-CC after Ga-complexation might influence the binding properties of the whole molecule. The reaction temperature influences the proportional distribution of the three diastereomers. Typically, the GMP-compliant synthesis is realised at 100 °C resulting in the predominant formation of the thermodynamically more stable configuration of Ga-HBED-CC whereby the composition proved to be stable for at least 3 h in the injection buffer (Figure 4C). HPLC-MS measurements confirmed the identity of both diastereomers of the ^{nat}Ga-labelled complex (supporting information). If the reaction is carried out at RT, a fraction of about 50% of another diastereomer is formed (Figure 4A). This diastereomer converts into the thermodynamically more stable one quite rapidly in a few hours at pH 4 (Figure 4D). However, neutralising the reaction mixture resulted in a much slower interconversion. As shown in Figure 4E the percentage composition remains nearly unchanged for hours which is in agreement with the observation of Schuhmacher *et al.*, who reported that the interconversion into the most stable configuration at pH 7 took several days [23].

From the *in vivo* point of view, the distribution of the diastereomers might be of high impact if one configuration of Ga-HBED-CC would not interact with the binding site and therefore would hamper the overall functionality of the PSMA inhibitor. Since the quality of the PET/CT images would be affected by the presence of a potentially non-functional diastereomer, it is important to elucidate their influence on the PSMA binding characteristics. Therefore, the cell binding properties of [^{68}Ga]Ga-PSMA-HBED-CC labelled at ambient temperature and 95 °C, respectively, were evaluated in cell-based assays. Figure 5A shows that the PSMA-specific cell surface binding and internalisation of the mixture of diastereomers (RT labelling) and the thermodynamically most stable diastereomer (95 °C labelling) were comparable. In addition, the affinity related IC_{50}-values of the reaction mixtures of both labelling conditions were determined on the PSMA expressing cell line LNCaP (Figure 5B). Indeed, both the RT-labelled fraction and the 95 °C-labelled fraction bound PSMA with identical affinities (IC_{50} values: 27.4 ± 1.3 nm and 24.8 ± 1.2 nm, respectively). It has to be concluded that the presence of a thermodynamically less stable diastereomer does not have any negative influence on the PSMA-binding properties indicating a robust stereochemical independence of the pharmacophore Glu-NH-CO-NH-Lys sidechain.

Figure 4. Radio-HPLC traces of RT (**A**) and 95 °C (**B**) labelled Glu-urea-Lys(Ahx)-HBED-CC. The peaks correspond to (1), the thermodynamically more stable, and (2), the thermodynamically less stable diastereomer, respectively. Graphs **C–E** show the radiochromatograms after various storage and labelling conditions: 95 °C labelled Glu-urea-Lys(Ahx)-HBED-CC stored for 3 h in injection buffer (**C**); RT labelled Glu-urea-Lys(Ahx)-HBED-CC after 3 h incubation in labelling reaction buffer at (**D**) pH 4, and (**E**) pH 7.

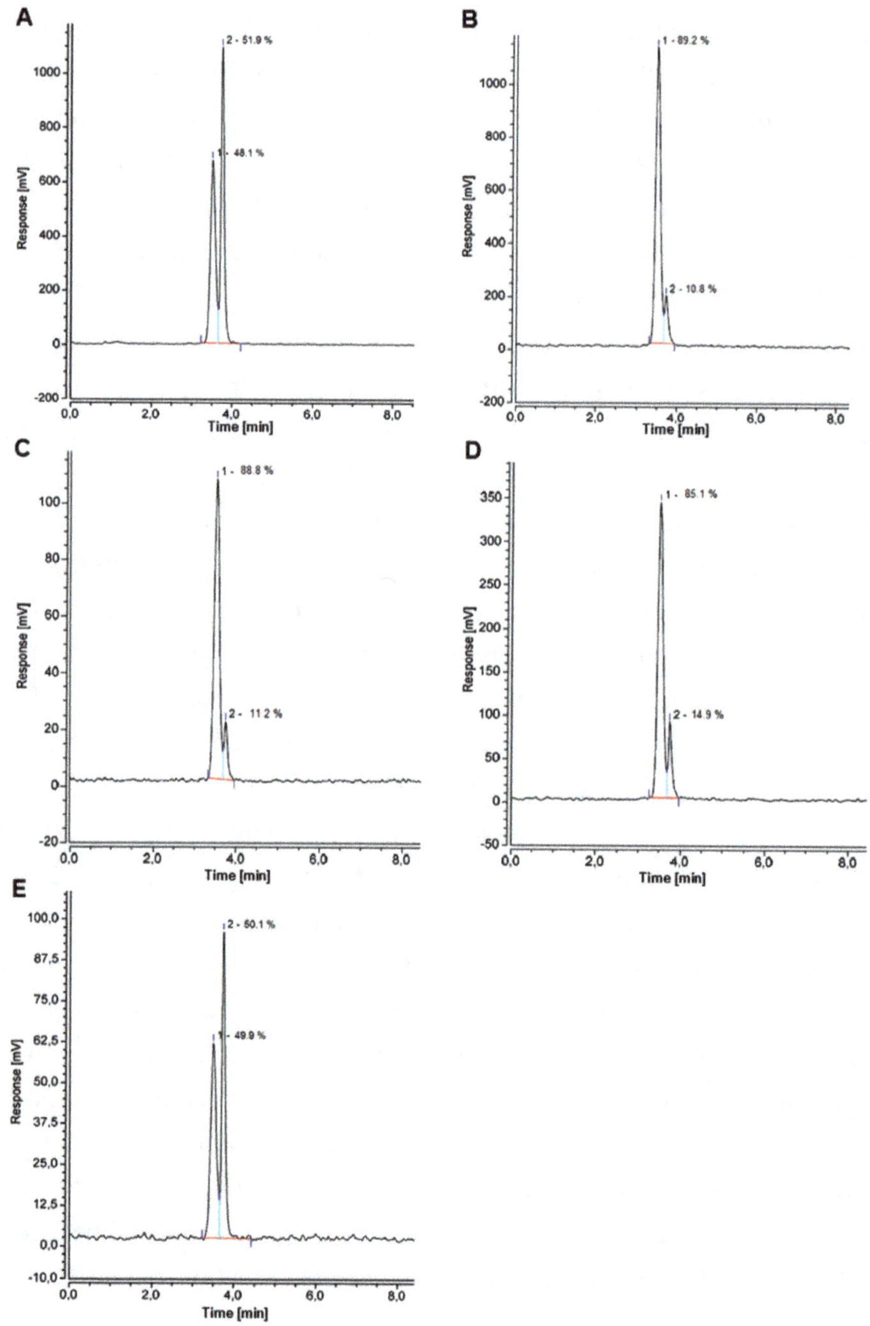

Figure 5. (**A**) LNCaP-cell binding and internalisation of [^{68}Ga]Ga-PSMA-HBED-CC labelled at RT or 95 °C, respectively. Specific cell uptake was determined by competitive blockade with 500 µM of the PSMA inhibitor 2-PMPA. Values are expressed as percentage of applied radioactivity bound to 10^6 cells [%IA/10^6 cells]. Data are expressed as mean ± SD (n = 3); (**B**) Determination of binding affinity of [^{nat}Ga]Ga-PSMA-HBED-CC to LNCaP cells as a function of the labelling temperature. The cells (10^5 per well) were incubated with the radioligand (^{68}Ga-labelled Glu-urea-Lys(Ahx)-HBED-CC) in the presence of different concentrations of ^{nat}Ga-analyte (0–5000 nM, 100 µL/well).

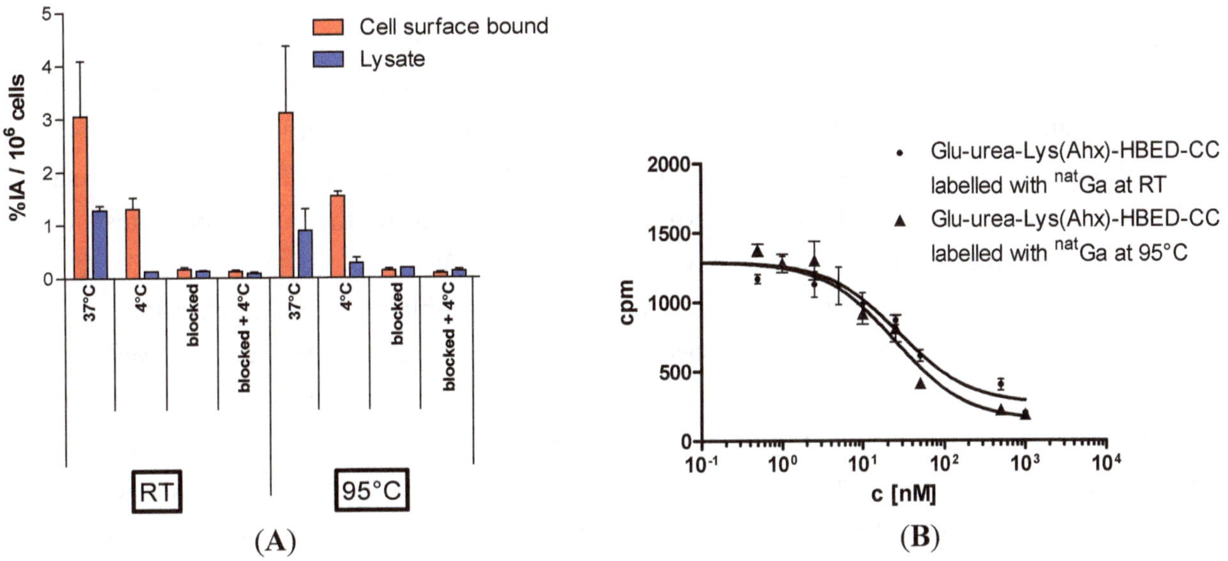

This information is important with regard to the radiopharmaceutical production process as a small fraction of one of the thermodynamically less stable diastereomers is still present in the labelling reaction mixture even at 95 °C labelling condition (Figure 4B) and would be part of the final formulation prepared for the patient. According to our results, a fraction of approx. 50% of the thermodynamically less stable diastereomer does not reduce the PSMA-specific cellular uptake and should therefore not have any negative influence on the quality of the PET images. However, it has to be considered that our conclusions are based on an indirect reasoning as the two major diastereomers were not separated chemically by HPLC for these experiments. A chemical separation via HPLC would result in an unknown concentration of unlabelled compound. As the cell binding directly depends on the used concentration it is crucial to know exactly the amount of analyte given to the cells. Since the proportional distribution of the observed two diastereomers can be easily controlled by pH and temperature of the labelling reaction mixture, the influence of the thermodynamically less stable diastereomer on the cell binding properties can be reliably determined by comparing RT-labelled and 95°C-labelled Glu-urea-Lys(Ahx)-HBED-CC. If the thermodynamically less stable diastereomer would not bind PSMA-presenting cell lines at all it would reduce the cell uptake considerably in the RT-labelled approach.

3.3. Automated Synthesis

The radiosynthesis of [^{68}Ga]Ga-PSMA-HBED-CC as described earlier [20] was reproduced reliably and slightly modified on a fully automated synthesis module in 80% ± 5% decay corrected radiochemical yield within 35 min applying single-use cassette-based kits. An audit trail was recorded for each radiosynthesis including all performed steps and courses of radioactivity on three gamma detectors, gas flow and temperature of the heating unit. The steps involved include conditioning of the purification cartridge, elution of the ^{68}Ge/^{68}Ga-generator, purification of the generator eluate, radiosynthesis and purification and sterile filtration of the final product. [^{68}Ga]Ga-PSMA-HBED-CC was obtained in >99% radiochemical purity as two diastereomers (Figure 4B) with a pH ranging between 6 and 8. Stability of [^{68}Ga]Ga-PSMA-HBED-CC in the final product solution was tested for up to 2 h after the end of radiosynthesis and yielded identical results for the radiochemical purity. The only residual solvent found in the final product solution was ethanol in less than 10% v/v taking the density at 20°C to be 0.79 g/mL. Bacterial endotoxin testing showed <2 IU/mL and all samples tested were sterile. Filter integrity of the sterile filter was tested using the bubble-point test. Gamma spectrometry showed characteristic peaks at 0.511 and 1.077 MeV.

For the production of radiopharmaceuticals using gallium-68 obtained from a generator system it is crucial that possible metal impurities washed off from the ^{68}Ge/^{68}Ga-generator as well as ^{68}Ge-breakthrough have to be eliminated prior the radiolabelling. Examples of methods for purification of the eluate are fractionated elution of the ^{68}Ge/^{68}Ga-generator or the trapping of the generator eluate on either a cationic or anionic exchange cartridge [31–33]. One of the most prominent methods has been described earlier by Zhernosekov *et al.* [33]. The drawback of this method for the purification of ^{68}Ga is the use of acetone, which has to be removed after synthesis and bares the risk of additional impurities [34]. Recently, a method based on the use of a strong NaCl solution to purify ^{68}Ga on a cation exchange cartridge has been reported [35,36]. For the radiosynthesis of [^{68}Ga]Ga-PSMA-HBED-CC we adapted the method from Martin *et al.* [36]. A volume of 1.2 mL of 5 M NaCl solution was confirmed to elute up to 85% of the trapped ^{68}Ga activity from the PS-H+ separation cartridge. As the majority of the ^{68}Ga activity was eluted with the last 200 μL of NaCl solution, a smaller volume than 1.2 mL could not be applied. Larger volumes did not lead to higher elution efficiency. Remaining ^{68}Ge was neither observed on the PS-H+ separation cartridge nor in the reaction vessel after elution with 5 M NaCl solution and neither in the final product preparation 48 h after purification of the generator eluate. This confirms the efficacy of this method to remove possible ^{68}Ge-breakthrough. We modified the reaction parameters due to the larger geometry of the reaction vessel on the synthesis module compared to the method described by Eder *et al.* [20]. To allow good mixing of ^{68}Ga and PSMA-HBED-CC in the reaction vessel, a minimum volume of 1 mL was necessary. Additionally, pH of the reaction mixture is seen to be a critical factor to obtain high radiochemical yields. HEPES (4-(2-hydroxyethyl)-1-piperazineethanesulfonic acid) is a well-known buffer in radiolabelling procedures using ^{68}Ga, but as we consider HEPES as a critical impurity for radiopharmaceutical applications we were looking for alternative buffer solutions. Firstly, citrate buffer was applied at different concentrations and at different pH but this was unsuccessful resulting in radiochemical yields <5%. We used different sodium acetate buffer solutions (pH 3.2–5.5) in concentrations ranging from 20 mM to 1.5 M and volumes ranging from 1 to 3 mL. The optimal reaction conditions with an average radiochemical yield of 80% were found using 1 mL of 1.5 M sodium acetate buffer solution with a pH of the reaction mixture ranging from 3.6 to 4.2. Lower or higher pH of the reaction mixture lead to a significant decrease in radiochemical yields. Although the ^{68}Ga-eluate was purified and concentrated using 5 M NaCl solution, sodium acetate buffer solutions with volumes smaller than 1 mL were not able to stabilise the pH of the reaction mixture sufficiently. Additionally, 10 µL of 1 M ascorbic acid was added to avoid the forming of side products when using a ^{68}Ge/^{68}Ga-generator with high starting activities [37]. We prolonged the reaction time to 10 min and heated to 100 °C because the resulting volume of the reaction mixture was by a factor 20 higher than previously reported [20]. High radiochemical yields were obtained reliably with only 1.9 µg (2 nmol) of PSMA-HBED-CC in our setup, different setups due to the properties of other synthesis modules might require slightly higher amounts (5–10 µg) of radiolabelling precursor. The crude reaction mixture was purified using a C18 cartridge which was then rinsed with ultrapure water to remove unreacted ^{68}Ga. After sterile filtration 10 mL of the final product solution were obtained and 1.5–2 mL taken for quality control and keeping of a retain sample. Batches of [^{68}Ga]Ga-PSMA-HBED-CC produced following this fully automated procedure are being released after passing quality control requirements according to a defined product specification (Table 1). The whole automated synthesis procedure was also successfully applied for the radiopharmaceutical production of [^{68}Ga]Ga-DOTA-TOC and is a useful tool for a quick clinical implementation of other novel ^{68}Ga-labelled compounds.

Table 1. Defined product specification of the final preparation of [^{68}Ga]Ga-PSMA-HBED-CC.

Appearance	Clear and Colourless
pH	4–8
Radioactivity concentration	10–200 MBq/mL
Radiochemical purity (HPLC)	≥95%
Chemical impurities (HPLC)	≤5 µg/mL PSMA-HBED-CC
Concentration ethanol (GC)	<10% v/v
Approximate half-life	68 ± 6 min
Bacterial endotoxins	<17.5 IU/mL
Filter integrity (bubble-point test)	>3.5 bar
Radionuclidic purity (γ-spectrometry)	^{68}Ga > 99.9% (γ-lines at 0.511 MeV and 1.077 MeV) ^{68}Ge: ≤0.001%
Sterility	Sterile

4. Conclusions

We have recently introduced HBED-CC in the PSMA inhibitor motif Glu-urea-Lys as radiometal chelator in order to optimise the interactions of the pharmacophore with the accessory hydrophobic pocket of the PSMA S1 binding site. In addition, HBED-CC represents a very effective and stable radiometal chelator allowing fast radiolabelling at room temperature while exhibiting an exceptionally high complex stability similar to the clinically used DOTA chelator. The formation of diastereomers can be controlled via distinct temperature conditions during the radiolabelling reaction and directed predominantly to the formation of the thermodynamically more stable one. In case of small fractions of other diastereomers, the biological functionality of the radiotracer [^{68}Ga]Ga-PSMA-HBED-CC is proven to be not affected. Taken together, the HBED-CC-conjugated PSMA inhibitor [^{68}Ga]Ga-PSMA-HBED-CC is suitable for being used in typical kit like radiochemical production processes for clinical use with high reproducibility and robustness.

Acknowledgments

There is no other financial relationship of the authors than a grant from the DFG (Deutsche Forschungsgemeinschaft) for M. Eder (ED234/2-1), which is gratefully acknowledged. HPLC-MS measurements were kindly performed and evaluated by Susanne Krämer (Department of Nuclear Medicine, University of Heidelberg, Heidelberg, Germany).

Author Contributions

Matthias Eder contributed in writing of the manuscript and data interpretation and analysis. Oliver Neels contributed in writing of the manuscript and the development of the GMP-compliant automated synthesis and quality control procedures. Miriam Müller contributed in the synthesis of peptides and chemicals, data interpretation and analysis and carried out the complex stability and labelling kinetics experiments. Ulrike Bauder-Wüst contributed in the data interpretation and analysis and carried out *in vitro* experiments. Yvonne Remde contributed to the development of the GMP-compliant automated synthesis. Martin Schäfer carried out and evaluated the synthesis of peptides and chemicals. Ute Hennrich contributed to the development of quality control procedures for the GMP-compliant automated synthesis. Michael Eisenhut contributed to the design of experiments for HBED-CC- and NOTA-conjugated model-peptide c(RGDyK). Ali Afshar-Oromieh gave scientific advice for the development of the GMP-compliant automated synthesis. Uwe Haberkorn gave scientific advice for the design of preclinical experiments. Klaus Kopka gave scientific advice, contributed to the design of experiments as well as in writing of the manuscript. All authors approved the manuscript.

References

1. Andriole, G.L.; Crawford, E.D.; Grubb, R.L., 3rd; Buys, S.S.; Chia, D.; Church, T.R.; Fouad, M.N.; Gelmann, E.P.; Kvale, P.A.; Reding, D.J.; *et al.* Mortality results from a randomized prostate-cancer screening trial. *N. Engl. J. Med.* **2009**, *360*, 1310–1319.
2. Beheshti, M.; Langsteger, W.; Fogelman, I. Prostate cancer: Role of SPECT and PET in imaging bone metastases. *Semin. Nucl. Med.* **2009**, *39*, 396–407.
3. Afshar-Oromieh, A.; Zechmann, C.M.; Malcher, A.; Eder, M.; Eisenhut, M.; Linhart, H.G.; Holland-Letz, T.; Hadaschik, B.A.; Giesel, F.L.; Debus, J.; *et al.* Comparison of PET imaging with a ^{68}Ga-labelled PSMA ligand and ^{18}F-choline-based PET/CT for the diagnosis of recurrent prostate cancer. *Eur. J. Nucl. Med. Mol. Imaging* **2014**, *41*, 11–20.

4. Afshar-Oromieh, A.; Malcher, A.; Eder, M.; Eisenhut, M.; Linhart, H.G.; Hadaschik, B.A.; Holland-Letz, T.; Giesel, F.L.; Kratochwil, C.; Haufe, S.; *et al.* PET imaging with a [^{68}Ga]Gallium-labelled PSMA ligand for the diagnosis of prostate cancer: Biodistribution in humans and first evaluation of tumour lesions. *Eur. J. Nucl. Med. Mol. Imaging* **2013**, *40*, 486–495.
5. Afshar-Oromieh, A.; Haberkorn, U.; Eder, M.; Eisenhut, M.; Zechmann, C.M. [^{68}Ga]Gallium-labelled PSMA ligand as superior PET tracer for the diagnosis of prostate cancer: Comparison with ^{18}F-FECh. *Eur. J. Nucl. Med. Mol. Imaging* **2012**, *39*, 1085–1086.
6. Barrett, J.A.; Coleman, R.E.; Goldsmith, S.J.; Vallabhajosula, S.; Petry, N.A.; Cho, S.; Armor, T.; Stubbs, J.B.; Maresca, K.P.; Stabin, M.G., *et al.* First-in-man evaluation of 2 high-affinity psma-avid small molecules for imaging prostate cancer. *J. Nucl. Med.* **2013**, *54*, 380–387.
7. Silver, D.A.; Pellicer, I.; Fair, W.R.; Heston, W.D.; Cordon-Cardo, C. Prostate-specific membrane antigen expression in normal and malignant human tissues. *Clin. Cancer Res.* **1997**, *3*, 81–85.
8. Schulke, N.; Varlamova, O.A.; Donovan, G.P.; Ma, D.; Gardner, J.P.; Morrissey, D.M.; Arrigale, R.R.; Zhan, C.; Chodera, A.J.; Surowitz, K.G.; *et al.* The homodimer of prostate-specific membrane antigen is a functional target for cancer therapy. *Proc. Natl. Acad. Sci. USA* **2003**, *100*, 12590–12595.
9. Fair, W.R.; Israeli, R.S.; Heston, W.D. Prostate-specific membrane antigen. *Prostate* **1997**, *32*, 140–148.
10. O'Keefe, D.S.; Bacich, D.J.; Heston, W.D. Comparative analysis of prostate-specific membrane antigen (PSMA) *versus* a prostate-specific membrane antigen-like gene. *Prostate* **2004**, *58*, 200–210.
11. Cunha, A.C.; Weigle, B.; Kiessling, A.; Bachmann, M.; Rieber, E.P. Tissue-specificity of prostate specific antigens: Comparative analysis of transcript levels in prostate and non-prostatic tissues. *Cancer Lett.* **2006**, *236*, 229–238.
12. Hillier, S.M.; Maresca, K.P.; Femia, F.J.; Marquis, J.C.; Foss, C.A.; Nguyen, N.; Zimmerman, C.N.; Barrett, J.A.; Eckelman, W.C.; Pomper, M.G.; *et al.* Preclinical evaluation of novel glutamate-urea-lysine analogues that target prostate-specific membrane antigen as molecular imaging pharmaceuticals for prostate cancer. *Cancer Res.* **2009**, *69*, 6932–6940.
13. Chen, Y.; Foss, C.A.; Byun, Y.; Nimmagadda, S.; Pullambhatla, M.; Fox, J.J.; Castanares, M.; Lupold, S.E.; Babich, J.W.; Mease, R.C.; *et al.* Radiohalogenated prostate-specific membrane antigen (PSMA)-based ureas as imaging agents for prostate cancer. *J. Med. Chem.* **2008**, *51*, 7933–7943.
14. Banerjee, S.R.; Foss, C.A.; Castanares, M.; Mease, R.C.; Byun, Y.; Fox, J.J.; Hilton, J.; Lupold, S.E.; Kozikowski, A.P.; Pomper, M.G. Synthesis and evaluation of Technetium-99m- and Rhenium-labeled inhibitors of the prostate-specific membrane antigen (PSMA). *J. Med. Chem.* **2008**, *51*, 4504–4517.
15. Kularatne, S.A.; Zhou, Z.; Yang, J.; Post, C.B.; Low, P.S. Design, synthesis, and preclinical evaluation of prostate-specific membrane antigen targeted ^{99m}Tc-radioimaging agents. *Mol. Pharm.* **2009**, *6*, 790–800.
16. Zaheer, A.; Cho, S.Y.; Pomper, M.G. New agents and techniques for imaging prostate cancer. *J. Nucl. Med.* **2009**, *50*, 1387–1390.

17. Banerjee, S.R.; Pullambhatla, M.; Byun, Y.; Nimmagadda, S.; Green, G.; Fox, J.J.; Horti, A.; Mease, R.C.; Pomper, M.G. ^{68}Ga-labeled inhibitors of prostate-specific membrane antigen (PSMA) for imaging prostate cancer. *J. Med. Chem.* **2010**, *53*, 5333–5341.
18. Eder, M.; Krivoshein, A.V.; Backer, M.; Backer, J.M.; Haberkorn, U.; Eisenhut, M. ScVEGF-PEG-HBED-CC and scVEGF-PEG-NOTA conjugates: Comparison of easy-to-label recombinant proteins for [^{68}Ga]PET imaging of VEGF receptors in angiogenic vasculature. *Nucl. Med. Biol.* **2010**, *37*, 405–412.
19. Eder, M.; Wangler, B.; Knackmuss, S.; Legall, F.; Little, M.; Haberkorn, U.; Mier, W.; Eisenhut, M. Tetrafluorophenolate of HBED-CC: A versatile conjugation agent for ^{68}Ga-labeled small recombinant antibodies. *Eur. J. Nucl. Med. Mol. Imaging* **2008**, *35*, 1878–1886.
20. Eder, M.; Schafer, M.; Bauder-Wust, U.; Hull, W.E.; Wangler, C.; Mier, W.; Haberkorn, U.; Eisenhut, M. ^{68}Ga-complex lipophilicity and the targeting property of a urea-based PSMA inhibitor for PET imaging. *Biocon. Chem.* **2012**, *23*, 688–697.
21. Liu, T.; Toriyabe, Y.; Kazak, M.; Berkman, C.E. Pseudoirreversible inhibition of prostate-specific membrane antigen by phosphoramidate peptidomimetics. *Biochemistry* **2008**, *47*, 12658–12660.
22. Taliaferro, C.H.; Martell, A.E. New multidentate ligands. Xxvi. *N,N′*-bis(2-hydroxybenzyl) ethylenediamine-*N,N′*-bis(methylenephosphonic acid monomethyl ester), and *N,N′*-bis(2-hydroxybenzyl)ethylenediamine-*N,N′*-bis(methylenephosphonic acid monoethyl ester): New chelating ligands for trivalent metal ions. *J. Coord. Chem.* **1984**, *13*, 249–264.
23. Schuhmacher, J.; Klivenyi, G.; Matys, R.; Stadler, M.; Regiert, T.; Hauser, H.; Doll, J.; Maier-Borst, W.; Zoller, M. Multistep tumor targeting in nude mice using bispecific antibodies and a gallium chelate suitable for immunoscintigraphy with positron emission tomography. *Cancer Res.* **1995**, *55*, 115–123.
24. Schuhmacher, J.; Klivenyi, G.; Hull, W.E.; Matys, R.; Hauser, H.; Kalthoff, H.; Schmiegel, W.H.; Maier-Borst, W.; Matzku, S. A bifunctional HBED-derivative for labeling of antibodies with ^{67}Ga, ^{111}In and ^{59}Fe. Comparative biodistribution with ^{111}In-DTPA and ^{131}I-labeled antibodies in mice bearing antibody internalizing and non-internalizing tumors. *Int. J. Rad. Appl. Instrum. B* **1992**, *19*, 809–824.
25. Eder, M.; Knackmuss, S.; Le Gall, F.; Reusch, U.; Rybin, V.; Little, M.; Haberkorn, U.; Mier, W.; Eisenhut, M. ^{68}Ga-labelled recombinant antibody variants for immuno-PET imaging of solid tumours. *Eur. J. Nucl. Med. Mol. Imaging* **2010**, *37*, 1397–1407.
26. Kubas, H.; Schafer, M.; Bauder-Wust, U.; Eder, M.; Oltmanns, D.; Haberkorn, U.; Mier, W.; Eisenhut, M. Multivalent cyclic RGD ligands: Influence of linker lengths on receptor binding. *Nucl. Med. Biol.* **2010**, *37*, 885–891.
27. Schuhmacher, J.; Maier-Borst, W. A new Ge-68/Ga-68 radioisotope generator system for production of Ga-68 in dilute HCl. *Int. J. Appl. Radiat. Isot.* **1981**, *32*, 31–36.
28. Schafer, M.; Bauder-Wust, U.; Leotta, K.; Zoller, F.; Mier, W.; Haberkorn, U.; Eisenhut, M.; Eder, M. A dimerized urea-based inhibitor of the prostate-specific membrane antigen for ^{68}Ga-PET imaging of prostate cancer. *EJNMMI Res.* **2012**, *2*, 23.
29. Zhang, A.X.; Murelli, R.P.; Barinka, C.; Michel, J.; Cocleaza, A.; Jorgensen, W.L.; Lubkowski, J.; Spiegel, D.A. A remote arene-binding site on prostate specific membrane antigen revealed by antibody-recruiting small molecules. *J. Am. Chem. Soc.* **2010**, *132*, 12711–12716.

30. Barinka, C.; Byun, Y.; Dusich, C.L.; Banerjee, S.R.; Chen, Y.; Castanares, M.; Kozikowski, A.P.; Mease, R.C.; Pomper, M.G.; Lubkowski, J. Interactions between human glutamate carboxypeptidase II and urea-based inhibitors: Structural characterization. *J. Med. Chem.* **2008**, *51*, 7737–7743.
31. Breeman, W.A.; de Jong, M.; de Blois, E.; Bernard, B.F.; Konijnenberg, M.; Krenning, E.P. Radiolabelling DOTA-peptides with ^{68}Ga. *Eur. J. Nucl. Med. Mol. Imaging* **2005**, *32*, 478–485.
32. Meyer, G.J.; Macke, H.; Schuhmacher, J.; Knapp, W.H.; Hofmann, M. ^{68}Ga-labelled DOTA-derivatised peptide ligands. *Eur. J. Nucl. Med. Mol. Imaging* **2004**, *31*, 1097–1104.
33. Zhernosekov, K.P.; Filosofov, D.V.; Baum, R.P.; Aschoff, P.; Bihl, H.; Razbash, A.A.; Jahn, M.; Jennewein, M.; Rosch, F. Processing of generator-produced ^{68}Ga for medical application. *J. Nucl. Med.* **2007**, *48*, 1741–1748.
34. Petrik, M.; Ocak, M.; Rupprich, M.; Decristoforo, C. Impurity in ^{68}Ga-peptide preparation using processed generator eluate. *J. Nucl. Med.* **2010**, *51*, 495–496.
35. Schultz, M.K.; Mueller, D.; Baum, R.P.; Leonard Watkins, G.; Breeman, W.A. A new automated NaCl based robust method for routine production of Gallium-68 labeled peptides. *Appl. Radiat. Isot.* **2013**, *76*, 46–54.
36. Martin, R.; Juttler, S.; Muller, M.; Wester, H.J. Cationic eluate pretreatment for automated synthesis of [^{68}Ga]CPCR4.2. *Nucl. Med. Biol.* **2014**, *41*, 84–89.
37. Mu, L.; Hesselmann, R.; Oezdemir, U.; Bertschi, L.; Blanc, A.; Dragic, M.; Loffler, D.; Smuda, C.; Johayem, A.; Schibli, R. Identification, characterization and suppression of side-products formed during the synthesis of high dose ^{68}Ga-DOTA-TATE. *Appl. Radiat. Isot.* **2013**, *76*, 63–69.

Appendix

HPLC-MS analysis

The ^{nat}Ga-labelled reference Glu-urea-Lys(Ahx)-[Ga(HBED-CC)] (DKFZ-GaPSMA-11) was purchased from ABX advanced biochemical compounds (Radeberg, Germany) and dissolved in 40 µL CH_3CN/H_2O (1:1). 2.6 µg were characterised at RT by mass spectrometry using a Agilent 1200 HPLC-MS system connected to an Orbitrap Mass Spectrometer (Exactive, Thermo Fisher Scientific) on a Hypersil Gold C18 column (2.1 × 200 mm, 1.9 µm; Thermo Scientific, Bremen, Germany) eluted with a linear gradient (eluent A: 0.05% TFA in water; eluent B: 0.05% TFA in acetonitrile; 0%–30% B in 30 min at RT, flow rate: 0.2 mL/min, absorbance: λ=214 nm). Full scan single mass spectra (positive mode) were obtained by scanning from m/z = 200−4000.

Figure S1. MS analysis of HPLC fractions of the mixture of diastereomers (fraction 23.84–27.00 min), of the thermodynamically more stable (fraction 23.95-25.04 min) and of the less stable diastereomer (fraction 26.58-26.88 min) of Ga-PSMA-HBED-CC, respectively.

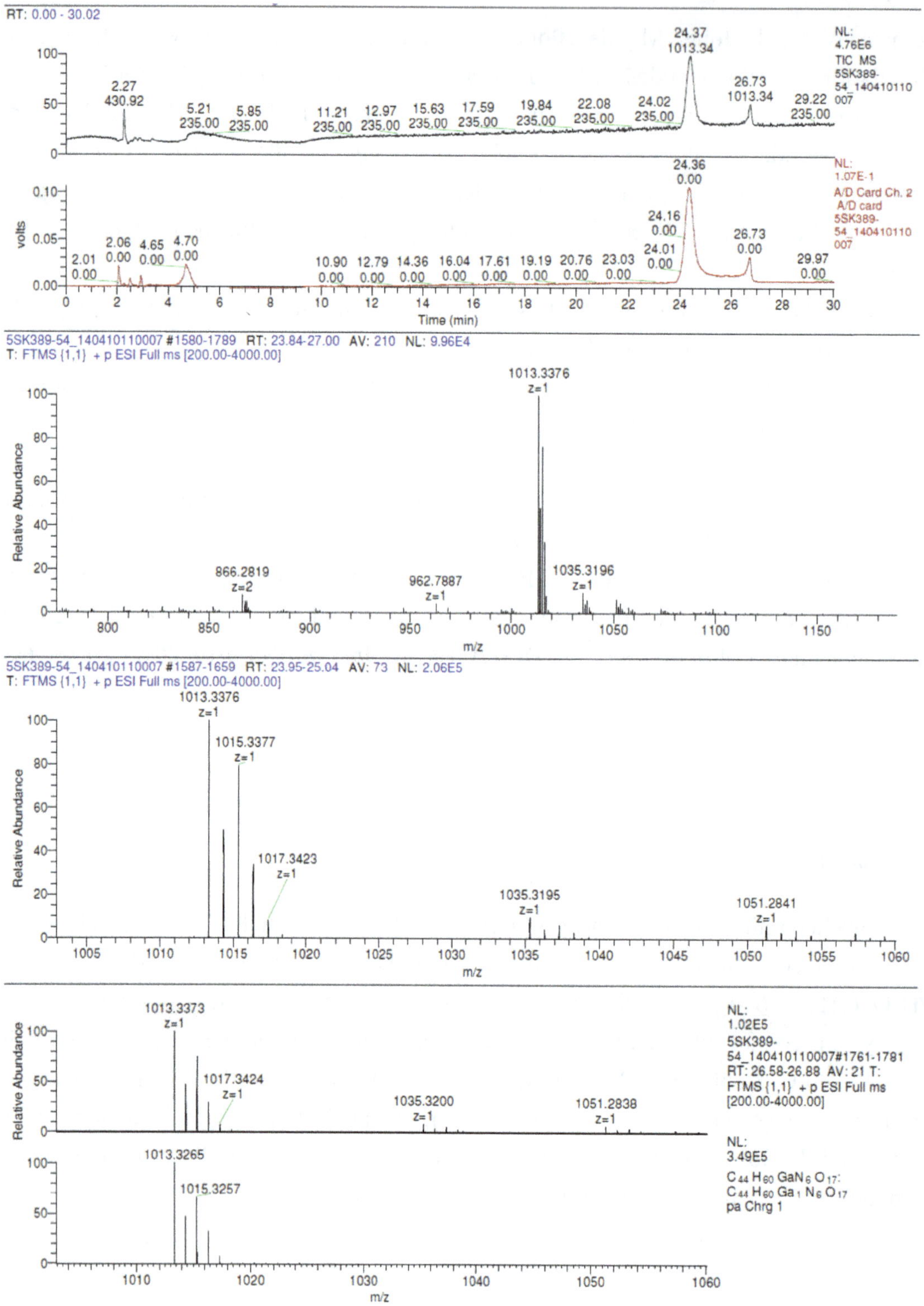

10

Imaging Biomarkers or Biomarker Imaging?

Markus Mitterhauser and Wolfgang Wadsak *

Radiochemistry and Biomarker Development Unit, Department of Biomedical Imaging and Image-guided Therapy, Division of Nuclear Medicine, Medical University of Vienna, A-1090 Vienna, Austria; E-Mail: markus.mitterhauser@meduniwien.ac.at

* Author to whom correspondence should be addressed; E-Mail: wolfgang.wadsak@meduniwien.ac.at

---

Abstract: Since biomarker imaging is traditionally understood as imaging of molecular probes, we highly recommend to avoid any confusion with the previously defined term "imaging biomarkers" and, therefore, only use "molecular probe imaging (MPI)" in that context. Molecular probes (MPs) comprise all kinds of molecules administered to an organism which inherently carry a signalling moiety. This review highlights the basic concepts and differences of molecular probe imaging using specific biomarkers. In particular, PET radiopharmaceuticals are discussed in more detail. Specific radiochemical and radiopharmacological aspects as well as some legal issues are presented.

Keywords: tracer; molecular probe; PET; radiopharmaceutical

---

1. Introduction

The terms "imaging biomarker" and biomarker imaging" are currently used in a variety of different contexts. Therefore, a clear definition of these terms is pivotal. "Biomarker" has already been defined by the National Institutes of Health (NIH, Bethesda, MD, USA) director's initiative on biomarkers and surrogate endpoints to be "a characteristic, that is objectively measured and evaluated as an indicator of normal biological processes, pathogenic processes, or pharmacologic responses to a therapeutic intervention" [1]. But this definition still gives room for a wide range of interpretations. On the one hand, it is evident that a biomarker has to be objectively measurable; on the other hand, it provides no information regarding the very nature of this measurable characteristic. From the given definition, a biomarker can be nearly every value associated with any process in any organism, even such trivial things as blood pressure, urinary pH or visual faculty. Going a bit further, a biomarker can be a molecular probe such as the calcium-score or levels of prostate specific antigen (PSA), or a functional indicator like extent of myocardial perfusion or renal clearance. Consequently, imaging biomarkers are all those biomarkers, which are determined by imaging techniques. Since there is no exclusivity to that term, examples are found in all methods: e.g., Nuchal translucency screening (ultrasound), sizing of adrenocortical incidentalomas (X-ray), BOLD-signal (magnetic resonance imaging—MRI), renal clearance (single photon emission computed tomography—SPECT).

Moreover, "imaging" is also a term with widespread use demanding for closer characterisation; coming from the Latin word *imago* meaning "picture". Hence, imaging is a tool enabling the operator to obtain a picture of the organism. It can enable the assessment of the biological basis of the body, including changes due to disease, response to therapeutic intervention. Nowadays, imaging is mostly used as a synonym for visualisation (derived from the Latin word *video* meaning "to see"), although visualising processes and conditions are only part of imaging these things. The aspect that distinguishes imaging from mere visualisation is quantitation. This brings us back to the definition of biomarker being a measurable signal. For that reason, a visualisation biomarker could not exist! Imaging (and therefore imaging biomarkers) can be characterised as structural, functional and molecular, respectively. Hence, one should distinguish truly molecular information from rather functional or even structural measurements and restrain from thoughtlessly terming everything "molecular imaging". So what makes imaging become molecular? The answer is simple: the visualisation and quantification of a molecular interaction between a molecular probe and a molecular target.

Recently, Lucignani strengthened the term "imaging biomarkers" and pointed out that they allow identifying measurable variables that are otherwise undetectable [2]. Furthermore, he stated that "moving the definition of an imaging biomarker from that of a technical probe to that of a biological variable" results in the recognition "that the use of imaging biomarkers transforms the role of molecular and anatomic imaging from technical to a fully clinical". Bringing this to a synopsis, an imaging biomarker is "not a tool or a method but a measureable variable".

Now, that we have defined imaging biomarkers can we simply rearrange these terms and consequently derive a definition of biomarker imaging as well? Unfortunately, it is not that simple and thus requires further reflection. Since biomarker imaging traditionally is understood as imaging of molecular probes, we highly recommend to avoid any confusion with the previously defined term "imaging biomarkers" and, therefore, only use "molecular probe imaging (MPI)" in that context. Molecular probes (MPs) comprise all kinds of molecules administered to an organism which inherently carry a signalling moiety. This moiety can for example be a radionuclide, a fluorescent chromophore, a paramagnetic core or a gas-filled or gas-producing nanostructure. The resulting signal has to be visualised and quantified by dedicated imaging procedures and technologies [3–8]. Hence, MPI always leads to an imaging biomarker; but imaging biomarkers do not necessarily require MPI! However, imaging biomarkers require a molecular imaging modality/technique in order to measure them (e.g., magnetic resonance spectroscopy doesn't use molecular probes but can detect imaging biomarkers and is considered a molecular imaging technique).

2. PET & MRI: Selected Examples

The blood-oxygen-level dependent (BOLD) signal is an indirect measure for the local oxygenation level in tissue [9]. It is quantifiable and derives from the application of MR imaging. Therefore, it follows the definition of an IB. But it's definitely not MPI: no MP is administered to achieve the resulting information.

Inorganic gadolinium (Gd) compounds as contrast enhancers for MRI are MPs [10]. Depending on physiological or pathophysiological status or changes in perfusion, these MPs can be quantified using MR technology. Thus, the imaging biomarker in that case is the extent of perfusion of the tissue measured through the Gd signal.

[^{18}F]FMISO ([^{18}F]fluoromisonidazole) is an example of an MP used in positron emission tomography (PET) for the assessment of hypoxia [11,12]. It is taken up by tissue and, in hypoxic cells, subsequently chemically changed and trapped. In this case, the biomarker is the extent of hypoxia in the investigated tissue indirectly measured through the uptake of [^{18}F]FMISO. Comparing these complementary techniques to assess information on oxygen levels, it is evident that the quality and depth of the information is different.

[^{18}F]FDG (2-deoxy-2-[^{18}F]fluoro-D-glucose) is a radiolabelled analogue of glucose. Like its parent compound it is transported through the blood stream and taken up by cells through specific glucose transporters (GLUT). GLUT is expressed by cells in correlation to its energy demand. Therefore, tumour cells, inflammatory tissue or myocytes as well as neurons exhibit up-regulated GLUT. After being taken up by the cell, the fate of [^{18}F]FDG and native glucose is different: due to the substitution of a hydroxyl moiety by the ^{18}F-label in the molecule the biochemical catabolism is altered. In the first step of glycolysis, both glucose and [^{18}F]FDG are phosphorylated by hexokinase enzyme. Subsequently, the glucose molecule is rearranged by an isomerase enzyme which is not able to use [^{18}F]FDG as substrate. The ^{18}F-substituent is hindering this transformation. Since hexokinase activity is the "driving force" in the cell to gain energy out of sugar molecules, it is—more or less—unidirectional allowing for almost no back-reaction. Hence, [^{18}F]FDG is trapped within the cell and its uptake correlates to the energy demand of the tissue [13–15]. In this case, the MP is [^{18}F]FDG; and the IB is a combination of hexokinase activity and GLUT expression, both representing a surrogate for energy demand.

^{68}Ga-DOTANOC (*i.e.*, ^{68}Ga-labelled L-cysteinamide, *N*-[[4,7,10-tris(carboxymethyl)-1,4,7,10-tetraazacyclododec-1-yl]acetyl]-D-phenylalanyl-L-cysteinyl-3-(1-naphthalenyl)-L-alanyl-D-tryptophyl-L-lysyl-L-threonyl-*N*-[(1*R*,2*R*)-2-hydroxy-1-(hydroxymethyl)propyl]-,cyclic(2-7)-disulfide), a radiolabelled peptide from the octreotide family, selectively targets somatostatin receptors [16,17]. In contrast to the endoligand, somatostatin (15 amino acids), ^{68}Ga-DOTANOC represents only the active binding sequence of 8 amino acids connected to a DOTA chelator which enables the complexation of radiometals such as ^{68}Ga. In contrast to "traditional" PET radionuclides (*i.e.*, ^{18}F, ^{11}C, ^{13}N,) that are produced in a cyclotron, ^{68}Ga is produced in a ^{68}Ge/^{68}Ga-radionuclide generator [18]. The somatostatin receptors are over-expressed in a variety of neuroendocrine tumours (NETs) and, therefore, represent an interesting and important target for clinical diagnosis and treatment [19,20]. Binding of ^{68}Ga-DOTANOC to these receptors enables visualisation and quantification of their extent of expression. Since the expression rate of somatostatin receptors can help to assess the dignity of the tissue and peripheral tissue involvement (staging) it represents a prospective surrogate marker for clinical outcome in many cases. Thus, in this case ^{68}Ga-DOTANOC is the MP; and the IB is the somatostatin receptor expression rate.

From these selected examples, it is obvious that MPs allow for more streamlined information. Since this information derives from a distinct interaction of the MP with a molecular structure or mechanism it represents—and should therefore be called—"molecular imaging". Of course, molecular imaging is not restricted to the field of nuclear medicine methods. Several new approaches (e.g., multi-modal nanoparticles, optical nano-tubes, functionalizes micro-bubbles) also fulfil the definition of a molecular signal; and of course, fluorescent, bioluminescent, ultrasound-, photoacoustic-, and MRI-compatible molecular imaging probes are also available.

Currently, there is great enthusiasm for the simultaneous acquisition of different modalities [21]. The combination of PET and CT entered clinical routine some years back [22] and is nowadays a common state-of-the-art technique. New PET scanners are not available without a CT any more. Lately, PET/MRI hybrid technology was pushed both by researchers and companies and has entered the commercial market within the last 2 years. Especially, the combination of PET and MRI techniques is very promising since the different types of quantitative information or contrasts from MR Imaging and spectroscopy, respectively [23], can be fused with those deriving from the tracer specific PET signal. Bringing these IBs together may lead to a better description—or even understanding—of (patho-)physiological processes on a molecular level. This could be the basis for true prospective and personalized diagnostics.

3. The Role of Radiopharmaceuticals in PET and PET/MRI

Essentially, molecular probes consist of two functional entities: (1) a chemical backbone which is responsible for the *in vivo* interactions within the organism and (2) a signalling functionality which enables the accurate detection from outside of the organism with dedicated instrumentation that subsequently allows the visualisation and quantification for MPI [24]. The signalling moiety can be a radionuclide, a paramagnetic functionality or any other group that evinces a detectable and quantifiable signal. For a connection between the signalling core and the vehicle part of the molecule, a linker may be necessary for (chemical) stabilisation. An illustrative scheme is presented in Figure 1.

Figure 1. Schematic design of a molecular probe and its interaction with the target site.

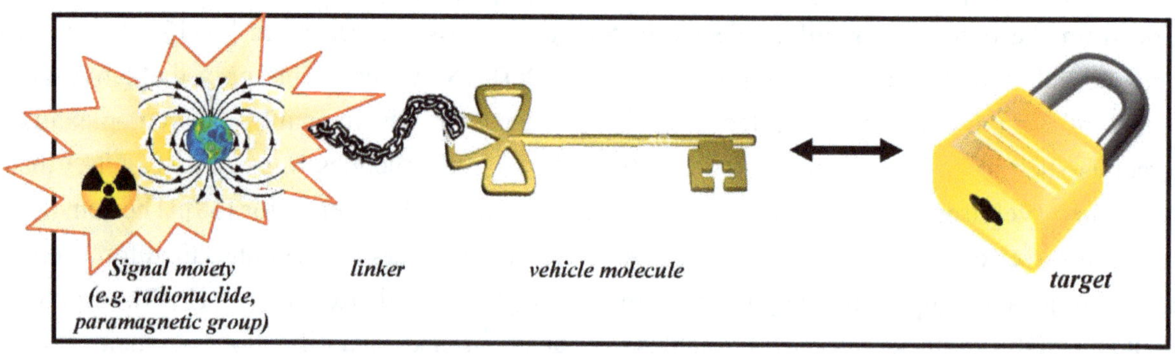

A radiopharmaceutical is a special MP bearing a radionuclide as signalling moiety. In the case of PET, the radionuclide has to belong to the class of positron emitters—examples are given in Table 1.

Table 1. Important PET radionuclides and their common way of production.

Nuclide	Production	Half-Life
^{18}F (F^-)	$^{18}O(p,n)^{18}F$	109.7 min
^{18}F (F_2)	$^{20}Ne(d,\alpha)^{18}F$	109.7 min
^{11}C	$^{14}N(p,\alpha)^{11}C$	20.4 min
^{13}N	$^{16}O(p,\alpha)^{13}N$	10.0 min
^{15}O	$^{14}N(d,n)^{15}O$	2.0 min
^{64}Cu	$^{64}Ni(p,n)^{64}Cu$	12.7 h
^{86}Y	$^{86}Sr(p,n)^{86}Y$	14.7 h
^{76}Br	$^{76}Se(p,n)^{76}Br$	16.0 h
^{68}Ga	$^{68}Ge/^{68}Ga$ generator	67.6 min
^{82}Rb	$^{82}Sr/^{82}Rb$-Generator	1.3 min
^{124}I	$^{124}Te(p,n)^{124}I$	4.2 days

The history of radiopharmaceuticals is rather short, since radioactivity was not detected before the end of the 19th century. The first nuclear medical examinations of the thyroid were conducted in the 1940s and in 1958 the first clinical application of a positron emitting nuclide (*i.e.*, O-15) was described [25]. But only after considerable improvements in the instrumentation were implemented, PET became of interest as a diagnostic technique for the community. Ido *et al.* presented the first synthesis of FDG in 1978 [26] but only the significant improvements made by Hamacher and Coenen at the research centre Juelich (Germany) [27] led to the unrivalled success of this compound. Even today, FDG is the by far most important PET radiopharmaceutical accounting for approximately 90% of all clinical PET examinations worldwide [28]. In recent years, more specific and selective tracers have been developed, labelled with different PET nuclides, providing further insight in oncological, cardiac and neurological relationships. Radiopharmaceuticals are by definition radiolabelled drugs for *in vivo* application. They have been referred to as drugs as early as in 1960 [29].

The most widely used PET-nuclides are fluorine-18, gallium-68 and carbon-11. Since gallium-68 can be produced through a radionuclide generator its application can be implemented in radio-pharmacies without direct access to an on-site cyclotron facility. A radionuclide generator requires only limited shielding and allows preparing ^{68}Ga-labelled radiopharmaceuticals directly in small facilities.

Due to its rather longer half-life, fluorine-18 can also be used in remote PET centres without their own cyclotron unit after shipping (satellite principle). In this manner, both ready-to-use ^{18}F-labelled radiopharmaceuticals as well as the radionuclide solution itself for subsequent radiosyntheses can be obtained. Therefore, the use of ^{18}F-labelled PET tracers is not strictly limited to facilities with an on-site cyclotron.

In contrast to that, Carbon-11 can only be used directly on site since its short half-life (20 min) does not allow any shipping to remote PET imaging units even if they are close by. This restriction derives from radiochemical yields and specific radioactivities which both decrease with time. Nevertheless,

Carbon-11 is of great importance because it enables the preparation of unchanged, so called authentic, molecular probes.

Until now, the clinical application of other PET nuclides is limited to research and scientific purposes and has not yet found its way into broad clinical routine. This fact can be explained either by their short half-lives (^{82}Rb, ^{13}N, ^{15}O) or their complex way of production (^{124}I, ^{76}Br, ^{64}Cu, ^{86}Y). Nevertheless, some of these nuclides will gain importance in the future since they have an isotope with suitable characteristics for therapeutic use ("theranostics"; e.g., ^{124}I–^{131}I, ^{86}Y–^{90}Y, ^{64}Cu–^{67}Cu) [30]. These theranostics enable the direct translation of a prospective diagnostic signal into a therapeutic application. It may even become possible to discriminate prospectively patients responding to nuclear medical treatment (curative and palliative) from non-responders. This concept is a clear example for personalized (nuclear) medicine.

Since radioactive molecular probes are chemically indistinguishable from their stable (*i.e.*, non-radioactive) parent compounds the organism is not able to differentiate between these two forms of the same compound. But this is only true for the exact identical substances—one with a radionuclide and the other with a non-radioactive isotope (belonging to the same element); e.g., [^{18}F]FDG *vs.* ^{19}F-FDG, [^{11}C]methionine *vs.* ^{12}C-methionine. It should be of note that [^{18}F]FDG and glucose are not strictly the same chemical compound and therefore a distinct difference in their biochemical behaviour is observed!

Essentially, three major disciplines have to interact and cooperate closely to enable a successful application of MPs in PET, PET/CT and PET/MRI, respectively, to gain IBs in a clinical setting: (medical) physics and technology, radiopharmaceutical sciences (radiochemistry and biomarker development) and (clinical) molecular imaging (see Figure 2). All experts and scientists involved in the whole process—regardless of their profession and provenience—have to invest in understanding of the basic principles and comprehension of the different scientific languages used by the different disciplines. Hence, understanding of radiopharmaceutical issues is as important as understanding of medical physics or molecular imaging as such. Overall, the molecular imaging probe (e.g., the PET tracer) plays THE central role in the whole process because it determines the achievable information and, hence, the subsequent processing through modelling techniques and its scientific and clinical interpretation. On the one hand, signal detection, resolution and computational processing are based—although not exclusively—on the chosen radionuclide with its particular physical characteristics: the selection of the PET radionuclide should focus on the following presumptions:

- Availability of the radionuclide;
- Physical characteristics of the radionuclide;
- Radiochemical issues; and
- Radiopharmacological issues.

On the other hand, it is pivotal to comprehend the (bio-)chemical properties of the molecular vehicle, especially for molecular modelling and dosimetry. Of particular interest is the deep understanding of:

- Binding and/or uptake characteristics in terms of affinity, selectivity and unspecific binding;
- Pharmacokinetics yielding information on input function, elimination rate and principal fate of the compound;

- Metabolic issues with respect to formation of metabolites potentially interfering with the original signal and stability considerations;
- Involvement in different (patho-)physiological processes such as parallel representation of both vital tumour tissue and inflammation or combined information on perfusion and hypoxia; and
- Pharmaceutical issues referring to interactions of molecular probes and co-medication as well as influence of the pharmaceutical formulation of the molecular probe (pharmacokinetic and pharmacodynamic considerations; *nota bene*: pharmacodynamic effects are in general of no interest in molecular imaging using radiopharmaceuticals because of the minuscule mass of compounds that is administered. Therefore, pharmacodynamics are not considered herein).

Even a basic understanding of radiochemical issues and preparation techniques is required for the application of PET/MRI in a scientific or clinical setting (e.g., formation of potential side-products, interaction patterns of both labelled and unlabelled compounds with the target structure, specific radioactivity and its time dependence).

Figure 2. Necessary interplay of the three major disciplines involved in successful application of PET/MRI—the central role of the molecular probe is highlighted.

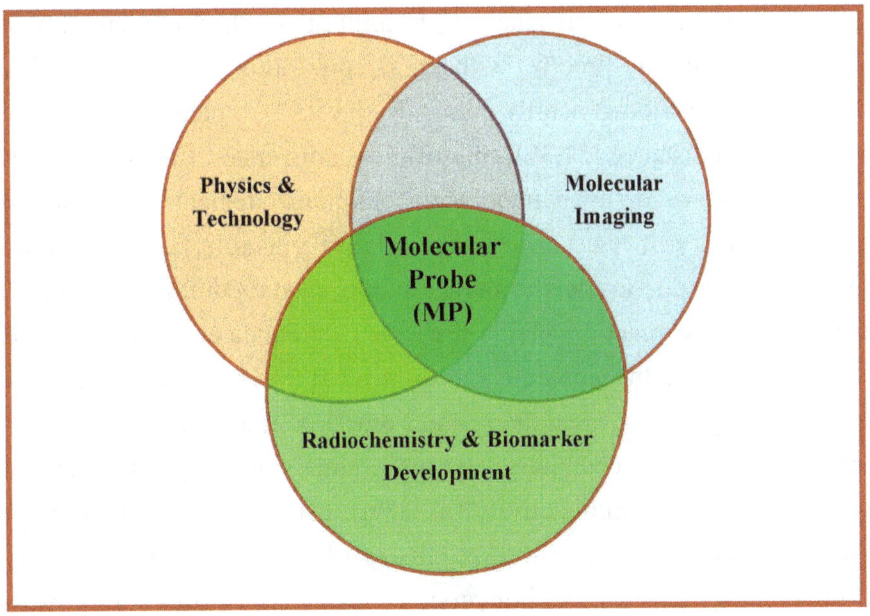

The molecular probe—and especially the targeting component—has to display a high degree of specificity and selectivity towards the target site. Important targets are:

- Receptor systems and their subtypes;
- Transporter proteins;
- Antigens;
- Specific intra- or extracellular enzymes;
- Alterations in gene and protein expression;
- Changes in physiology and metabolism, such as hypoxia or differences in vascularisation and perfusion;
- Energy turnover.

The molecular probes either interact directly with the aforementioned targets and processes or enable an indirect assessment of imaging biomarkers.

In a pathophysiological state, these targets and/or processes may be altered distinctively in comparison to their baseline status. Hence, the quantifiable signal resulting from the interaction of the MP with these molecular targets may also be changed considerably. For example, in many tumours the expression rate of some receptors or transporters as well as enzymatic activity and representation of antigens on the cell surface is modified and these changes may serve as a suitable predictor for stage and allocation of these tumours (IB).

4. Specific Radiochemical Considerations

Radiopharmaceutical chemistry focuses on activation of the radionuclide, radiolabelling procedures and purification and formulation of the product. Since the chemical form of the radionuclide (coming from the cyclotron or a generator system) is normally not predisposed for direct labelling reactions, the first step in the labelling sequence is an activation reaction. For instance, [^{18}F]fluoride delivered from the target is received as an aqueous solution that is chemically inactivated due to its shell of water molecules and therefore has to be removed from its aqueous environment. This is achieved by azeotropic drying with acetonitrile in presence of an aminopolyether as phase transfer catalyst. The next step is a coupling reaction directly with or incorporation into the predesigned precursor compound. This substitution reaction generally demands elevated temperature or other ways of chemical activation (e.g., microwave assistance [31,32], microfluidic conversion [33,34], high pressures). Due to the very nature of these micro- or even nano-scale reactions, dedicated equipment is required. In contrast to traditional chemistry, it is usual to waive relative yields in favour of reduction of reaction time [24]. As a matter of fact, due to the short-lived nature of the commonly used PET-radionuclides (*cf.* Table 1) increased relative reaction yields are often outbalanced by the physical decay during longer reaction durations. Thus, the absolute radiochemical yields (at the end of synthesis (EOS); measured in GBq) are usually higher when using short reaction times (*i.e.*, 1–20 min). This means that, in contrast to conventional organic chemistry, the main aim is not a quantitative conversion but the maximum achievable total yield of radioactivity (in GBq). It is therefore sometimes the better choice to sacrifice chemical conversion output (in %). This is of particular interest for Carbon-11: if for example in a ^{11}C-methylation reaction the conversion yield is 15% after 1 min at room temperature (which is ridiculously low and an unacceptable value for an organic chemist) and increases to 50% after 35 min under heating at 80 °C (which means that for heating up and cooling down an other 5 min are required) the total achievable yield is lower for the latter conditions! Other differences to conventional chemistry are:

- There is no stoichiometry between the reaction partners (*i.e.*, the radionuclide and the precursor molecule)! A huge excess of the precursor is present in the reaction solution compared to the amount of radionuclide. An illustrative extrapolation reflecting this imbalance would be to react a whole shipload of precursor material with as little as one single sugar cube of radionuclide!
- Reactions that are unsuccessful under normal chemical circumstances are sometimes successful in radiochemistry and *vice versa*.

- Due to the very low mass of reaction partners (often 1 mg precursor or less), the use of special miniature equipment is demanded.

- Working with high amounts of radioactivity (several tens of GBq) requires powerful radiation protection devices. All radiolabelling procedures have to take place in a fully lead shielded environment (dedicated hot cells) under remote control using special equipment for manipulation like tele-tongs or robotic arms.

- For the routine delivery of radiopharmaceuticals with maximum quality, the radiosyntheses are performed in automated synthesis modules which can be remotely controlled from outside the shielded hot cells (quality assurance). The production sequences are programmed in advance based on optimization procedures and performed automatically with constant and reproducible quality.

- Any carrier (stable isotope of the radionuclide taking part in the reactions) influences the radiochemical conversion leading to a significant amount of indistinguishable, non-radioactive product that "dilutes" the final radiopharmaceutical. This is followed by a significant change in stoichiometry. This carrier also determines the maximum achievable specific radioactivity which is a measure for the radioactivity per mass unit (e.g., GBq/µmol or MBq/nmol) [35,36]. Such carrier is introduced into the radiosynthetic procedure either on purpose (due to production obligations) or by unwanted "contamination" of reaction partners or solvents. [36,37] In case of Carbon-11, even the $^{12}C\text{-}CO_2$ always present in air may contribute significantly to a reduction in specific activity. In case of fluorine-18, the isotopically enriched target material (water, >98% ^{18}O) also contains traces of non-radioactive fluorine-19 as dissolved fluoride anions. Typically, the content of ^{19}F-fluoride is specified as <0.1 mg/L (=100 ppb) [38–40] and the total target volume usually is 2–5 mL. Hence, up to 0.2–0.5 ng of ^{19}F-fluoride are present—that equals 10–26 pmol. However, 100 GBq of [^{18}F]fluoride equal only 30.0 pg (=1.6 pmol) Therefore, up to a 16-fold excess of non-radioactive fluoride may be present in terms of amount of substance!

- When working with solutions with high radioactivity concentrations, one has to consider radiolysis as a major factor reducing product purity leading to formation of unwanted by-products. Especially when dealing with batches that are to be shipped (e.g., [^{18}F]FDG and [^{18}F]fluoride for labelling) concentrations up to 35 GBq/mL (700 GBq in 20 mL) can be reached [41]! In these cases, addition of stabilizers to the product matrix may be indicated.

Radiolysis may also occur during the production process (also for carbon-11), particularly when applying excessive heating and evaporation to dryness *under vacuo* for product purification [42]. Hence, alternative methods under mild conditions are usually applied in radiopharmaceutical chemistry, such as heating under microwave conditions or reduction of residual solvents by solid phase extraction (SPE) techniques [43]. Overall, high starting activities (leading to satisfactory final activities) and measures to suppress radiolysis have to be thoughtfully balanced.

5. Specific Radiopharmacological Considerations

With respect to the short-lived nature of the used radionuclides, also some distinct differences in the (radio-)pharmacological behaviour of the MPs occur that have to be taken into consideration when dealing with radiopharmaceuticals.

- As already mentioned earlier in this review, the specific radioactivity is an essential parameter for the quantification and visualisation of the MP's signal—the imaging biomarker. In many (patho-)physiological imaging procedures the actual number of target sites is limited and the process of binding between the MP and the specific target (e.g., receptor subtype, transporter, antigen binding pocket) is saturable. Then, the maximum available binding sites (B_{max}) determine the maximum achievable signal. Specific radioactivity (as the measure for the ratio of non-radioactive to radioactive molecules with the identical structure and binding characteristics) therefore allows predicting the amount of detectable signal, reflecting the ratio of signal-evincing to signal-erasing binding. Consequently, the required specific radioactivity has to be higher when the density of the target sites is lower. *Nota bene*, the specific radioactivity should be kept constant throughout a (quantified) clinical study and should always be included as a co-variable in statistical analysis of the data (e.g., binding potential).
- The radionuclide as the signalling function of the MP only allows for the allocation and quantification of the annihilation events. But it does not reflect the integrity of the MP. Thus, it might occur that the radionuclide (or a small part of the molecule which includes the signalling radionuclide) is cleaved from the intact parent molecule through active metabolism. Subsequently, the measured signal would be wrongly assigned and quantification would be systematically biased. Therefore, knowledge on and quantification of the metabolic stability of the MP (both in target tissue and blood stream) are pivotal.
- The availability of the desired radionuclide and the potential alterations in the *in vivo* behaviour of the MP due to the insertion of this radionuclide unfortunately point into opposite directions. (*cf.* Figure 3) For example, gallium-68 is readily available through a radionuclide-generator system but, since it is a radiometal, has to be integrated into the MP's backbone by addition of a bulky chelating group and complexation. This leads to a drastic change in the molecular structure and therefore the MP's *in vivo* behaviour becomes unpredictable. This is true not only for gallium-68 but for all radiometals and leads to probable changes in pharmacokinetics of the so-labelled radiopharmaceuticals. As a consequence, there is—despite significant efforts throughout many years—only one MP labelled with a radiometal targeting a receptor system in the brain that found its way into clinical application, namely ^{99m}Tc-TRODAT [44,45]. Moreover, interactions between radiometal and chelator within a complex are usually much weaker than covalent binding. On the other hand, carbon-11 labelled radiotracers represent the authentic (unchanged) molecule. carbon-11 is always bound covalently within the vehicle molecule, most often as a [^{11}C]methyl group attached to an amine, hydroxyl or carboxyl moiety. No isotopic effect can be observed and, consequently, organisms are not able to distinguish between the original compound and its ^{11}C-labelled analogue. Finally, fluorine-18 is also attached covalently to the parent molecule. Since normally the target molecules do not bear a fluorine atom in their chemical structure the label has to be added (and not substituted).

Although the structural change may appear small it can not be excluded that this will lead to pronounced changes in the MP's characteristics—both, *in vitro* and *in vivo*. This could be in both directions: it might lead to reduced affinity, stability or selectivity but could also lead to ameliorated *in vivo* behaviour [24].

Figure 3. The radiochemist's dilemma: availability of radionuclides *vs.* potential changes of *in vivo* behaviour. Usually, the better the availability of the radionuclide (e.g., Tc-99m > F-18 > C-11) the more pronounced the observed changes of the MP's properties regarding e.g., uptake, binding characteristics and pharmacokinetics.

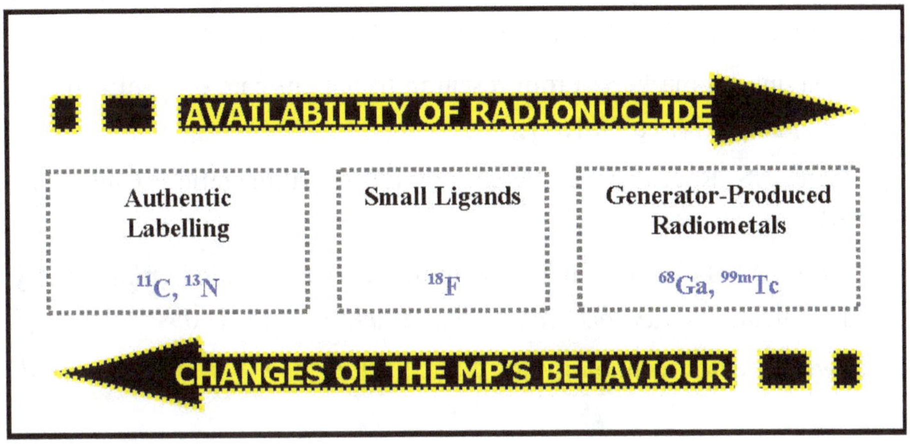

The choice of the used radionuclide (and MP) will therefore always be a compromise between availability and economical considerations on the one hand, and physical properties, radiolabelling possibilities and radiopharmacological issues on the other hand.

6. Regulatory Aspects and Quality Assessment

By law in most countries, PET-radiopharmaceuticals are drugs. Hence, a manifold of regulatory aspects have to be addressed prior to release for human. Since the majority of radiopharmaceuticals are administered intravenously, these parenteral drugs have to follow even stricter regulations. A specific monograph in the European Pharmacopoiea has been established to generally cover radiopharmaceutical preparations [46]. Furthermore, there are more than 50 specific monographs for radiopharmaceuticals, with growing numbers with every new edition. These monographs provide details on preparation, precursors, and tests of identity, purity, chemical purity, radionuclidic purity, radiochemical purity, and measurement of radioactivity, residual solvents, sterility, endotoxines and even labelling of the containers. The short half-life especially of PET radionuclides allows for "parametric" release of the product under specific circumstances (=the final product may be released by a radiopharmacist before completion of the whole QC procedure). This implicates that the methods used for the preparation of the radiopharmaceutical have to be safe and robust and included in a general quality management system.

Finally, the time for multi-modal molecular imaging probes has finally come and the simultaneous gathering of molecular information on the basis of imaging biomarkers and hybrid systems has already started, paving its way into personalized medical diagnosis and treatment.

Author Contributions

Both Markus Mitterhauser and Wolfgang Wadsak contributed equally to the whole content of this review. They conducted writing, formatting, revising and design.

References

1. Biomarkers Definitions Working Group. Biomarkers and surrogate endpoints: Preferred definitions and conceptual framework. *Clin. Pharmacol. Ther.* **2001**, *69*, 89–95.
2. Lucignani, G. Imaging biomarkers: From research to patient care—A shift in view. *Eur. J. Nucl. Med. Mol. Imaging* **2001**, *34*, 1693–1697.
3. Peng, B.H.; Levin, C.S. Recent development in PET instrumentation. *Curr. Pharm. Biotechnol.* **2010**, *11*, 555–571.
4. Mittra, E.; Quon, A. Positron emission tomography/computed tomography: The current technology and applications. *Radiol. Clin. N. Am.* **2009**, *47*, 147–160.
5. Lecomte, R. Novel detector technology for clinical PET. *Eur. J. Nucl. Med. Mol. Imaging* **2009**, *36*, S69–S85.
6. Lewellen, T.K. Recent developments in PET detector technology. *Phys. Med. Biol.* **2008**, *53*, 287–317.
7. Spanoudaki, V.C.; Ziegler, S.I. PET & SPECT instrumentation. *Handb. Exp. Pharmacol.* **2008**, *185*, 53–74.
8. Townsend, D.W. Positron emission tomography/computed tomography. *Semin. Nucl. Med.* **2008**, *38*, 152–166.
9. Forster, B.B.; MacKay, A.L.; Whittall, K.P.; Kiehl, K.A.; Smith, A.M.; Hare, R.D.; Liddle, P.F. Functional magnetic resonance imaging: The basics of blood-oxygen-level dependent (BOLD) imaging. *Can. Assoc. Radiol. J.* **1998**, *49*, 320–329.
10. Hermann, P.; Kotek, J.; Kubícek, V.; Lukes, I. Gadolinium(III) complexes as MRI contrast agents: Ligand design and properties of the complexes. *Dalton Trans.* **2008**, *21*, 3027–3047.
11. Lee, S.T.; Scott, A.M. Hypoxia positron emission tomography imaging with 18f-fluoromisonidazole. *Semin. Nucl. Med.* **2007**, *37*, 451–461.
12. Padhani, A. PET imaging of tumour hypoxia. *Cancer Imaging* **2006**, *31*, S117–S121.
13. Smith, T.A. FDG uptake, tumour characteristics and response to therapy: A review. *Nucl. Med. Commun.* **1998**, *19*, 97–105.
14. Abouzied, M.M.; Crawford, E.S.; Nabi, H.A. 18F-FDG imaging: Pitfalls and artifacts. *J. Nucl. Med. Technol.* **2005**, *33*, 145–155.
15. Pauwels, E.K.; Ribeiro, M.J.; Stoot, J.H.; McCready, V.R.; Bourguignon, M.; Mazière, B. FDG accumulation and tumor biology. *Nucl. Med. Biol.* **1998**, *25*, 317–322.

16. Breeman, W.A.; de Blois, E.; Sze Chan, H.; Konijnenberg, M.; Kwekkeboom, D.J.; Krenning, E.P. (68)Ga-labeled DOTA-peptides and (68)Ga-labeled radiopharmaceuticals for positron emission tomography: Current status of research, clinical applications, and future perspectives. *Semin. Nucl. Med.* **2011**, *41*, 314–321.
17. Lopci, E.; Nanni, C.; Rampin, L.; Rubello, D.; Fanti, S. Clinical applications of 68Ga-DOTANOC in neuroendocrine tumours. *Minerva Endocrinol.* **2008**, *33*, 277–281.
18. Prata, M.I. Gallium-68: A new trend in PET radiopharmacy. *Curr. Radiopharm.* **2012**, *5*, 142–149.
19. Reubi, J.C.; Laissue, J.; Waser, B.; Horisberger, U.; Schaer, J.C. Expression of somatostatin receptors in normal, inflamed, and neoplastic human gastrointestinal tissues. *Ann. N. Y. Acad. Sci.* **1994**, *733*, 122–137.
20. Reubi, J.C.; Krenning, E.; Lamberts, S.W.; Kvols, L. Somatostatin receptors in malignant tissues. *J. Steroid Biochem. Mol. Biol.* **1990**, *37*, 1073–1077.
21. Zaidi, H.; Montandon, M.L.; Alavi, A. The clinical role of fusion imaging using PET, CT, and MR imaging. *Magn. Reson. Imaging Clin. N. Am.* **2010**, *18*, 133–149.
22. Beyer, T.; Townsend, D.W.; Brun, T.; Kinahan, P.E.; Charron, M.; Roddy, R.; Jerin, J.; Young, J.; Byars, L.; Nutt, R. A combined PET/CT scanner for clinical oncology. *J. Nucl. Med.* **2000**, *41*, 1369–1379.
23. Moser, E.; Stadlbauer, A.; Windischberger, C.; Quick, H.H.; Ladd, M.E. Magnetic resonance imaging methodology. *Eur. J. Nucl. Med. Mol. Imaging* **2009**, *36*, S30–S41.
24. Wadsak, W.; Mitterhauser, M. Basics and principles of radiopharmaceuticals for PET/CT. *Eur. J. Radiol.* **2010**, *73*, 461–469.
25. Ter-Pogossian, M.M.; Powers, W.E. *Radioisotopes in Scientific Research*; Pergamon Press: London, UK, 1958.
26. Ido, T.; Wan, C.N.; Casella, V.; Fowler, J.S.; Wolf, A.P.; Reivich, M.; Kuhl, D.E. Labeled 2-deoxy-D-glucose analogs. 18F-labeled 2-deoxy-2-fluoro-D-glucose, 2-deoxy-2-fluoro-D-mannose and ^{14}C-2-deoxy-2-fluoro-D-glucose. *J. Label. Compd. Radiopharm.* **1978**, *14*, 175–184.
27. Hamacher, K.; Coenen, H.H.; Stoecklin, G. Efficient stereospecific synthesis of no-carrier-added 2-[^{18}F]-fluoro-2-deoxy-D-glucose using aminopolyether supported nucleophilic substitution. *J. Nucl. Med.* **1986**, *27*, 235–238.
28. Rowe, C.; Keefe, G.O.; Scott, A.M.; Tochon-Danguy, H.T. Positron emission tomography in neuroscience. *Medicamundi* **2005**, *44*, 9–16.
29. Briner, W.H. Radiopharmaceuticals are drugs. *Mod. Hosp.* **1960**, *95*, 110–114.
30. Del Vecchio, S.; Zannetti, A.; Fonti, R.; Pace, L.; Salvatore, M. Nuclear imaging in cancer theranostics. *Q. J. Nucl. Med. Mol. Imaging* **2007**, *51*, 152–163.
31. Kallmerten, A.E.; Alexander, A.; Wager, K.M.; Jones, G.B. Microwave accelerated labeling methods in the synthesis of radioligands for positron emission tomography imaging. *Curr. Radiopharm.* **2011**, *4*, 343–354.
32. Velikyan, I.; Beyer, G.J.; Långström, B. Microwave-supported preparation of (68)Ga bioconjugates with high specific radioactivity. *Bioconjug. Chem.* **2004**, *15*, 554–560.
33. Wang, M.W.; Lin, W.Y.; Liu, K.; Masterman-Smith, M.; Kwang-Fu Shen, C. Microfluidics for positron emission tomography probe development. *Mol. Imaging* **2010**, *9*, 175–191.
34. Elizarov, A.M. Microreactors for radiopharmaceutical synthesis. *Lab Chip* **2009**, *9*, 1326–1333.

35. Zeevaart, J.R.; Olsen, S. Recent trends in the concept of specific activity: Impact on radiochemical and radiopharmaceutical producers. *Appl. Radiat. Isot.* **2009**, *64*, 812–814.
36. De Goeij, J.J.M.; Bonardi, M.L. How to define the concepts specific activity, radioactive concentration, carrier, carrier-free and no-carrier added. *J. Radioanal. Nucl. Chem.* **2005**, *263*, 13–18.
37. *Handbook of Radiopharmaceuticals: Radiochemistry and Applications*, 1st ed.; Welch, M.J., Redvanly, C.S., Eds., John Wiley & Sons: Chichester, UK, 2002; p. 43.
38. Rotem Industries. Hyox 18 Enriched Water. Available online: http://www.rotem-medical.com/hyox18/ (accessed on 4 May 2012).
39. Huayi Isotopes Co. Oxygen 18 Water 95 atom %. Specifications. Available online: http://www.huayi-isotopes.com/EnProductShow.asp?ID=136 (accessed on 4 May 2012).
40. Isoflex. Oxygen-18 Enriched Water—98 atom %. Product Specifications. Available online: http://www.isoflex.com/imaging/O-18_wt-98.html (accessed on 4 May 2012).
41. Eberl, S.; Eriksson, T.; Svedberg, O.; Norling, J.; Henderson, D.; Lam, P.; Fulham, M. High beam current operation of a PETtrace™ cyclotron for $18F^-$ production. *Appl. Radiat. Isot.* **2012**, *70*, 922–930.
42. Fukumura, T.; Nakao, R.; Yamaguchi, M.; Suzuki, K. Stability of 11C-labeled PET radiopharmaceuticals. *Appl. Radiat. Isot.* **2004**, *61*, 1279–1287.
43. Lemaire, C.; Plenevaux, A.; Aerts, J.; del Fiore, G.; Brihaye, C.; le Bars, D.; Comar, D.; Luxen, A. Solid phase extraction—An alternative to the use of rotary evaporators for solvent removal in the rapid formulation of PET radiopharmaceuticals. *J. Label. Compd. Radiopharm.* **1999**, *42*, 63–75.
44. Meegalla, S.K.; Plössl, K.; Kung, M.-P.; Chumpradit, S.; Stevenson, D.A.; Kushner, S.A.; McElgin, W.T.; Mozley, P.D.; Kung, H.I.E. Synthesis and characterization of Tc-99m labeled tropanes as dopamine transporter imaging agents. *J. Med. Chem.* **1997**, *40*, 9–17.
45. Kung, H.F.; Kim, H.-J.; Kung, M.-R.; Meegalla, S.K.; Plössl, K.; Lee, H.-K. Imaging of dopamine transporters in humans with technetium-99m TRODAT-1. *Eur. J. Nucl. Med.* **1996**, *23*, 1527–1530.
46. Radiopharmaceutical Preparations. Radiopharmaceutica, 5.0/0125. In *European Pharmacopoeia (Europaeisches Arzneibuch)*, 5th ed.; (5. Ausgabe Grundwerk); Official Austrian version; Verlag Oesterreich GmbH: Vienna, Germany, 2005; pp. 823–831.

11

Radiolabeling of Nanoparticles and Polymers for PET Imaging

Katharina Stockhofe, Johannes M. Postema, Hanno Schieferstein and Tobias L. Ross [†,*]

Institute of Nuclear Chemistry, Johannes Gutenberg-University Mainz, Fritz-Strassmann-Weg 2, 55128 Mainz, Germany; E-Mails: stockhofe@uni-mainz.de (K.S.); postema@uni-mainz.de (J.M.P.); schiefe@uni-mainz.de (H.S.)

[†] Present address: Radiopharmaceutical Chemistry, Department of Nuclear Medicine, Hannover Medical School, Carl-Neuberg-Strasse 1, 30625 Hannover, Germany

* Author to whom correspondence should be addressed; E-Mail: ross.tobias@mh-hannover.de or ross@uni-mainz.de

---

Abstract: Nanomedicine has become an emerging field in imaging and therapy of malignancies. Nanodimensional drug delivery systems have already been used in the clinic, as carriers for sensitive chemotherapeutics or highly toxic substances. In addition, those nanodimensional structures are further able to carry and deliver radionuclides. In the development process, non-invasive imaging by means of positron emission tomography (PET) represents an ideal tool for investigations of pharmacological profiles and to find the optimal nanodimensional architecture of the aimed-at drug delivery system. Furthermore, in a personalized therapy approach, molecular imaging modalities are essential for patient screening/selection and monitoring. Hence, labeling methods for potential drug delivery systems are an indispensable need to provide the radiolabeled analog. In this review, we describe and discuss various approaches and methods for the labeling of potential drug delivery systems using positron emitters.

Keywords: positron emitter; radiolabeling; nanoparticles; polymers; drug delivery; PET; imaging; nanomedicine

---

1. Introduction

The field of nanomedicine has attracted more and more interest over the last decades, as nanoparticles (NPs) and polymeric structures have been related to biological and pathophysiological questions. Originally, NPs or polymers were designed and used for various purposes, like magnetic resonance imaging (MRI), computed tomography (CT) and optical imaging or simply drug delivery [1,2]. Therefore, these materials had to meet different requirements with respect to their applications. On the other hand, NPs and polymers provide an almost ideal platform to combine different modalities such as the combination of drug delivery with functional imaging techniques such as positron emission tomography (PET) or single photon computed tomography (SPECT). In this line, molecular imaging modalities are essential for patient screening/selection and monitoring in personalized therapy approaches. Furthermore, non-invasive molecular imaging techniques are excellent tools to investigate pharmacological profiles and to identify the optimal nanodimensional architecture of the aimed-at drug delivery system. Multimodal hybrid technologies such as PET/CT or PET/MRI were developed giving the chance to examine the pharmacological profiles of NPs or polymers [3]. Additionally, polymer-drug conjugates, which have already been applied for chemotherapy approaches, were radiolabeled to investigate their biodistribution via PET imaging [4]. PET, with its possibility to detect and quantify picomolar amounts of a radiotracer, has emerged as one of the most powerful imaging techniques, which underlines its outstanding role for functional imaging of physiological and/or pathophysiological processes.

Thus, novel strategies were explored for the radiolabeling of NPs (inorganic and organic) or polymers to investigate their pharmacodynamics and pharmacokinetics *in vivo* in dependence on their architecture, size and structure. To investigate the *in vivo* characteristics of NPs and polymers, it has to be considered how they are interacting with tissues and cells, and especially which time frame allows a suitable visualization of certain effects and functions, like the enhanced permeability and retention (EPR) effect (Figure 1), which is a passive targeting phenomenon and the mostly used mechanism for the uptake of NP or polymers at oncological target sites in pre-clinical and clinical studies [5,6].

Figure 1. Illustration of the Enhanced Permeation and Retention (EPR) effect of macromolecular structures as drug delivery systems in malignant tissue.

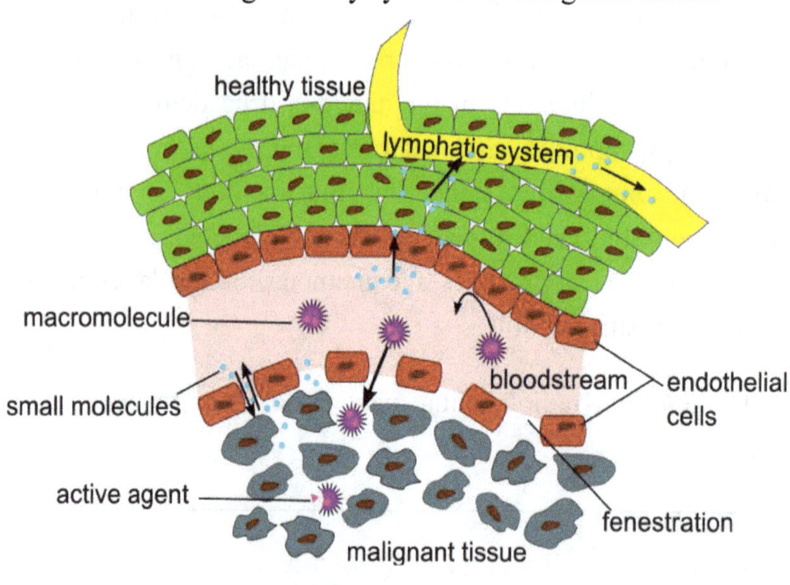

The EPR effect describes the accumulation of NPs in tumor tissues, due to fenestrations in the blood vessel's endothelial layer and a significantly reduced lymphatic drainage in the tumor tissue [7].

Since this review focuses on radiolabeling strategies for polymers and NPs for PET imaging, the radionuclides discussed are positron emitters. Radiolabeling strategies for NPs and polymers using other radionuclides for SPECT or endoradiotherapy are reviewed elsewhere [8,9].

The physical half-life ($T_{½}$) of the radionuclide plays a crucial role for measurements in the desired time frame, and it has to be considered which radionuclide or half-life, respectively, is suitable for the investigated question and pharmacokinetic profile (*c.f.* Figure 2).

Figure 2. The *Clock-Of-Nuclides* showing the positron emitters used for radiolabeling of NPs or polymers, so far. Clockwise starting at ^{13}N (at noon) with the shortest physical half-life and ending at ^{74}As with the longest physical half-life.

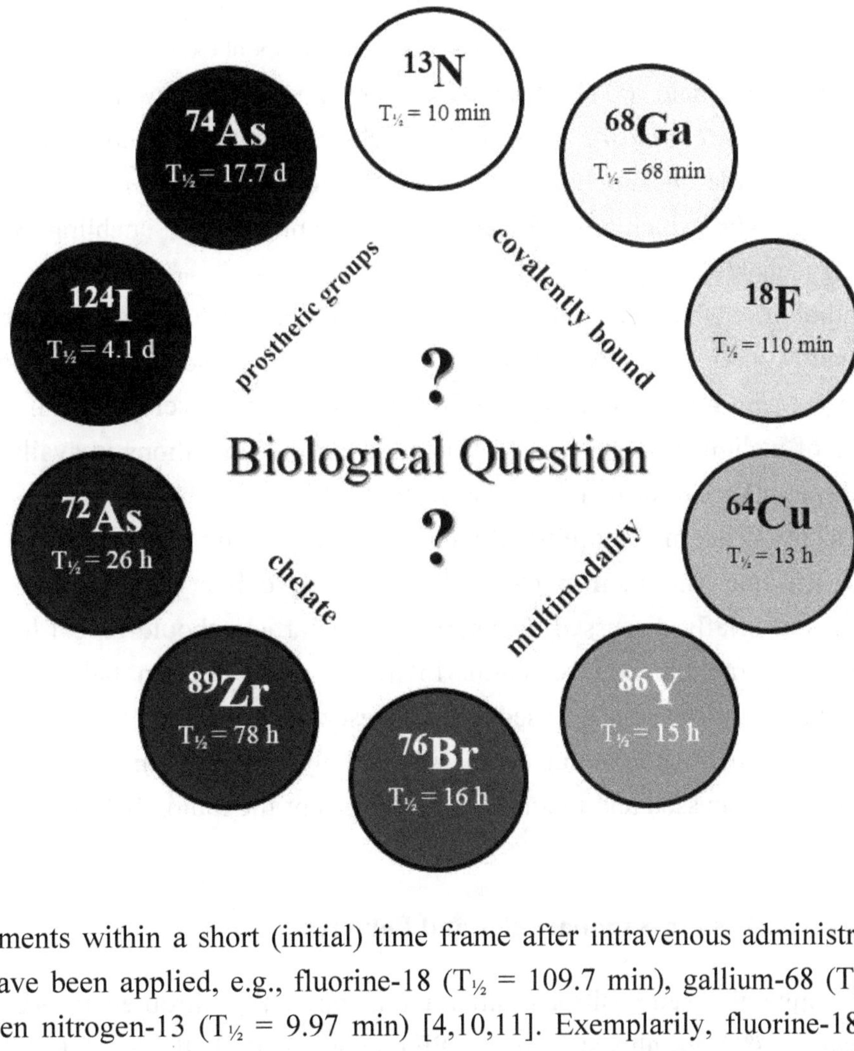

For measurements within a short (initial) time frame after intravenous administration, short-lived radionuclides have been applied, e.g., fluorine-18 ($T_{½}$ = 109.7 min), gallium-68 ($T_{½}$ = 67.7 min) or interestingly even nitrogen-13 ($T_{½}$ = 9.97 min) [4,10,11]. Exemplarily, fluorine-18, which asks for covalent attachment to the NPs or polymers, is the most widely used PET nuclide and therefore, ^{18}F-labeling strategies are of high interest. Due to its ideal imaging characteristics and good availability, ^{18}F is a very attractive radionuclide for radiolabeling of NPs and polymers. Even if the accumulation, using the EPR effect, is a relatively slow process, first indications about a potential renal clearance or fast metabolism of the NPs or polymers can be obtained by using short-lived radionuclides such as ^{18}F. On the other hand, the multifarious types of NPs and polymers require different coupling strategies, which guarantee fast, stable and high yielding of the respective radiosynthesis/radioconjugation. Numerous possibilities of how a radionuclide can be attached to these systems (either directly or via prosthetic group labeling) are available and essential. In case of ^{18}F, direct radiolabeling is often impossible or provides only low radiochemical yields (RCYs). Consequently, an alternative (indirect) labeling strategy has to be considered, frequently resulting in novel coupling reactions using (novel) ^{18}F-labeled prosthetic groups.

In contrast to the short-lived radionuclides, radiolabeling with longer-lived radionuclides allows a prolonged time frame for scanning. Examples are copper-64 ($T_{½}$ = 12.7 h), bromine-76 ($T_{½}$ = 16.2 h), iodine-124 ($T_{½}$ = 4.1 d) and arsenic-74 ($T_{½}$ = 17.8 d) [12–14]. Moreover, it has to be considered if the NP or polymer allows radiolabeling *via* covalent linkage (e.g., using radioiodine) or *via* a bifunctional chelator (BFC) (e.g., using radiometals). Thus, labeling with a radiometal requires a chelator, which forms stable complexes with the radiometal. The most widely used chelators are 1,4,7,10-tetra-azacyclododecane-1,4,7,10-tetraacetic acid (DOTA) and 1,4,7-triazacyclononane-1,4,7-triacetic acid (NOTA) as examples of macrocyclic chelating agents. Further prominent examples are acyclic chelators like diethylenetriaminepentaacetic acid (DTPA) and deferoxamine (DFO). Additionally, some of the chelating systems enable a *theranostic* approach by substituting the diagnostic radionuclide with a therapeutic one, whereas the chelator and the nanodimensional structure remain. Furthermore, it is possible to couple, e.g., NPs, which are MR-active to a chelating system enabling *in vivo* tracking by multimodal imaging techniques (e.g., PET/MRI).

Most of the radiolabeled NPs and polymers were subsequently tested *in vivo* to explore which systems can ultimately serve as for which imaging modality in personalized/individualized therapy approaches. So far, the aim of predominantly preclinical studies is to develop several tools for potential therapy approaches of malignancies and to overcome the current limitations in availability of suitable and individualized (radiolabeled) drug delivery systems.

This review article will summarize information about radiolabeling procedures of NPs or polymers intended for PET imaging and their potential use as drug delivery systems. Additionally, first *in vitro*/*in vivo* data are briefly discussed. Furthermore, this article should reveal how the biological question determines the radionuclide selection. In detail, every section has a short introduction followed by a summary table of already used approaches, which includes the type of nanostructure, material, size range of nanostructure, obtained specific activity, reaction time and RCY. Subsequently, the summarized data are discussed and unique characteristics of the radiolabeling and *in vivo* behavior are highlighted.

2. ^{18}F-Labeling Approaches for Nanoparticles and Polymers

^{18}F is the most commonly used positron emitter and its optimal positron energy ($E_{\beta+,max}$) (635 keV) and high β^+ intensity (97%) are almost ideal for PET imaging. Its half-life of 109.8 min allows for even extensive radiosyntheses and enables shipment of ^{18}F-radiopharmaceuticals or ^{18}F itself. In spite of all these benefits, in the clinics, ^{18}F is mostly used in the form of 2-[^{18}F]fluoro-2-deoxy-D-glucose ([^{18}F]FDG). Recently, ^{18}F has been used as a suitable PET nuclide to track NPs, quantum dots (QDs) or polymers, *in vivo* [4,15–24]. Section 2 will give a short overview of the research carried out using ^{18}F-labeling in combination with polymers and NPs and their most important characteristics.

As shown in Table 1, several different systems have been radiolabeled with ^{18}F over the last years. The short half-life of ^{18}F has, however, undoubtedly limited the number of labeling studies performed. Nevertheless, the early biodistribution data of the first four hours post-injection (p.i.) are crucial with respect to the initial excretion routes and seem to give a good idea of the general pharmacokinetic profile and the potential as a drug delivery system.

Table 1. An overview of ^{18}F-labeled nanoparticles, polymers and their important characteristics. (n.d. = no data, RCY = radiochemical yield, h.r. = hydrodynamic radii, HPMA = *N*-(2-hydroxypropyl)methacrylamide, DSPE-PEG2000-NH_2 = 1,2-distearoyl-*sn*-glycero-3-phosphoethanolamine-*N*-[amino(polyethylene glycol)-2000], Cd = cadmium, Se = selenium, Zn = zinc, S = sulfur, Na = sodium, Y = yttrium, F = fluorine, Yb = ytterbium, Er = erbium, Tm = terbium, Gd = gadolinium, Ce = cerium, O = oxygen, Al = aluminium, Si = silicium).

Nanostructure/system	Material	Size [nm]	Specific activity	Reaction time [min]	RCY [%]	Ref.
phospholipid coated core/shell quantum dot	CdSe/CdZnS DSPE-PEG2000-NH_2	≥20	37–75 MBq/nmol	145	n.d	[15]
nanoparticles	$NaYF_4$ (co-doped with Yb, Er, Tm, Gd)	10–20	n.d.	10 (only labeling)	92	[16]
nanoparticle/peptide	gold/CLPFFD (peptide)	23 (h.r.)	27 atoms ^{18}F per NP *	60 (only labeling)	0.3–0.8	[17]
amino functionalized nanoparticle	CeO_2 (ceria)	5	n.d	n.d	17.7 ± 0.3	[18]
hydrophobin functionalized porous silicon	p-type porous silica	215 ± 54	73.4 ± 13.9 MBq/g	10 (only labeling)	40.2 ± 0.5	[19]
nanoparticles	Al_2O_3 (alumina)	n.d	2.3 ± 0.2 MBq/mg	6 (only irradiation)	n.d	[20]
nanoparticles	gold	n.d	n.d	n.d	n.d	[21]
nanoparticles	mesoporous SiO_2 (silica)	100–150	n.d	n.d	70	[22]
polymers	HPMA-based block copolymers	n.d	1.5–2.5 MBq/μmol	n.d	≥50	[4]
polymers	HPMA-based block copolymers	n.d	n.d	n.d	10–37	[23]
polymers	HPMA-based block copolymers	38–113 (h.r.)	n.d	n.d	5–18	[24]

* The authors calculated this value from the radioactivity-to-mass-ratio.

2.1. ^{18}F-Labeled Quantum Dots

QDs are well known for their versatile optical properties and currently, extensive research is focused on new methods to exploit these particles. One unique property for biochemical applications is the fact that QDs often luminesce brightly in the visible area of the spectrum when exposed to UV. Therefore, these particles could be used for multimodality imaging purposes. However, their applicability so far has been very limited due to their composition of toxic metals.

In 2008 Ducongé *et al.* [15] described a novel method for the ^{18}F-labeling of core/shell QDs. The CdSe/CdZnS QDs are well known for their luminescent properties [25,26] and the authors described the use of their labeled QDs for PET and optical whole body imaging. After preparation, the QDs were encapsulated with polyethylene glycol (PEG-phospholipid micelles) and this coating was further functionalized with thiol groups. To these functionalities a coupling *via* a maleimido-based prosthetic group was performed, which was recently developed for the ^{18}F-labeling of peptides. The maleimido reagent 1-[3(2-[^{18}F]fluoropyridin-3-xyloxy)propyl]pyrrole-2,5-dione ([^{18}F]FPyME) [27] has been synthesized within 110 min in 20% yield (not decay corrected). The coupling of the QDs was performed by adding QDs in phosphate buffered saline (PBS) to the dried ^{18}F-labeled maleimido reagent and subsequent vortexing for 15 min. The QDs were purified by gel filtration on a NAP-10 G25 sephadex cartridge, which yielded a 1.5 mL solution of ^{18}F-labeled QDs. The total synthesis took 145 min and a activity concentration of 555–1110 MBq/mL was obtained when the reaction was started with 37 GBq of [^{18}F]fluoride. The *in vivo* experiments showed a long blood circulation time of the QDs with a plasma half-life of 2 h and only small amounts of radioactivity in urine. In comparison to non-PEG-coated QDs, the uptake in liver and spleen could significantly be reduced. In *ex vivo* studies, no cadmium was detected in urine, indicating that the small amount of radiation found in the urine correspond to a low-molecular-weight degradation product under the renal threshold, implying that the QDs are not cleared from the body via the renal pathway.

2.2. ^{18}F-Labeled Nanoparticles

NPs exist in a wide variety of sizes and materials, which is advantageous compared to the QDs. They can also be functionalized with different organic groups. These groups can be used to extend circulation time (e.g., PEG) or to conjugate a targeting moiety or a labeling agent. It is further possible to dope NPs with rare earth elements, which are known for their optical and magnetic properties, allowing the particles to luminesce or be used in MRI. Modification of these NPs allows them to serve as multimodality imaging agents.

In 2011 Liu *et al.* [16] developed ^{18}F-labeled rare earth containing NPs. As a basis for their NPs Liu *et al.* used $NaYF_4$, the particles were surface-modified with Gd^{3+} by cation exchange for Y^{3+} for use in MRI and different rare earth elements (Yb, Er) for use in luminescence studies. [^{18}F]Fluoride was incorporated into the NPs through interactions with the rare earth ions in an aqueous [^{18}F]fluoride (170 MBq) solution under sonication for 10 min. The NPs were separated by centrifugation and washed with water (3 times). Radio-TLC indicated an excellent labeling yield of 92%. Surface-modification of the NPs was carried out by coordination of carboxylic acid functions of different (bio)molecules to the surface of the NP. Thus, folic acid for active targeting was bound to the NP as well as oleic acid and aminocaproic acid. *In vitro* cell experiments demonstrated low cytotoxicity, *in vivo* studies showed a high uptake almost exclusively in the liver (80.9% ID/g) and spleen (36.6% ID/g) already after 10 min showing a decrease in the liver (53.5% ID/g) and further increase in the spleen (89.9% ID/g) 2 h p.i.. The rapid accumulation in spleen and liver was confirmed by MRI and optical imaging studies, furthermore, MRI studies showed a significant contrast enhancement due to the presence of the NPs. Considering the simple labeling method by just mixing [^{18}F]fluoride with metallic (rare earth) NPs, the *in vivo*-stability is remarkable. An early, but stable bone uptake of ~13% ID/g revealed an initial loss of [^{18}F]fluoride from the particles.

Guerrero *et al.* [17] synthesized and studied ^{18}F-labeled gold-peptide conjugates. Gold NPs were conjugated to an amphipathic peptide CLPFFD, which showed in a previous study the ability to remove β-amyloid aggregates, which are involved in Alzheimer's disease [28,29]. *N*-Succinimidyl-4-[^{18}F]fluorobenzoate ([^{18}F]SFB) was prepared as prosthetic group and used to radiolabel the NPs. [^{18}F]SFB was synthesized starting with drying and activating of ^{18}F in the presence of the amino polyether 1,10-diaza-4,7,13,16,21,24-hexaoxabicyclo[8.8.8]hexacosane (Kryptofix© K2.2.2) and K_2CO_3. After azeotropic drying, the precursor 4-(*tert*-butoxycarbonylmethyl)phenyl trimethylamonium trifluoromethanesulfonate, dissolved in acetonitrile, was added and heated to 90 °C for 10 min. Final deprotection was facilitated by 1M HCl (100 °C, 5 min). [^{18}F]SFB was purified on a C18-HELA cartridge. The eluate was treated with 25% methanolic tetramethylammonium hydroxide solution. After drying, the activated ester was formed by addition of *N,N,N',N,'*-tetramethyl-*O*-(*N*-succinimidyl)uronium tetrafluoroborate (TSTU). The product was purified by semipreparative HPLC with a RCY of 37%, a radiochemical purity (RCP) of ≥99% and specific activity of 110 ± 15 GBq/µmol. The labeling of the NPs was performed by first drying the NPs by centrifugation and re-dissolving them in DMSO/sodium citrate, followed by the addition of the NPs to 4.44 ± 1.11 GBq of dry [^{18}F]SFB. This mixture was stirred for 1 h before sodium citrate was added and centrifugation of the whole mixture was performed. Subsequent washing was repeated until no more radioactivity was released. The residual solid was re-dissolved in a mixture of sodium citrate and Tween80. Guerrero *et al.* reported for the final product an average of 27 ^{18}F atoms per NP (derived from calculation from the radioactivity-to-mass-ratio) with a labeling yield of 0.8% ± 0.3%. During *in vivo* studies it was observed that 120 min p.i. a considerable amount of the NPs was trapped by the reticuloendothelial system (RES) in the spleen. Furthermore, a fast renal clearance was observed leading to a rapid blood concentration drop during the first minutes p.i.

Ceria based NPs carrying an amino functionality were studied by Rojas *et al.* [18] Ceria-NPs were surface modified by silylation with 3-(aminopropyl)triethoxysilane to enable subsequent coupling to [^{18}F]SFB. The [^{18}F]SFB was prepared using the standard method already used by Guerrero *et al.*, with almost identical results, a RCY of 37% ± 5%, a RCP of 98% and a specific activity of 102 ± 7 GBq/µmol. The ceria-NPs (2.0 mg ± 0.3 mg) were labeled by stirring them for 1 h in a DMSO (150 µL) phosphate buffer (100 µL; pH = 7.4) mixture with ~2.6 GBq of [^{18}F]SFB. After the reaction additional phosphate buffer was added and the mixture was centrifuged. The solid was then washed twice with phosphate buffer by centrifugation and the supernatant was checked for radioactivity, leading to a RCY of 18%. After suspension of the NPs in phosphate buffer, they were injected intravenously in Sprague-Dawley rats. High uptake values in liver, spleen and lungs were immediately observed after administration. At 2 h p.i., almost all particles were cleared from the blood. The remaining particles in the blood pool were further cleared *via* renal excretion. Only a very limited uptake in the brain was observed.

Sarparante *et al.* [19] functionalized porous silica NPs with hydrophobin as a self-assembled protein coating to study the *in vitro* and *in vivo* behavior using PET. Thermally hydrocarbonized porous silicon (THCPSi) NPs were synthesized and labeled with ^{18}F. Labeling was facilitated *via* a direct ^{18}F-fluorination using the Si-F-bond formation as driving force. Dry cryptate complex (K.2.2.2./K_2CO_3-system) was dissolved in anhydrous DMF containing 4% (*v/v*) acetic acid. The solution was added to 1 mg of the NPs suspended in DMF and the mixture was heated to 120 °C for 10 min. The particles were separated by centrifugation and repeatedly washed in ethanol and water using sonication. Finally, the particles were suspended in ethanol. The radiolabeled particles were covered with HBFII (which is a fungal protein class II hydrophobin). In *in vivo* studies (rat model, RAW 264.7 macrophages and HepG2 liver cells), the ^{18}F-HFBII-THCPSi NPs accumulated mainly in liver and spleen. The HFBII coating improved the pharmacokinetics and biodistribution compared to the uncoated variant ^{18}F-THCPSi. However, a slow HFBII-leaching from the coated NPs reduced the benefit of the HFBII coating and restored a fast renal clearance of the NPs.

An elegant direct way of labeling Al_2O_3-NPs with ^{18}F was developed by Pérez-Campaña *et al.* [20]. Al_2O_3-NPs were directly activated in a cyclotron via the nuclear reaction $^{18}O(p,n)^{18}F$. [^{18}O]Al_2O_3-NPs were obtained by reacting $AlCl_3$ in ammonia and ^{18}O-enriched (100%) water. A short irradiation time (beam time 6 min, current 5 μA) yielded high amounts of radioactivity (2.3 ± 0.2 MBq/mg, saturation yield = 225.45 MBq/μA) of which 71% ± 4% could be attributed to ^{18}F, the residue being assigned to ^{13}N, which is always formed during ^{18}F-production in a cyclotron *via* the $^{16}O(p,\alpha)^{13}N$ reaction. Due to the much shorter half-life of ^{13}N (9.7 min) the samples could be left for the ^{13}N to decay without a significant loss of ^{18}F. A second irradiation experiment was carried out with pure Al_2O_3, after irradiation only trace amounts of ^{18}F could be detected as was expected from the natural abundance of ^{18}O (0.201%), showing that there are no side reactions on the alumina. PET scans were carried out in dynamic mode and showed a renal excretion of the NPs, while a long retention of radioactivity in the heart indicated a long blood circulation half-life. PET imaging further revealed a minimal uptake in bones, suggesting that ^{18}F might slowly leak from the NPs. Stability tests in rat serum at 37 °C, however, confirmed a stable ^{18}F-label on the NPs with no degradation over a period of 8 h.

Unak *et al.* [21] worked on radiolabeled gold NPs. However, they only tested them *in vitro* in cancer cell cultures (MCF7, human breast adenocarcinoma cell line). Gold NPs were labeled with modified [^{18}F]FDG. The cysteamine derivative [^{18}F]FDG-CA was synthesized from a mannose-triflate cysteamine (Man-CA) precursor. Man-CA was produced according to standard methods, which entailed the addition of mannose-triflate to a mixture of cysteamine and $NaCNBH_3$. Direct ^{18}F-labeling of Man-CA was performed with [^{18}F]fluoride (7.4 GBq) in the K2.2.2./K_2CO_3 system and DMF at 90 °C for 20 min. Purification was facilitated by elution from different ion exchange columns and a C18 cartridge. Labeling and synthesis of the gold NPs was carried out by mixing the previous prepared [^{18}F]FDG-CA with 20 mM $HAuCl_4$ solution and the addition of a $NaBH_4$ solution (Figure 3). The mixture was stirred at 60 °C for 2 h, giving the desired ^{18}F-labeled gold NPs. anti-metadherin (anti-MTDH) was conjugated to the particles for an active targeting of metadherin, which is overexpressed in many breast cancer cell-lines. Coupling of anti-MTDH was done by using 1,1'-carbonyldiimidazole as a reagent, involving multiple shaking steps, whereof two were 45 min each. The incorporation of these NPs into MCF7 breast cancer cells was higher than that of free ^{18}F (2%) or [^{18}F]FDG-CA alone (3%), 30% and 33% respectively for NPs without and with anti-MTDH. Additional apoptosis studies showed the expected decrease *in* the apoptotic effect for the NPs (20%), when compared to [^{18}F]FDG-CA with 30% apoptotic effect, which is known for cysteamine in combination with radiation.

Figure 3. Radiolabeling of thiol-functionalized Au-NPs using a maleimido-[^{18}F]FDG. [^{18}F]FDG was produced in accordance with the standard protocol [21].

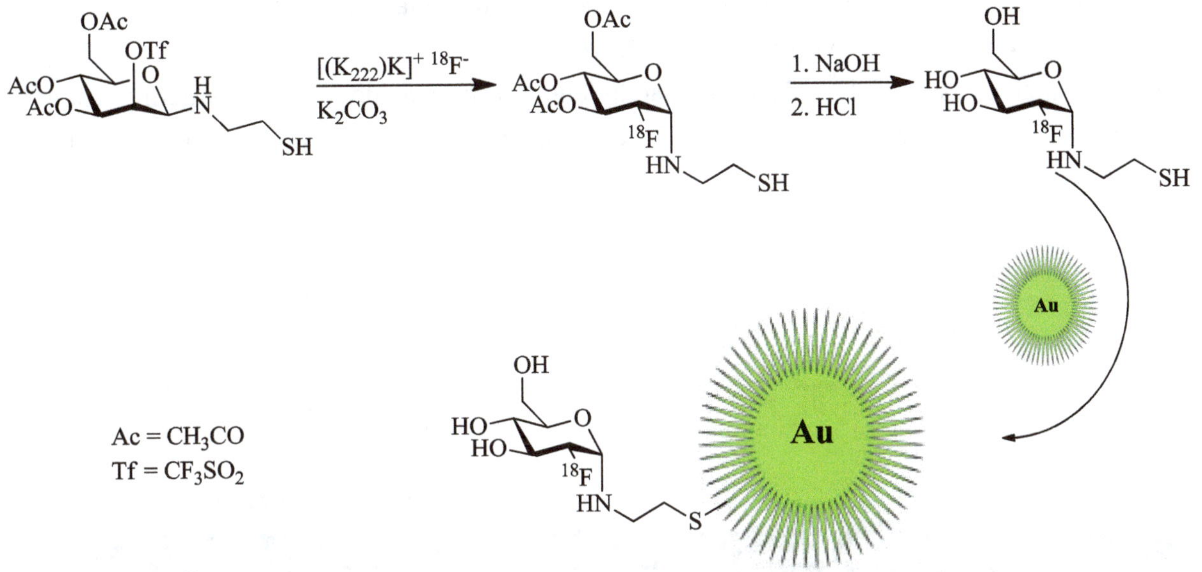

Recently, Lee *et al.* [22] described a bioorthogonal labeling strategy where they applied a copper-free click reaction *in vivo* for ^{18}F-(pre)labeling of NPs (Figure 4). The radiotracer used in this experiment consisted of ω-[^{18}F]fluoropentaethylene glycolic azide with a specific activity of 42 GBq/µmol. NPs where modified with azadibenzocyclooctyne (DBCO) and PEG. The reaction was first tested in PBS at 36.7 °C to test if the copper-free click reaction has a chance to work *in vivo*, this gave almost quantitative yields within 15–20 min. The modified NPs were injected and allowed 24 h to accumulate in tumors via the EPR effect. After 24 h, the radiotracer was injected and PET images were acquired. A control group was measured, which was given only the radiolabeled product and not the NPs. The comparison between the two groups showed similar uptake in all tissues except for the tumor, whereas the pre-targeted animals showed a much higher tumor uptake than the non-targeted animals which confirms that the copper-free click reaction proceeds efficiently *in vivo*. Furthermore, it was found that increasing the amount of radiolabeled compound also increased the tumor uptake and thereby the signal-to-noise ratio.

2.3. ^{18}F-Labeled Polymers

Polymers can appear in many different compositions and architectures. The fact that polymers are derived from organic materials means that they can easily be modified using organic chemistry techniques and that ^{18}F is covalently bound to the molecule, limiting the possibility of leaching. Polymers can be modified to carry targeting agents and/or their architecture can be varied. Some of the known polymers are biodegradable *in vivo* with no toxicity at all. Furthermore, several different polymer/drug conjugates are known, e.g., pHPMA-doxorubicin [30], and about twelve have been approved for the market and about fifteen additional conjugates have entered clinical trials to treat different diseases [31].

Figure 4. (**A**) Pre-targeting/labeling protocol for *in vivo* click reaction. (**B**) 3D PET images (upper row) and transversal slides (lower row) of a U87 MG tumor-bearing mouse injected with ω-[^{18}F]fluoro-pentaethylene glycolic azide without pretargeting. (**C**) 3D PET images (**upper row**) and transversal slides (**lower row**) of a U87 MG tumor-bearing mouse injected with ω-[^{18}F]fluoro-pentaethylene glycolic azide with pretargeting using DBCO-PEG-NPs. Reprinted with permission from S.B. Lee *et al.* [22]; Copyright 2013 John Wiley and Sons.

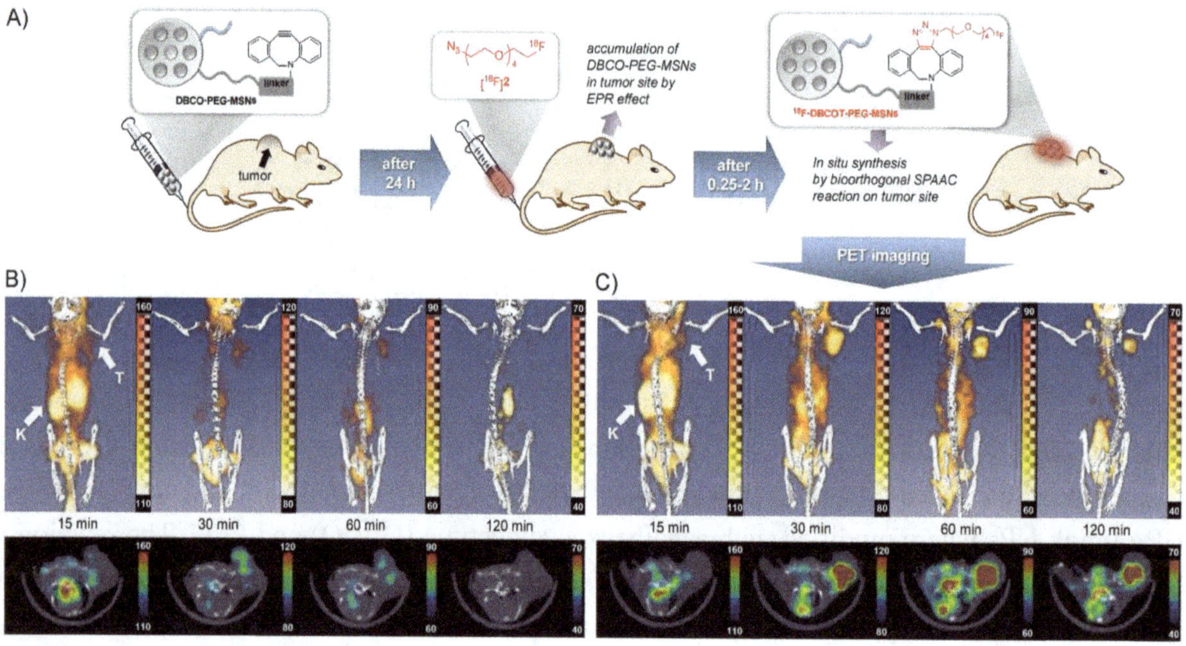

The polymers discussed in the following section were all labeled using the prosthetic group radiolabeling method for HPMA-based polymers described by Herth *et al.* in 2009 [4]. Generally, for the radiolabeling ^{18}F was first dried and activatedas cryptate complex (K2.2.2/K_2CO_3-system). The precursor ethylene-1,2-ditosylate was added in acetonitrile and heated for 3 min in a sealed vial to complete the ^{18}F-labeling. Purification from crude mixture was facilitated by HPLC (Lichrosphere RP18-EC5, acetonitrile/water). The HPLC-fraction containing the 2-[^{18}F]fluoroethyl-1-tosylate ([^{18}F]FETos) was diluted with water (1:4 HPLC fraction/water) and loaded on a C18-Sep-Pak cartridge (Waters, Milford, MA, USA), dried by a nitrogen stream and eluted with DMSO, ready for further coupling reactions. The whole preparation takes around 40 min with a RCY from 60% to 80%. Labeling of the polymer was typically done by dissolving about 3 mg of polymer in DMSO followed by the addition of 1 μL of 5N NaOH solution and addition to the [^{18}F]FETos solution. The coupling reaction was performed at temperatures between 80 and 150 °C for 20 min. Radio-size exclusion chromatography (SEC) was used to separate the smaller compounds from the labeled polymer. The SEC is performed with physiological saline solution and hence, the collected polymer fraction is directly available for *in vivo* studies.

Herth and co-workers described the labeling of an HPMA-polymer by using [^{18}F]FETos, which was coupled to the hydroxyl group of a tyramine moiety which was previously incorporated in the polymer during the polymer analogous reaction [4]. Several polymers of different molecular weights were labeled with ^{18}F and a systematic study was done to find the optimal ^{18}F-labeling conditions. Best results were obtained using 120 °C for 10 min in DMSO. Moreover, at 60 °C 20% RCY could be obtained within 20 min leading the authors to conclude that labeling at room temperature would be possible. The authors further reported that the compound was cleared from the body predominantly via the urine and that initially after injection some metabolism was visible.

In 2011 a follow-up was made to this study by Allmeroth and Moderegger *et al.* [23] where different polymers were synthesized and ^{18}F-labeled. The polymers were either HPMA homopolymers or HPMA-*ran*-LMA (LMA = lauryl methacrylate) copolymers. Different molecular weight (M_W) polymers were synthesized with sizes ranging from 12,000 to 130,000 g/mol. The obtained RCY in this study varied and a trend was noticeable that the RCY decreased with increasing M_W, the RCY also decreased when HPMA-*ran*-LMA copolymer was used instead of the HPMA-homopolymer. During *in vivo* studies, a clear difference was noticeable between the high and low M_W polymers. Expectedly, the low M_W polymers tended to renal excretion with 12% ID/g in kidneys while for the high M_W polymers this was reduced to 6.4% ID/g. The authors found a difference in circulation time between the homo- and *ran*-LMA-co-polymer with a similar M_W. The HPMA-*ran*-LMA copolymer had a much longer blood circulation time with around 30% ID/g for the low M_W and 60% ID/g for the high M_W polymer still present in the blood at 2 h p.i.

HPMA-*b*-LMA block-copolymers were employed in 2013 [24] to study the effect of different grades of PEGylation. This work was specifically focused on trying to avoid aggregate formation and reducing protein interactions by coating the polymer with amino-functionalized PEG_{2000} fragments. ^{18}F-Labeling of the polymers was again carried out with [^{18}F]FETos, however, this time Cs_2CO_3 was used as base instead of K2.2.2/K_2CO_3. The authors came to the conclusion that the introduction of the PEG_{2000} as well as the degree of PEGylation has a great influence on the pharmacokinetics of the polymer. Thus, the polymer with only a small percentage of PEGylation still showed a fast clearance via the liver and a short blood circulation time. An increase in the PEGylation grade correlated with an increase in the blood circulation time and an increased tumor uptake in the Walker-256 carcinoma (rat model).

^{18}F-Labeling of NPs and polymers is just at the very beginning, but the first examples have already shown their potential in both the suitability of the radiochemistry and the benefit of the pharmacological information from PET imaging. There is still a broad range of methods for the ^{18}F-introduction to be explored for their applicability to macromolecular drug delivery systems and further studies and research will quickly follow.

In the next section, the radiolabeling for NPs and polymers and their preliminary preclinical evaluation using the metallic PET nuclides ^{68}Ga and ^{64}Cu is summarized and discussed.

3. Labeling of Polymers and Nanoparticles with ^{64}Cu and ^{68}Ga

There are only a few radiometals suitable for PET, including ^{64}Cu, ^{68}Ga and ^{89}Zr, which are attached to (polymeric and nanodimensional) molecules via BFCs. Thus, the chemistry is quite different from that of covalently bound radionuclides. There are two main roots to label a polymeric or nanodimensional system (Figure 5). Either the label is attached to the whole polymer/particle, which has been synthesized in advance, or one compound (in the case of metals this is a BFC) is labeled first and subsequently the polymer/particle is formed. Whether to use the so called pre- or postradiolabeling [32,33] is dependent on several factors, above all the half-life of the chosen radionuclide. In this section, the approaches in ^{64}Cu and ^{68}Ga-(nano)chemistry are discussed.

Figure 5. Three general radiolabeling approaches using metallic radionuclides and nanoparticles.

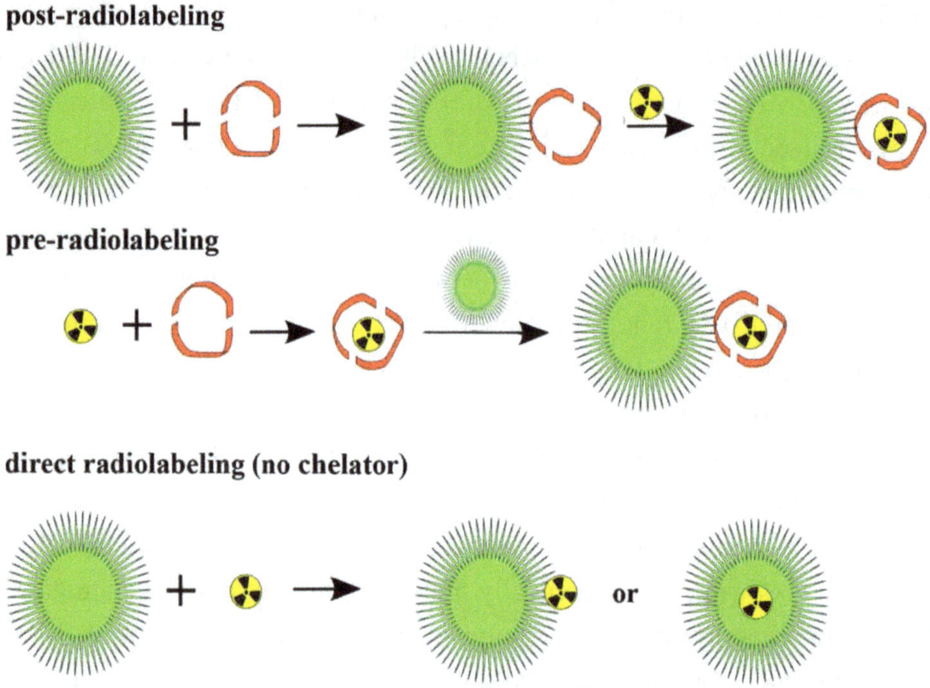

3.1. Radiolabeling with ^{64}Cu

Copper-64 with a half-life of 12.7 h, its a positron energy $E_{\beta+,max}$ of 655 keV and an β^+ intensity of 17% [34] is a frequently used PET nuclide which is available via different production routes. The most common one is the ^{64}Ni(p,n)^{64}Cu nuclear reaction providing good yields of up to 241MBq/μAh [33–35].

As a radiometal, copper-64 requires a BFC for attaching it to biomolecules and forming stable complexes. The most popular one is DOTA or derivatives of this macrocycle. Originally, DOTA was designed for lanthanides (e.g., Gd^{3+}), but it can be used for a wide range of (radio)metals as well. Since DOTA has four carboxylic functions on the side-chains of the macrocycle bearing four nitrogens, leading to a deformed octahedral complexation of the Cu^{2+}-ion, which is preferred due to the Jahn-Teller effect [36] thereby leaving two of the acidic functions "free". Thus, one is available for the coupling to a molecule (in our case NPs or polymers) and the other one allows further derivatization or acts as additional hydrophilic group. Additional macrocyclic chelators are TETA (1,4,8,11-tetraazacyclotetradecane-*N,N',N'',N'''*-tetraacetic acid) and NOTA or derivatives of those.

The general ^{64}Cu-labeling conditions in literature are very similar: Since the product of the bombardment at the accelerator (after target dissolving and work-up) in every case is $CuCl_2$ in hydrochloric acid, this species is transferred into the copper(II)acetate by adding ammonium acetate buffer. Subsequently, the solution of the polymer/particle is added and the mixture is heated for 30–240 min [32,37] to 40–43 °C [32,37–42] or to 80–95 °C [43–47]. The pH-value varies from nearly neutral (7.4 [40]) to slightly acidic 5.5 [47–51].

In the same manner, purification methods of crude labeling mixtures are quite similar. The excess of copper is removed by either adding another chelating agent (in most cases DTPA [37,40–43,46,50], but also EDTA is used [44,48,50]), bySEC (with PD10 [38,40] or by a filter centrifugation [47,49–51]).

Table 2 gives an overview on the different approaches in radiolabeling NPs and polymers with ^{64}Cu and ^{68}Ga.

Table 2. An overview of different approaches of ^{64}Cu-labeled nanoparticles and polymers and important parameters. (n.d. = no data, RCY = radiochemical yield, RCP = radiochemical purity, PAA-PMA = polyacrylic acid – polymethacrylic acid, PS-PAA = polystyrene – polyacrylic acid, PMMA = polymethylmethacrylic acid, PMASI = polymethacryloxy-succinimide).

Nanostructure/ system	Material	Size [nm]	Chelator	Labeling time	T [°C]	pH	RCY (RCP) [%]	Specific activity	Ref.
organic polymer (star or arm)	mPEG (metoxy-terminated PEG)	25–70	DOTA	n.d.	n.d.	n.d.	n.d. (≥95%)	≥3700 kBq/μg	[52]
core-shell arm or star copolymers	PEG, *N,N*-dimethylacrylamide, *N*-acryloxysuccinimide	5–70	DOTA	1 h	80	n.d.	n.d. (≥95%)	185-370 GBq/mg	[43]
organic polymers	PAA-PMA, PEG (folic acid)	20	TETA	2.5 h	43	7.4	15%–20% (95%)	n.d.	[40]
inorganic QDs	silicone	15	DOTA	n.d.	n.d.	5.5	78%	n.d.	[48]
inorganic NPs	iron oxide	30	DOTA	1 h	40	6.5	n.d.	n.d.	[39]
organic polymers	PS-PAA	13–47	DOTA	2 h	43	n.d.	n.d.	n.d.	[42]
organic polymers	poly(*t*-butyl acrylate), PEG, methyl acrylate, styrene	18–37	TETA	2–4 h	43	n.d.	n.d.	n.d.	[37]
organic polymers	PMMA, PMASI, PEG	10–20	DOTA	1 h	80	n.d.	n.d. (≥95%)	0.4–0.8 MBq/μg	[46]
organic polymer	CANF (C-atrial natriuretic factor) comb	20, 22	DOTA	1 h	80	n.d.	60:5% ± 7.3%	n.d	[45]
organic polymer	CANF (C-atrial natriuretic factor) comb	n.d.	DOTA	1 h	80	n.d.	n.d.	n.d.	[44]
inorganic NPs	iron oxide	68	NOTA	40 min	40	6.5	n.d.	n.d.	[40]
inorganic NPs	silicone	77	DOTA	1 h		5.5	n.d.	n.d.	[49]
organic polymers	glycol chitosan	300	DOTA	30 min	40	n.d.	≥98%	11 MBq/mg	[32]
QDs	CdSe	12; 21	DOTA	1 h	37	5.5	≥95%	≥37 GBq/μmol	[51]
inorganic NP	dextranated iron oxide	20	DTPA	25 min	95	5.5	n.d.	370 MBq/mg Fe	[47]
QDs	CdSe and InAs	2; 12	DOTA	1 h	37	0.1 5.5	n.d.	n.d.	[53]
inorganic NPs	iron oxide	20	DOTA	1 h	37	5.5	94% (≥95%)	2–4 GBq/mmol	[40,50]

As mentioned before, two general radiolabeling approaches are available, pre- and postradiolabeling. Several examples are described and discussed below.

3.1.1. Post-Radiolabeling

Most of the labeling procedures described here, are "post-radiolabeling" processes [32,33], meaning that the polymeric or nanoparticular system is formed first, a chelator is coupled to this system and in the last step the radiolabel is introduced. This procedure has been applied to various nanodimensional structures, for organic polymers as well as for inorganic NPs.

^{64}Cu-Labeled Organic Polymers

Pressly and coworkers attached DOTA to a C-type atrial natriuretic factor (CANF) functionalized Comb-copolymer for targeting the natriuretic peptide clearance receptor in prostate cancer [44,45]. After the self-assembly of the DOTA-CANF-Comb-copolymer to a particle, ^{64}Cu-radiolabeling was done by adding approximately 5 pmol of the readily prepared particles to a solution of 185 MBq ^{64}Cu at pH 5.5 at 80 °C. Subsequently, both purification methods were applied, EDTA-challenge as well as a desalting column. The ^{64}Cu-labeled CANF-Comb-copolymers were tested in CWR22 tumor mice and compared with a non-targeted version, ^{64}Cu-Comb-copolymer. The targeted version showed significantly higher tumor uptake of ˜9% ID/g (24 h) than ^{64}Cu-Comb-copolymer (~3% ID/g, 24 h). Moreover, the uptake of the ^{64}Cu-CANF-Comb-copolymers decreased in all non-targeted tissues and organs over time (1-24 h), while the tumor accumulation increased over time from ~4% to ~9% ID/g. Under blockade conditions (100-fold excess of inactiveCANF-Comb-copolymer) the tumor uptake was significantly reduced, and thus CANF-specificity was confirmed [44].

Welch *et al.* have chosen a similar root, by coupling DOTA to a polymer via amide formation, and performed radiolabeling with ^{64}Cu after self-assembling [52]. It was demonstrated that the shape of the polymer (*star*- or *arm-shaped*) has a stronger influence on its biodistribution in BLAB/C mice than the size or molecular weight, respectively. Thus, in contrast to the arm polymer, the star polymer was found to have an extended blood circulation time. Additionally, the arm polymer showed a greater uptake in liver and spleen than the star polymer [52].

Rossin *et al.* combined the passive targeting that NPs automatically undergo with active targeting by attaching folic acid to their shell-cross-linked micelles. Thus, they could ratify the EPR-effect, but at the same time they could not see a clear difference between the folate-conjugated tracer and the polymer without targeting-vector [40]. TETA was used as chelating agent and conjugated to shell-cross-linked nanoparticles (SCKs) composed from an amphiphilic block-copolymer. The SCKs were mixed with 185 MBq ^{64}Cu and reacted at slightly increased temperatures for 2.5 h, before free copper was removed by a DTPA-challenge, giving a RCP of ≥95%. Although there was no obvious difference between the targeted and the non-targeted micelles in tumor uptake (human KB cells, female nu/nu mice), the liver uptake increased due to the functionalization with folic acid [40].

^{64}Cu-Labeled Inorganic Nanoparticles

In most cases, the inorganic substances that are described are silicon-based or iron-based NPs. In addition, some groups exploit the physical properties of the metals, such as their magnetic behavior or their suitability as MRI or CT contrast agents. Such NPs show potential as dual modality imaging agents. A combination of a morphological imaging technique (MRI/CT) and PET as a functional imaging technique is one of the most potent imaging systems.

Tu *et al.* coated manganese-doped silicon QDs with dextrane and coupled a DO3A-derivative as chelator. ^{64}Cu-Radiolabeling was facilitated in acetate buffer (pH 5.5), followed by an EDTA-challenge. After centrifuge filtration, a RCY of 78% was achieved. *In vivo* PET images show that the QDs were retained in the bladder and liver for over 1 h p.i. and can still be found in the liver at 48 h p.i. In general, a rapid blood clearance was observed (<2.5% ID/g 10 min p.i. in the blood) [48]. Originally, DOTA-NHS-ester was applied as chelator, but the activated ester did not couple to the particles' surface. The authors assumed that the side chain was slightly too short and designed a DO3A-derivative with a propylamine chain. As a result, the coupling worked in satisfying yields and enabled radiolabeling [48].

Huang *et al.* loaded mesoporous silica nanoprobes with a near infrared (NIR)-dye, and labeled the nanostructures with two different metal ions, which were Gd^{3+} (T_1-contrast agent in MRI) and $^{64}Cu^{2+}$ for PET imaging, respectively. As a chelating agent DOTA was employed on the one hand, and on the other hand the authors exploited the fact that both the copper and the gadolinium embed into the surface pores. The labeling conditions were 1 h of constant shaking at a pH of 5.5 and 40 °C. Stability tests showed that the procedure delivers a highly stable radiotracer, which exhibits excellent uptakes in the sentinel lymph node (SLN), which could be demonstrated in PET imaging using BALB/C mice carrying 4T1 tumors [49,54].

Non-iron and non-silica-based inorganic particles have been radiolabeled by Schipper *et al.* to investigate the biodistribution in living mice of CdSe-QDs, which carry DOTA at their surfaces. They labeled the particles at a pH of 5.5, 37 °C and for 1 h and gained excellent RCYs of ≥95% and quite high specific activities of ≥37 GBq/µmol. *In vivo* microPET images and biodistribution data showed a delayed uptake in the organs of the RES (liver and spleen) if the QDs are coated with PEG or peptide(s). Additionally, the group could show that hydrodynamic diameters of their QDs (12 nm and 21 nm) had no influence on the biodistribution [51,53].

3.1.2. Pre-Radiolabeling

Recently, Dong-Eun Lee *et al.* followed a very interesting approach to radiolabel glycol chitosan nanoparticles (CNPs) [32]. Copper-free click chemistry was applied to attach a ^{64}Cu-radiolabeled alkyne complex to azide-functionalized CNPs *in vivo*. The general labeling procedure was (due to DOTA as chelator) 30 min at 40 °C, where a DOTA-DBCO-conjugate was labeled with excellent RCYs of more than 98% within 30 min at 40 °C. PET imaging in SCC/-tumor-bearing mice showed promising results with an excellent tumor-to-background contrast. Furthermore, a significant uptake in liver and kidneys was observed.

3.2. Radiolabeling with ^{68}Ga

The amount of reports about ^{68}Ga-labeled polymers and NPs is much smaller than for ^{64}Cu. Table 3 gives an overview. Gallium-68 decays with a half-life of 67.71 min under β^+-decay into stable zinc-68. It has 89% positron branching accompanied by 3.22% γ-emission [55]. Its positron energy $E_{\beta+,mean}$ of 740 keV [55] is ideal for PET imaging and provides a high spatial resolution.

Table 3. An overview of the different approaches of ^{68}Ga-labeled nanoparticles and polymers and crucial parameters. (n.d. = no data, RCY = radiochemical yield, RCP = radiochemical purity, CAN = cerium-ammonium-nitrate).

Nanostructure/ system	Material	Size [nm]	Chelator	Labeling time [min]	T [°C]	pH	RCY (RCP) [%]	Specific activity	Ref.
organic nanogels	PEG	250–270	NODAGA	15	RT	4.5	≥99%	≥1500 GBq/g	[56]
inorganic NP	iron oxide, oleanic acid	60	NOTA	20	RT	5.0–5.5	n.d.	n.d.	[57]
inorganic NP	γ-Fe_2O_3, CAN; PEG-coat	44–55	NODAGA	30	60	3.5	84% ± 6%	n.d.	[11]
superparamagnetic NPs	iron oxide amino-silane coated	100	none	20	70	n.d.	(≥95%)	358 MBq/nmol	[58]
organic polymer	poly-glycidyl-methacrylate (poly-2,3-epoxy-propylmethacrylate)	144	none	15	82–60	n.d.	n.d.	0.2 MBq/mg	[59]

In contrast to copper-64, gallium-68 is a generator-produced nuclide. It is the daughter of germanium-68 which has a half-life of 270.8 d and decays under electron capture into gallium-68 [55]. Thus, as a major advantage no on-site cyclotron is required and the costs for nuclide production are much lower.

Gallium, as well as copper, requires a chelating agent, which can be DOTA (frequently used for copper), but also NOTA which is a highly potent chelator for the smaller gallium(III)-cation. So far, only NOTA and its derivatives have been used to radiolabel organic and inorganic nanodimensional systems with gallium-68.

Due to the fact that the chelator is the same (or at least a derivative of NOTA) the quite different labeling methods are surprising. Sing *et al.* nearly had quantitative RCYs by labeling nanogels after 15 min at room temperature [56], whereas Locatelli and coworkers used much higher temperatures and twice as much time and did not reach more than 90% RCY [11]. Both used NODAGA as chelating system. Noteworthy, the labeled structures are of fundamental difference. Locatelli *et al.* described inorganic NPs composed of γ-Fe_3O_4 and cerium ammonium nitrate, whereas Singh *et al.* investigated (organic) polymeric nanogels.

Locatelli *et al.* also performed PET imaging studies with male Sprague Dawley rats to find out that the uptake in liver, spleen and lungs is quite high. A high uptake and long retention in the heart indicates a long blood circulation time [11].

In contrast to the radiocopper chemistry, in the radiogallium labeling chemistry methods like DTPA-challenge are rather exotic. Purification methods and procedures for ^{68}Ga-radiotracers are commonly based on SPE (solid phase extraction) cartridges as well as SEC. Due to the time-consuming procedure, the latter is unfavorable. However, Singh *et al.* employed PD10-columns to separate the ^{68}Ga-labeled product from the crude reaction mixture, and Locatelli *et al.* used ultracentrifugation for purification [11,56].

Kim *et al.* applied very mild labeling conditions. By adjusting the pH to 5.0–5.5 [57] they are at the upper limit of the suitable pH-range for ^{68}Ga-labeling reactions. Oleanic acid conjugated iron oxide NPs (IONPs) (carrying again NOTA) were successfully radiolabeled within 20 min at room temperature. As a result, a potent dual imaging agent for MRI and PET was prepared. They show very nicely a significant uptake in the tumor for both imaging systems, MRI and PET [57].

A quite interesting work was reported by Stelter *et al.*, where they did not use any chelating agent at all. They simply utilized the fact that primary amines can form stable complexes with gallium(III) and coated their particles with aminosilanes. For radiolabeling, 130 MBq ^{68}Ga were added for 20 min at 70 °C. Afterwards a DTPA-challenge which is common in copper-radiochemistry was employed. Hence, they could on the one hand eliminate the surplus ^{68}Ga and on the other hand ensure the stability of their compound against transchelation. They gained excellent RCPs (≥95%) and demonstrated feasibility in *in vivo* small animal PET studies in Wistar rats. The compound only accumulated in liver and spleen [58].

A similar approach, *i.e.*, without chelator, was published by Cartier *et al.* in 2007. They used EPMA-particles (poly-2,3-epoxypropylmethacrylate) and 300 MBq ^{68}Ga for radiolabeling and started at temperatures of about 82 °C and let it drop to 60 °C during a period of 15 min. After purification via PD10, the specific activities were 0.2 MBq/mg lattice. Injection into Wistar rats and PET imaging showed that this compound accumulates in the liver 1 h p.i [59].

In gallium-chemistry, no pre-radiolabeling approach like in copper-chemistry has been published, yet. Of course, the much shorter half-life of the gallium-68 plays the predominant role, here. However, only the development of faster labeling methods and rapid coupling/conjugation chemistry would enable radiolabeling via the pre-radiolabeling approach for ^{68}Ga. On the other hand, the existing labeling strategies enable the development of pre-targeting approaches based on ^{68}Ga, which is particularly suitable for the application with NPs and polymers.

4. Labeling of Polymers and Nanoparticles with Other Positron Emitters

As already mentioned before, a broad variety of different radionuclides with a wide range of half-lives available for NPs and polymers is of paramount interest. Such a pool of nuclides is crucial to meet the imaging requirements for following a slow pharmacological process like the EPR effect with PET measurements over a longer period (*i.e.*, days). On the other hand, data about the initial biodistribution and pharmacokinetics have already proven a high significance for the applicability of a potential drug delivery system. Besides, the major radionuclides ^{18}F, ^{64}Cu and ^{68}Ga, several other positron emitters have been applied for radiolabeling of NPs and polymers (Table 4). Remarkably, the corresponding half-lives are spread over a very wide range from minutes to weeks, and thus offer very interesting possibilities with a great flexibility.

Table 4. Further positron emitters used for radiolabeling of polymers and nanoparticles and their decay properties [13,60–62].

Positron Emitter	Half-life	Decay Properties (%)	$\beta^{+,max\text{-}energy}$ [MeV]	Production Route	Daughter ($T_{½}$)
^{13}N	9.97 min	β^+ (100)	1.19	$^{16}O(p,\alpha)^{13}N$	^{13}C (stable)
^{11}C	20.4 min	β^+ (99.8)/EC (0.2)/	0.96	$^{14}N(p,\alpha)^{11}C$	^{11}B (stable)
^{86}Y	14.7 h	β^+ (33)/EC (66)/γ	3.14	$^{86}Sr(p,n)^{86}Y$	^{86}Sr (stable)
^{76}Br	16.2 h	β^+ (55)/EC (45)/γ	3.94	$^{76}Se(p,n)^{76}Br$ $^{76}Se(d,2n)^{76}Br$	^{76}Se (stable)
^{72}As	26.0 h	β^+ (88)/EC (22)	3.33	$^{72}Se/^{72}As$ (generator)	^{72}Ge (stable)
^{89}Zr	3.3 d	β^+ (23)/EC (77)/γ	1.81	$^{89}Y(p,n)^{89}Zr$	^{89}Y (stable)
^{124}I	4.18 d	β^+ (23)/EC (77)/γ	0.901	$^{124}Te(p,n)^{124}I$	^{124}Te (stable)
^{74}As	17.8 d	β^+ (29)/β^- (61)	1.54	$^{74}Ge(p,n)^{74}As$	^{74}Ge (stable)

The PET radionuclides discussed in this section are quite different in their half-lives, and they are similarly diverse in their (radio)chemistry. Consequently, the following examples show nicely how the choice of the radionuclide/-chemistry and nanostructures interact. Furthermore, the broad range of half-lives provides *in vivo* data from the first initial minutes up to several days. Table 5 gives an overview on the different combinations of radionuclides and NPs or polymers discussed in this section.

Table 5. An overview of radiolabeled nanoparticles and polymers using various positron emitters. (n.d. = no data, RCY = radiochemical yield (decay corrected), HPMA = *N*-(2-hydroxypropyl)-methacrylamide, PEO = polyethyleneoxide, h.d. = hydrodynamic radii).

Positron Emitter ($T_{½}$)	Nanostructure/ System	Material	Size [nm]	Labeling Time [min]	T [°C]	RCY (RCP) [%]	Specific Activity	Ref.
^{13}N (9.97 min)	nanoparticle	Al_2O_3 (alumina)	10–10,000	6 (beam time)	n.d.	1.9 MBq/mg	1.9 MBq/mg	[10]
^{11}C (20.4 min)	nanoparticle	iron oxide-COOH iron oxide-NH_2 silica-NH_2 platinum-COOH	16 16 32 2.5	5 min (methylation)	125	0.3 2.3 3.2 7.6	n.d.	[63]
^{86}Y (14.7 h)	nanotube	carbon	47 ± 17	30	60	n.d. (90)	555 GBq/g	[64]
^{76}Br (16.2 h)	polymer/dendrimer	PEO	12 (h.r)	20	RT	n.d. (95)	190 kBq/µg	[65]
^{72}As (26.0 h) ^{74}As (17.8 d)	polymer	HPMA	n.d.	60–120	30–70	20–90	100 kBq/µmol	[12]
^{89}Zr (3.3 d)	nanoparticle						592 GBq/g	[66]
^{124}I (4.18 d)	nanoparticle	iron oxide						[67]

Pérez-Campaña *et al.* irradiated commercial Al_2O_3-NPs with a proton beam (16 MeV) and utilized the $^{16}O(p,\alpha)^{13}N$ nuclear reaction to produce ^{13}N-labeled NPs [10]. In the same manner, they already produced ^{18}F-labeled NPs via the $^{18}O(p,n)^{18}F$ nuclear reaction on ^{18}O-enriched Al_2O_3-NPs and demonstrated the feasibility of this approach [20]. Furthermore, the *in vivo* data (Sprague-Dawley rats) revealed an uptake plateau of the ^{18}F-labeled NPs in organs after 1 h. Consequently, the cost-intensive ^{18}O-enrichment of Al_2O_3-NPs can be avoided by facilitating the $^{16}O(p,\alpha)^{13}N$ nuclear reaction and the shorter-lived radionuclide ^{13}N (9.97 min). NPs of 10, 40, 150 nm and 10 μm were applied. The short half-life of 9.97 min enabled an *in vivo* PET imaging over a period of 68 min, thus, sufficient to track the pharmacokinetics and biodistribution of those NPs. The NPs were irradiated as solid in an aluminum capsule for 6 min with a 16 MeV proton beam of 5 μA. Subsequent suspension of the NPs into physiological saline and centrifugation already gave the injectable solution. *In vivo* PET studies in Sprague-Dawley rats show an expected biodistribution in strong dependence on the particles' size (Figure 6). Accordingly, the smallest NPs of 10 nm exhibited an exclusively renal excretion with all radioactivity in kidneys and bladder/urine. With increasing size, the renal glomerular filtration cut-off was quickly reached and ^{13}N-NPs of 40 nm still showed a renal fraction, but already a high uptake in liver. The tendency to lung accumulation increased with the larger particles, hence, 10 μm NPs were only found in lungs.

Figure 6. **(A–D)** PET images of ^{13}N-nanoparticles of different size in Sprague-Dawley rats (60 min p.i.). **(A)** 10 nm, **(B)** 40 nm, **(C)** 150 nm, **(D)** 10 μm. **(E)** Schematic anatomical overview with localization of important organs. **(F)** The corresponding particles size distribution of the employed NPs. Reprinted with permission from Pérez-Campaña C. *et al.* [10]; Copyright 2013 American Chemical Society.

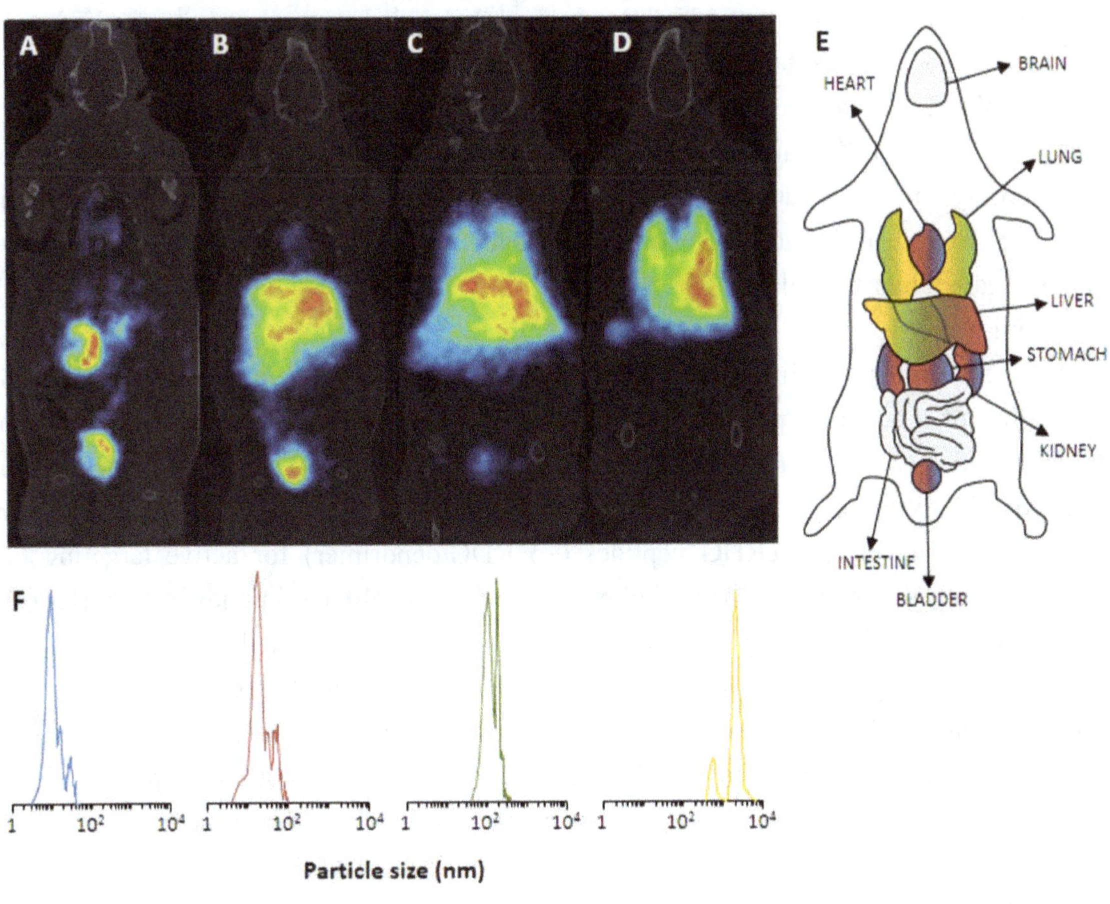

For the development of NPs for dual imaging (PET and MRI), Sharma *et al.* radiolabeled iron oxide NPs with the short-lived PET-radionuclide carbon-11 ($T_{½}$ = 20.4) [63]. Additionally, they used silica and platinum NPs to establish the ^{11}C-labeling procedure. The radiolabeling was based on the commonly used ^{11}C-methylation via [^{11}C]methyl iodide, which was produced on a commercial radiosynthesis module (Microlab, GE Medical Systems, Wauwatosa, WI, USA). ^{11}C-methylation of the different NPs was enabled by surface modification with either amino functionalities or carboxylic acids, leading to the NPs (size) iron oxide-COOH (16 nm), iron oxide-NH2 (16 nm), silica-NH_2 (32 nm) and platinum-COOH (2.5 nm). The ^{11}C-methylation was facilitated by heating to 125 °C in DMF or DMSO for 5 min. RCY were varying from 0.3% to 7.6% in dependence of the NPs (see Table 5). The ^{11}C-labeled NPs were purified only by washing and centrifugation. The low RCY for iron oxide NPs was assumed to be a result of particle agglomeration and low ligand density on the NP's surface. However, the ^{11}C-labeled NPs were stable (>95%) in plasma at 37 °C for at least 120 min. In proof of concept *in vivo* studies using the ^{11}C-labeled magnetic iron oxide NPs in mice, dual imaging of the liver showed perfect matches for PET and MRI in fused images.

A PET radionuclide with a convenient half-life of 14.7 h is ^{86}Y. McDevitt and co-workers used ^{86}Y for the radiolabeling of carbon nanotubes (CNT) and studied the *in vivo* behavior in nude mice [64]. The surface of single walled carbon nanotubes was amino-functionalized and derivatized using *p*-NCS-DOTA for a stable thiourea formation with primary amino functions. The DOTA-CNT were mixed with a [^{86}Y]YCl_3-solution (296 MBq) for 30 min (60 °C, pH 5.5). The ^{86}Y-DOTA-CNT was isolated via SEC (P6 resin (BioRad)). ^{86}Y-DOTA-CNT was obtained in good radiochemical purities of ≥90% and with a specific activity of 555 GBq/g. The ^{86}Y-labeled nanotubes were applied to healthy nude mice to study their *in vivo* behavior. *In vivo* PET imaging at 3 h p.i. showed major uptake in liver, kidneys and spleen, which was confirmed by *ex vivo* biodistribution studies 24 h p.i. giving 15.2% ± 1.5%, 5.96% ± 1.20% and 0.82% ± 0.04% ID/g, respectively. No further background activity was observed, only a minor accumulation in bones was detectable. Interestingly, the authors compared the *in vivo* data of two different administration protocols, intravenous and intraperitoneal injection. Both methods gave almost similar results in kidneys and spleen, only the liver uptake being higher after i.v. administration.

With an almost similar half-life (16.2 h), the radiohalogen ^{76}Br was employed by Almutairi *et al.* for radiolabeling of a dendritic polymer [65]. Based on a core-shell architecture, an eight-branched polyethylene oxide (PEO) dendrimer was synthesized via NHS-esters. The dendrimer was functionalized with tyrosine moieties for a direct electrophilic radiobromination. Furthermore, the PEO-branches were coupled to cRDG peptides (~5 RDG/dendrimer) for active targeting the $\alpha_v\beta_3$ intergin for angiogenesis imaging. ^{76}Br-Radiobromination was facilitated in phosphate buffer (pH 7) in the presence of chloramine-T (CAT). After 20 min radiolabeling, purification via SEC (HiTrap cartridge, GE healthcare) gave the product in high radiochemical purities of ≥95%. In *in vitro* cell assays, the multivalent cRDG-dendrimer provided a 50fold increase in affinity (avidity) due to the multivalency with an IC_{50} value of 0.18 nM instead of 10.4 nM (mono-cRDG peptide). Similarly, a 6-fold increase in endocytosis was observed using the multivalent dendrimers. The ^{76}Br-labeled dendrimers were further applied to mice with a hind limb ischemia. *In vivo* PET imaging 24 h p.i. showed high uptake in the diseased regions and *ex vivo* biodistribution studies 4 h, 24 h and 48 h p.i.

indicated a relatively fast renal clearance, whereby a prolonged retention in kidneys was assigned to a specific binding/uptake of the RDG-groups.

Herth *et al.* developed the radiolabeling of HPMA-based polymers for $^{72/74}$As (Figure 7) [12]. Radioarsenic was achieved from a proton (15 MeV) irradiation of a natural germanium target leading to 4 GBq ^{72}As (30 μA beam current) and 400 MBq ^{74}As (200 μA beam current), respectively. To enable the radiolabeling of four different HPMA-based polymers, the polymers were functionalized with dithiobenzoic ester end groups which can be reduced to free thiol moieties by tris(2-carboxyethyl)phosphine (TCEP) and covalently bind to arsenic (Figure 7).

Figure 7. Thiol-functionalization of HPMA-based polymers and radiolabeling strategy for $^{72/74}$As-labeled HPMA-based polymers.

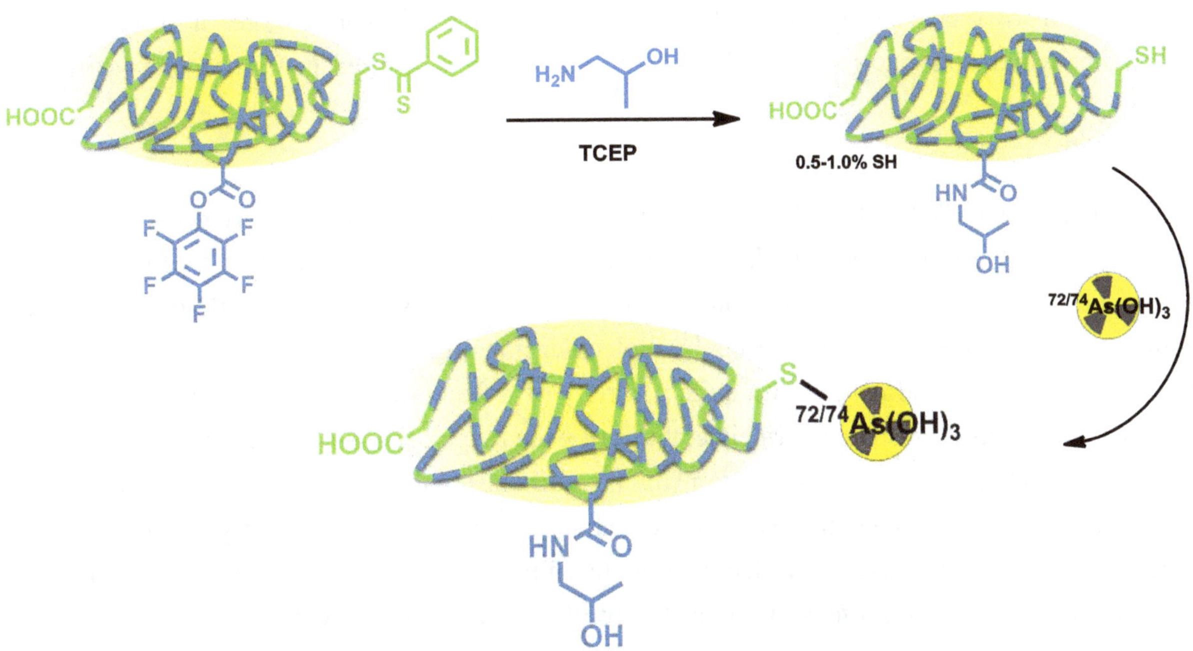

Four different HPMA-based polymers were modified, three of them with a thiol content of 0.5%–1.0%. Another HPMA-polymer was especially designed to exhibit a higher thiol content of 10% by introducing additional disulfide sidechains (Figure 7). For radiolabeling, the radioarsenic was separated from the germanium target by distillation and after further work-up, $^{72/74}$As was available in PBS solution (pH 7) [62]. The different polymers were radiolabeled in aqueous solutions at 70 °C (low thiol) or 30 °C (high-thiol) and gave RCYs of ~20% for low-thiol-content polymers and up to 90% for the high-thiol-content polymer. The $^{72/74}$As-labeled HPMA-polymers were tested *in vitro* towards their stability. All new $^{72/74}$As-labeled HPMA-polymers showed an excellent stability in physiological saline over a time period of 48 h. The radiolabeled polymers were not further investigated or evaluated.

In similarity to McDevitt *et al.* [64], single walled nanotubes (SWNTs) were employed in combination with the longer-lived ^{89}Zr by Ruggiero *et al.* [66]. The SWNTs were amino-functionalized and further derivatized with the chelator DFO for ^{89}Zr-radiolabeling. Moreover, the SWNTs were coupled to an antiVE-cad (vascular endothelial cadherin) antibody (E4G10) for active targeting of neo-vascularization (angiogenesis). ^{89}Zr-Radiolabeling was facilitated using ^{89}Zr-oxalate at pH 5 for 60 min at 60 °C. The ^{89}Zr-SWNTs were isolated via SEC. The new ^{89}Zr-nanotubes were applied to *in vivo* PET studies using a human colon adenocarcinoma model (LS174T) in mice. PET imaging was performed daily over one week. The imaging studies revealed a fast blood clearance within one hour and a specific and high uptake in the targeted sites.

Choi *et al.* applied ^{124}I to iron oxide NPs [67]. The magnetic radiolabeled NPs are intended to act as a dual-modality imaging agent for MRI/PET imaging of SLNs. Synthesized magnetic iron oxide NPs were highly monodispersed ($\sigma < 5\%$) with a size of 15 nm. To facilitate the radioiodination, the surface of the NP was coated with serum albumin, of which the tyrosine groups offer the possibility of direct electrophilic iodination in the *ortho*-position. The hydrodynamic size of the albumin-coated particles was 32 nm. The radiolabeling was performed using [^{124}I]NaI in presence of Iodo-Beads as oxidant. The ^{124}I-labeled NPs were evaluated in Sprague-Dawley rats applying PET and MRI imaging with the focus on SLN detection. Using both modalities for functional and morphological information, a clear visualization of two brachial lymph nodes in rats was achieved. Furthermore, a dissection of the corresponding lymph node ducts in which the radiolabeled NPs were detected, confirmed the imaging results.

5. Conclusions

Radiolabeling approaches for NPs and polymers are essential tools in the development of potential drug delivery systems. In this regard, positron emitters are of special interest as they allow PET imaging. Furthermore, a radiolabeled analog of a drug delivery system for PET enables patient selection, therapy planning and monitoring by molecular imaging.

Several radiolabeling strategies with quite a variety of different PET isotopes have been developed and show very promising results. In principle, the very wide range of half-lives (see "*Clock-Of-Nuclides*", Figure 2) allows tracking and detection of nanodimensional probes from the time point of administration to several days and even weeks p.i. Interestingly, several examples with short-lived isotopes (*i.e.*, ^{18}F, ^{68}Ga and even ^{13}N) demonstrate the fundamental importance of the initial few hours. Moreover, short-lived isotopes have been used in pre-targeting concepts, which offer a great flexibility regarding the time point of imaging.

However, there are quite a number of problems one has to deal with during the evaluation of nanoparticular and polymeric systems for PET imaging. It starts with the synthesis of the structures and the decision of what labeling approach should be investigated or is suitable for the biological question asked (half-life; biological target). Subsequently, the radiosynthesis comes to the fore, meaning how to get the NPs or polymers labeled (direct labeling, prosthetic group labeling or *in situ* generation of the radionuclide) in sufficient RCYs and in the right formulation, like volume activity and/or purification. If all the physicochemical properties can be fulfilled, the *in vitro* and *in vivo* testing begins. *In vitro* tests of some QDs showed an increased toxicity, which could be decreased by using the known concept of PEGylation. It has also been shown that coating NPs with biocompatible/biodegradable structures has a positive effect on the *in vitro*/*in vivo* behavior. If the toxicity of the NPs and polymers could be excluded micro-PET studies were conducted.

The next step is the use of the radiolabeling and PET imaging platform for systematic optimization of NPs and polymers towards specific applications. A major aspect, which repeats throughout all *in vivo* evaluations of NPs or polymeric structures, is their accumulation in either the liver/spleen (large sizes) or the kidneys (small sizes). Noticeable is that not only the size of the particles matters, rather its architecture, which significantly determines the biodistribution. However, as long as new nanomaterials for potential drug delivery systems are developed, there is still a demand for new methods and strategies in radiolabeling of NPs and polymers to provide a suitable (dual)system for the asked biological question. Further research in this exciting field can be expected, ideally with a NP or polymer which accumulates specifically at target sites and can be tracked *in vivo*, and/or can transport a therapeutic agent.

Author Contributions

Katharina Stockhofe: ^{68}Ga- & ^{64}Cu-chapter, Figures 1 and 5, Tables 2 and 3; Johan Postema: ^{18}F-chapter, Figure 3 and Table 1; Hanno Schieferstein: Abstract, Introduction, Conclusions, Figure 2 and proof-reading; Tobias L. Ross: Chapter about other positron emitters, Figures 2 and 7, Tables 4 and 5, and proof-reading.

References

1. Weissleder, R.; Pittet, M.J. Imaging in the era of molecular oncology. *Nature* **2008**, *452*, 580–589.
2. Duncan, R. Polymer conjugates as anticancer nanomedicines. *Nat. Rev. Cancer* **2006**, *6*, 688–701.
3. Hagooly, A.; Rossin, R.; Welch, M.J. Small Molecule Receptors as Imaging Targets. In *Handbook of Experimental Pharmacology*; Springer: Berlin, Germany, 2008; pp. 93–129.
4. Herth, M.M.; Barz, M.; Moderegger, D.; Allmeroth, M.; Jahn, M.; Thews, O.; Zentel, R.; Rösch, F. Radioactive labeling of defined HPMA-based polymeric structures using [18F]FETos for *in vivo* imaging by positron emission tomography. *Biomacromolecules* **2009**, *10*, 1697–1703.
5. Matsumura, Y.; Maeda, H. A New Concept for Macromolecular Therapeutics in Cancer Chemotherapy : Mechanism of Tumoritropic Accumulation of Proteins and the Antitumor Agent Smancs A New Concept for Macromolecular Therapeutics in Cancer Chemotherapy: Mechanism of Tumoritropic Accum. *Cancer Res.* **1986**, *46*, 6387–6392.
6. Duncan, R. The dawning era of polymer therapeutics. *Nat. Rev. Drug Discov.* **2003**, *2*, 347–360.
7. Iyer, A.K.; Khaled, G.; Fang, J.; Maeda, H. Exploiting the enhanced permeability and retention effect for tumor targeting. *Drug Discov. Today* **2006**, *11*, 812–818.
8. Morales-avila, E.; Ferro-Flores, G.; Ocampo-Gracia, B.E.; de Maria Ramírez, F. Radiolabeled Nanoparticles for Molecular Imaging. In *Molecular Imaging*; Schaller, B., Ed.; IntechOpen: Rijeka, Croatia, 2012.
9. De Barros, A.B.; Tsourkas, A.; Saboury, B.; Cardoso, V.N.; Alavi, A. Emerging role of radiolabeled nanoparticles as an effective diagnostic technique. *EJNMMI Res.* **2012**, *2*, 39.
10. Pérez-Campaña, C.; Gómez-Vallejo, V.; Puigivila, M.; Martín, A.; Calvo-Fernández, T.; Moya, S.E.; Ziolo, R.F.; Reese, T.; Llop, J. Biodistribution of different sized nanoparticles assessed by positron emission tomography: A general strategy for direct activation of metal oxide particles. *ACS Nano* **2013**, *7*, 3498–3505.

11. Locatelli, E.; Gil, L.; Israel, L.L.; Passoni, L.; Naddaka, M.; Pucci, A.; Reese, T.; Gomez-Vallejo, V.; Milani, P.; Matteoli, M.; *et al.* Biocompatible nanocomposite for PET/MRI hybrid imaging. *Int. J. Nanomed.* **2012**, *7*, 6021–6033.
12. Herth, M.M.; Barz, M.; Jahn, M.; Zentel, R.; Rösch, F. 72/74As-labeling of HPMA based polymers for long-term *in vivo* PET imaging. *Bioorg. Med. Chem. Lett.* **2010**, *20*, 5454–5458.
13. Koehler, L.; Gagnon, K.; McQuarrie, S.; Wuest, F. Iodine-124: A promising positron emitter for organic PET chemistry. *Molecules* **2010**, *15*, 2686–2718.
14. Xie, H.; Wang, Z.J.; Bao, A.; Goins, B.; Phillips, W.T. *In vivo* PET imaging and biodistribution of radiolabeled gold nanoshells in rats with tumor xenografts. *Int. J. Pharm.* **2010**, *395*, 324–330.
15. Ducongé, F.; Pons, T.; Pestourie, C.; Hérin, L.; Thézé, B.; Gombert, K.; Mahler, B.; Hinnen, F.; Kühnast, B.; Dollé, F.; *et al.* Fluorine-18-labeled phospholipid quantum dot micelles for *in vivo* multimodal imaging from whole body to cellular scales. *Bioconjug. Chem.* **2008**, *19*, 1921–1926.
16. Liu, Q.; Sun, Y.; Li, C.; Zhou, J.; Li, C.; Yang, T.; Zhang, X.; Yi, T. ^{18}F-Labeled Magnetic-Upconversion. *ACS Nano* **2011**, *5*, 3146–3157.
17. Guerrero, S.; Herance, J.R.; Rojas, S.; Mena, J.F.; Gispert, J.D.; Acosta, G.A; Albericio, F.; Kogan, M.J. Synthesis and *in vivo* evaluation of the biodistribution of a 18F-labeled conjugate gold-nanoparticle-peptide with potential biomedical application. *Bioconjug. Chem.* **2012**, *23*, 399–408.
18. Rojas, S.; Gispert, J.D.; Abad, S.; Buaki-Sogo, M.; Victor, V.M.; Garcia, H.; Herance, J.R. *In Vivo* Biodistribution of Amino-Functionalized Ceria Nanoparticles in Rats Using Positron Emission Tomography. *Mol. Pharm.* **2012**, *9*, 3543–3550.
19. Sarparanta, M.; Bimbo, L.M.; Rytkönen, J.; Mäkilä, E.; Laaksonen, T.J.; Laaksonen, P.; Nyman, M.; Salonen, J.; Linder, M.B.; Hirvonen, J.; *et al.* Intravenous delivery of hydrophobin-functionalized porous silicon nanoparticles: Stability, plasma protein adsorption and biodistribution. *Mol. Pharm.* **2012**, *9*, 654–663.
20. Pérez-Campaña, C.; Gómez-Vallejo, V.; Martin, A.; San Sebastián, E.; Moya, S.E.; Reese, T.; Ziolo, R.F.; Llop, J. Tracing nanoparticles *in vivo*: A new general synthesis of positron emitting metal oxide nanoparticles by proton beam activation. *Analyst* **2012**, *137*, 4902–4906.
21. Unak, G.; Ozkaya, F.; Medine, E.I.; Kozgus, O.; Sakarya, S.; Bekis, R.; Unak, P.; Timur, S. Gold nanoparticle probes: Design and in vitro applications in cancer cell culture. *Colloids Surf. B Biointerfaces* **2012**, *90*, 217–226.
22. Lee, S.B.; Kim, H.L.; Jeong, H.-J.; Lim, S.T.; Sohn, M.-H.; Kim, D.W. Mesoporous silica nanoparticle pretargeting for PET imaging based on a rapid bioorthogonal reaction in a living body. *Angew. Chem. Int. Ed. Engl.* **2013**, *52*, 10549–10552.
23. Allmeroth, M.; Moderegger, D.; Biesalski, B.; Koynov, K.; Rösch, F.; Thews, O.; Zentel, R. Modifying the body distribution of HPMA-based copolymers by molecular weight and aggregate formation. *Biomacromolecules* **2011**, *12*, 2841–2849.
24. Allmeroth, M.; Moderegger, D.; Gündel, D.; Buchholz, H.-G.; Mohr, N.; Koynov, K.; Rösch, F.; Thews, O.; Zentel, R. PEGylation of HPMA-based block copolymers enhances tumor accumulation *in vivo*: A quantitative study using radiolabeling and positron emission tomography. *J. Control. Release* **2013**, *172*, 77–85.

25. Zhu, H.; Prakash, A.; Benoit, D.N.; Jones, C.J.; Colvin, V.L. Low temperature synthesis of ZnS and CdZnS shells on CdSe quantum dots. *Nanotechnology* **2010**, *21*, 255604.
26. Yang, P.; Ando, M.; Murase, N. Facile synthesis of highly luminescent CdSe/CdxZn1−xS quantum dots with widely tunable emission spectra. *Colloids Surfaces A Physicochem. Eng. Asp.* **2011**, *390*, 207–211.
27. De Bruin, B.; Kuhnast, B.; Hinnen, F.; Yaouancq, L.; Amessou, M.; Johannes, L.; Samson, A.; Boisgard, R.; Tavitian, B.; Dollé, F. 1-[3-(2-[18F]fluoropyridin-3-yloxy)propyl]pyrrole-2,5-dione: Design, synthesis, and radiosynthesis of a new [18F]fluoropyridine-based maleimide reagent for the labeling of peptides and proteins. *Bioconjug. Chem.* **2005**, *16*, 406–420.
28. Araya, E.; Olmedo, I.; Bastus, N.G.; Guerrero, S.; Puntes, V.F.; Giralt, E.; Kogan, M.J. Gold Nanoparticles and Microwave Irradiation Inhibit Beta-Amyloid Amyloidogenesis. *Nanoscale Res. Lett.* **2008**, *3*, 435–443.
29. Kogan, M.J.; Bastus, N.G.; Amigo, R.; Grillo-Bosch, D.; Araya, E.; Turiel, A.; Labarta, A.; Giralt, E.; Puntes, V.F. Nanoparticle-mediated local and remote manipulation of protein aggregation. *Nano Lett.* **2006**, *6*, 110–115.
30. Lu, Z.-R. Molecular imaging of HPMA copolymers: Visualizing drug delivery in cell, mouse and man. *Adv. Drug Deliv. Rev.* **2010**, *62*, 246–257.
31. Duncan, R.; Vicent, M.J. Polymer therapeutics-prospects for 21st century: The end of the beginning. *Adv. Drug Deliv. Rev.* **2013**, *65*, 60–70.
32. Lee, D.-E.; Na, J.H.; Lee, S.; Kang, C.M.; Kim, H.N.; Han, S.J.; Kim, H.; Choe, Y.S.; Jung, K.-H.; Lee, K.C.; *et al.* Facile method to radiolabel glycol chitosan nanoparticles with (64)Cu via copper-free click chemistry for MicroPET imaging. *Mol. Pharm.* **2013**, *10*, 2190–2198.
33. Liu, Y.; Welch, M.J. Nanoparticles labeled with positron emitting nuclides: Advantages, methods, and applications. *Bioconjug. Chem.* **2012**, *23*, 671–682.
34. Welch, M.J., Redvanly, C.S. *Handbook of Radiopharmaceuticals: Radiochemistry and Applications*; Wiley: Hoboken, NJ, USA, 2003; pp. 1–471.
35. Smith, S.V. Molecular imaging with copper-64. *J. Inorg. Biochem.* **2004**, *98*, 1874–1901.
36. Riedel, E. *Anorganische Chemie*, 5th ed.; de Gruyter: Berlin, Germany, 2002; p. 736.
37. Sun, X.; Rossin, R.; Turner, J.L.; Becker, M.L.; Joralemon, M.J.; Welch, M.J.; Wooley, K.L. An assessment of the effects of shell cross-linked nanoparticle size, core composition, and surface PEGylation on *in vivo* biodistribution. *Biomacromolecules* **2005**, *6*, 2541–2554.
38. Cai, W.; Wu, Y.; Chen, K.; Cao, Q.; Tice, D.A.; Chen, X. In vitro and *in vivo* characterization of ^{64}Cu-labeled Abegrin, a humanized monoclonal antibody against integrin alpha v beta 3. *Cancer Res.* **2006**, *66*, 9673–9681.
39. Xie, J.; Chen, K.; Huang, J.; Lee, S.; Wang, J.; Gao, J.; Li, X.; Chen, X. PET/NIRF/MRI triple functional iron oxide nanoparticles. *Biomaterials* **2010**, *31*, 3016–3022.
40. Yang, X.; Hong, H.; Grailer, J.J.; Rowland, I.J.; Javadi, A.; Hurley, S.A.; Xiao, Y.; Yang, Y.; Zhang, Y.; Nickles, R.J.; *et al.* cRGD-functionalized, DOX-conjugated, and ^{64}Cu-labeled superparamagnetic iron oxide nanoparticles for targeted anticancer drug delivery and PET/MR imaging. *Biomaterials* **2011**, *32*, 4151–4160.
41. Rossin, R.; Pan, D.; Qi, K.; Turner, J.L.; Sun, X.; Wooley, K.L.; Welch, M.J. Radio2herapy: Synthesis, Radiolabeling, and Biologic Evaluation. *J. Nucl. Med.* **2005**, *46*, 1210–1218.

42. Sun, G.; Xu, J.; Hagooly, A.; Rossin, R.; Li, Z.; Moore, D.A.; Hawker, C.J.; Welch, M.J.; Wooley, K.L. Strategies for Optimized Radiolabeling of Nanoparticles for *in vivo* PET Imaging. *Adv. Mater.* **2007**, *19*, 3157–3162.
43. Fukukawa, K.; Rossin, R.; Hagooly, A.; Pressly, E.D.; Hunt, J.N.; Messmore, B.W.; Wooley, K.L.; Welch, M.J.; Hawker, C.J. Synthesis and characterization of core-shell star copolymers for *in vivo* PET imaging applications. *Biomacromolecules* **2008**, *9*, 1329–1339.
44. Pressly, E.D.; Pierce, R.A; Connal, L.A; Hawker, C.J.; Liu, Y. Nanoparticle PET/CT imaging of natriuretic peptide clearance receptor in prostate cancer. *Bioconjug. Chem.* **2013**, *24*, 196–204.
45. Liu, Y.; Pressly, E.D.; Abendschein, D.R.; Hawker, C.J.; Woodard, G.E.; Woodard, P.K.; Welch, M.J. Targeting angiogenesis using a C-type atrial natriuretic factor-conjugated nanoprobe and PET. *J. Nucl. Med.* **2011**, *52*, 1956–1963.
46. Pressly, E.D.; Rossin, R.; Hagooly, A.; Fukukawa, K.; Messmore, B.W.; Welch, M.J.; Wooley, K.L.; Lamm, M.S.; Hule, R.A.; Pochan, D.J.; *et al.* Structural Effects on the Biodistribution and Positron Emission Nanoparticles Comprised of Amphiphilic Block Graft Copolymers. *Biomacromolecules* **2007**, *8*, 3126–3134.
47. Nahrendorf, M.; Zhang, H.; Hembrador, S.; Panizzi, P.; Sosnovik, D.E.; Aikawa, E.; Libby, P.; Swirski, F.K.; Weissleder, R. Nanoparticle PET-CT imaging of macrophages in inflammatory atherosclerosis. *Circulation* **2008**, *117*, 379–387.
48. Tu, C.; Ma, X.; House, A.; Kauzlarich, S.M.; Louie, A.Y. PET Imaging and Biodistribution of Silicon Quantum Dots in Mice. *ACS Med. Chem. Lett.* **2011**, *2*, 285–288.
49. Huang, X.; Zhang, F.; Lee, S.; Swierczewska, M.; Kiesewetter, D.O.; Lang, L.; Zhang, G.; Zhu, L.; Gao, H.; Choi, H.S.; *et al.* Long-term multimodal imaging of tumor draining sentinel lymph nodes using mesoporous silica-based nanoprobes. *Biomaterials* **2012**, *33*, 4370–4378.
50. Glaus, C.; Rossin, R.; Welch, M.J.; Bao, G. *In vivo* evaluation of (64)Cu-labeled magnetic nanoparticles as a dual-modality PET/MR imaging agent. *Bioconjug. Chem.* **2010**, *21*, 715–722.
51. Schipper, M.L.; Cheng, Z.; Lee, S.-W.; Bentolila, L.A; Iyer, G.; Rao, J.; Chen, X.; Wu, A.M.; Weiss, S.; Gambhir, S.S. microPET-based biodistribution of quantum dots in living mice. *J. Nucl. Med.* **2007**, *48*, 1511–1518.
52. Welch, M.J.; Hawker, C.J.; Wooley, K.L. The advantages of nanoparticles for PET. *J. Nucl. Med.* **2009**, *50*, 1743–1746.
53. Schipper, M.L.; Iyer, G.; Koh, A.L.; Cheng, Z.; Ebenstein, Y.; Aharoni, A.; Keren, S.; Bentolila, L.A; Li, J.; Rao, J.; *et al.* Particle size, surface coating, and PEGylation influence the biodistribution of quantum dots in living mice. *Small* **2009**, *5*, 126–134.
54. Hooker, J.M. Modular strategies for PET imaging agents. *Curr. Opin. Chem. Biol.* **2010**, *14*, 105–111.
55. Roesch, F. Maturation of a key resource—The germanium-68/gallium-68 generator: Development and new insights. *Curr. Radiopharm.* **2012**, *5*, 202–211.
56. Singh, S.; Bingöl, B.; Morgenroth, A.; Mottaghy, F.M.; Möller, M.; Schmaljohann, J. Radiolabeled nanogels for nuclear molecular imaging. *Macromol. Rapid Commun.* **2013**, *34*, 562–567.

57. Kim, S.-M.; Chae, M.K.; Yim, M.S.; Jeong, I.H.; Cho, J.; Lee, C.; Ryu, E.K. Hybrid PET/MR imaging of tumors using an oleanolic acid-conjugated nanoparticle. *Biomaterials* **2013**, *34*, 8114–8121.
58. Stelter, L.; Pinkernelle, J.G.; Michel, R.; Schwartländer, R.; Raschzok, N.; Morgul, M.H.; Koch, M.; Denecke, T.; Ruf, J.; Bäumler, H.; *et al.* Modification of aminosilanized superparamagnetic nanoparticles: Feasibility of multimodal detection using 3T MRI, small animal PET, and fluorescence imaging. *Mol. Imaging Biol.* **2010**, *12*, 25–34.
59. Cartier, R.; Kaufner, L.; Paulke, B.R.; Wüstneck, R.; Pietschmann, S.; Michel, R.; Bruhn, H.; Pison, U. Latex nanoparticles for multimodal imaging and detection *in vivo*. *Nanotechnology* **2007**, *18*, 195102.
60. Qaim, S.M. Development of novel positron emitters for medical applications: Nuclear and radiochemical aspects. *Radiochim. Acta* **2011**, *99*, 611–625.
61. Qaim, S.M. The present and future of medical radionuclide production. *Radiochim. Acta* **2012**, *100*, 635–651.
62. Jahn, M.; Radchenko, V.; Filosofov, D.V.; Hauser, H.; Eisenhut, M.; Rösch, F.; Jennewein, M. Separation and purification of no-carrier-added arsenic from bulk amounts of germanium for use in radiopharmaceutical labelling. *Radiochim. Acta* **2010**, *98*, 807–812.
63. Sharma, R.; Xu, Y.; Kim, S.W.; Schueller, M.J.; Alexoff, D.; Smith, S.D.; Wang, W.; Schlyer, D. Carbon-11 radiolabeling of iron-oxide nanoparticles for dual-modality PET/MR imaging. *Nanoscale* **2013**, *5*, 7476–7483.
64. McDevitt, M.R.; Chattopadhyay, D.; Jaggi, J.S.; Finn, R.D.; Zanzonico, P.B.; Villa, C.; Rey, D.; Mendenhall, J.; Batt, C.A; Njardarson, J.T.; *et al.* a PET imaging of soluble yttrium-86-labeled carbon nanotubes in mice. *PLoS One* **2007**, *2*, e907.
65. Almutairi, A.; Rossin, R.; Shokeen, M.; Hagooly, A.; Ananth, A.; Capoccia, B.; Guillaudeu, S.; Abendschein, D.; Anderson, C.J.; Welch, M.J.; *et al.* Biodegradable dendritic positron-emitting nanoprobes for the noninvasive imaging of angiogenesis. *Proc. Natl. Acad. Sci. USA* **2009**, *106*, 685–690.
66. Ruggiero, A.; Villa, C.H.; Holland, J.P.; Sprinkle, S.R.; May, C.; Lewis, J.S.; Scheinberg, D.A; McDevitt, M.R. Imaging and treating tumor vasculature with targeted radiolabeled carbon nanotubes. *Int. J. Nanomed.* **2010**, *5*, 783–802.
67. Choi, J.; Park, J.C.; Nah, H.; Woo, S.; Oh, J.; Kim, K.M.; Cheon, G.J.; Chang, Y.; Yoo, J.; Cheon, J. A hybrid nanoparticle probe for dual-modality positron emission tomography and magnetic resonance imaging. *Angew. Chem. Int. Ed. Engl.* **2008**, *47*, 6259–6262.

12

Radiolabeled Cetuximab Conjugates for EGFR Targeted Cancer Diagnostics and Therapy †

Wiebke Sihver [1,*], Jens Pietzsch [1,2], Mechthild Krause [3,4,5,6], Michael Baumann [3,4,5,6], Jörg Steinbach [1,2] and Hans-Jürgen Pietzsch [1]

1. Helmholtz-Zentrum Dresden-Rossendorf (HZDR), Institute of Radiopharmaceutical Cancer Research, Bautzner Landstraße 400, Dresden 01328, Germany; E-Mails: j.pietzsch@hzdr.de (J.P.); j.steinbach@hzdr.de (J.S.); h.j.pietzsch@hzdr.de (H.-J.P)
2. Department of Chemistry and Food Chemistry, Technische Universität Dresden, Dresden 01062, Germany
3. Department of Radiation Oncology and OncoRay, Medical Faculty and University Hospital Carl Gustav Carus, Technische Universität Dresden, Dresden 01307, Germany; E-Mails: mechthild.krause@uniklinikum-dresden.de (M.K.); michael.baumann@uniklinikum-dresden.de (M.B.)
4. OncoRay—National Center for Radiation Research in Oncology, Medical Faculty and University Hospital Carl Gustav Carus, Technische Universität Dresden, Dresden 01307, Germany
5. German Cancer Consortium (DKTK) Dresden and German Cancer Research Center (DKFZ), Heidelberg 69120, Germany
6. HZDR, Institute of Radiation Oncology, Bautzner Landstraße 400, Dresden 01328, Germany

† Dedicated to Prof. Bernd Johannsen (Dresden-Rossendorf) on the occasion of his 75th birthday

* Author to whom correspondence should be addressed; E-Mail: w.sihver@hzdr.de

---

Abstract: The epidermal growth factor receptor (EGFR) has evolved over years into a main molecular target for the treatment of different cancer entities. In this regard, the anti-EGFR antibody cetuximab has been approved alone or in combination with: (a) chemotherapy for treatment of colorectal and head and neck squamous cell carcinoma and (b) with external radiotherapy for treatment of head and neck squamous cell carcinoma. The conjugation of radionuclides to cetuximab in combination with the specific targeting properties of this antibody might increase its therapeutic efficiency. This review article gives an overview of the preclinical studies that have been performed with radiolabeled cetuximab for imaging and/or treatment of different tumor models. A particularly promising approach seems to be the treatment with therapeutic radionuclide-labeled cetuximab in combination with external radiotherapy. Present data support an important impact of the tumor micromilieu on treatment response that needs to be further validated in patients. Another important challenge is the reduction of nonspecific uptake of the radioactive substance in metabolic organs like liver and radiosensitive organs like bone marrow and kidneys. Overall, the integration of diagnosis, treatment and monitoring as a theranostic approach appears to be a promising strategy for improvement of individualized cancer treatment.

Keywords: EGFR; radiolabeled cetuximab conjugates; radioimmunotherapy (RIT); cancer theranostics; external beam radiotherapy (EBRT); endoradionuclide therapy

---

1. Introduction

Worldwide, cancer is one of the most common causes of death. In general, patients will be treated with approaches comprising surgery or external beam radiotherapy (EBRT) alone, or surgery combined with EBRT or chemotherapy, that have been developed and improved in the last years [1–3]. In EBRT usually 1.8 to 2 Gy fractions are delivered from a linear accelerator over several weeks. Radioimmunotherapy (RIT) approaches are applying radioactive antibodies (Ab) or Ab fragments in patients either locally close to the tumor or systemically with the goal to bind to tumor specific targets, thereby inactivating cancer cells. Remarkably, the curative treatment of metastases by RIT might be a special chance of this method. For patients with advanced inoperable stages of cancer, particularly head and neck cancer, primary radiochemotherapy still offers curative potential that has increased over the last decades by improvement of techniques and combined radiochemotherapy treatment approaches. However, currently around 50%–70% of all patients with advanced head and neck squamous cell carcinoma (HNSCC) develop locoregional recurrences after primary radiochemotherapy [4,5]. Thus, it is of high importance to develop and prove novel therapeutic strategies that could improve locoregional tumor control. Currently, successful targeted approaches for cancer therapy focus on receptors located on the surface of cancer cells that are higher expressed in cancer than in normal tissue.

Over many years the epidermal growth factor receptor (EGFR) has been investigated as a major target for the treatment of uncontrolled tumor growth. The EGFR, a glycosylated transmembrane protein, one of four members of closely related receptor tyrosine kinases (EGFR = ErbB1/HER1; ErbB2/HER2; ErbB3/HER3; ErbB4/HER4), is involved in regulating cell growth, differentiation and survival of cells. It is composed of an extracellular ligand binding region, a transmembrane region and an intracellular tyrosine kinase domain. The cytosine-rich extracellular domain binds endogenous growth factors, like epidermal growth factor (EGF), transforming growth factor alpha (TGF-α) [6], heparin-binding growth factor [7], amphiregulin [8]and betacellulin [9]. Binding of one of the endogenous ligands results in the formation of receptor homodimers (EGFR-EGFR) or receptor heterodimers (EGFR—homolog ErbB receptor) [10]. Dimerization causes autophoshorylation of the tyrosine residues that in turn initiates activation of signaling cascades. One of the main downstream signaling pathways is the MAP kinase system [11]. Activation of the MAPKs via Ras is regulating transcription of molecules for cell proliferation, migration, adhesion and survival [12]. Another major target, the PI3K/Akt signaling pathway, is involved in control of biological processes like growth, proliferation, angiogenesis, senescence, apoptosis, and formations of genetic aberrations [13]. Furthermore, of particular importance is the signal transduction pathway JAK/STAT, that mediates motility, invasion, adhesion, immune tolerance, cell survival and also proliferation [14,15].

The EGFR is often overexpressed in human malignancies such as HNSCC, gastrointestinal and abdominal carcinomas, lung carcinomas, carcinomas of the reproductive tract, melanomas, glioblastomas and thyroid carcinomas [16]. Although data are heterogeneous, overexpression is often associated with an aggressive tumor phenotype and a poor clinical prognosis. To target tumor cell proliferation or growth via EGFR, monoclonal antibodies (mAb) against this receptor have been developed. A promising potential therapeutic possesses the chimeric human-murine IgG1 mAb cetuximab (C225; Erbitux®, ImClone LLC), that has been approved by the Food and Drug Administration (FDA) for treatment of colorectal cancer as single drug or in combination with chemotherapy and of HNSCC in combination with radiation therapy or as monotherapy after failure of platinum-based therapy (2004 approval). Cetuximab, a 152 kDa molecule, is composed of two 449-amino-acid heavy chains and of two 214-amino-acid light chains interfaced both by covalent (disulfide) and non-covalent bonds [17]. The competitive binding of the mAb at the extracellular domain of the EGFR prevents binding of the natural ligands. On the other hand, cetuximab binding to EGFR also leads to receptor dimerization and internalization of the antibody-receptor-complex [18], not necessarily causing downregulation of membraneous EGFR expression [19]. Furthermore, cetuximab can induce antibody-dependent cell-mediated cytotoxicity [20].

The affinity of cetuximab toward EGFR is about tenfold higher than that of the endogenous ligands EGF or α-TGF (cetuximab 0.1–0.2 nM *vs.* EGF, α-TGF 1–2 nM) [21,22]. Blocking of the EGFR also affects the cell cycle by inducing upregulation of the cell cycle inhibitor p27Kip1. Consequently, EGFR expressing cells remain in a G1 arrest, preventing DNA synthesis [23–25]. Inhibition of tumor growth with cetuximab has in many cases been confirmed *in vivo* [18,26].

There are several studies about treatment of, particularly, head and neck cancer or colorectal cancer with cetuximab combined with chemotherapy, that show prolonged median overall survival [27–29], whereas similar treatment of non-small cell lung cancer remained uncertain and was not recommended [30]. Similarly, cetuximab paired with various chemotherapeutic regimens and/or other biological agents failed to improve the outcome of patients with pancreatic cancer [31].

2. Cetuximab Combined with Radiotherapy

In a clinical phase III randomized trial the combination of cetuximab and radiotherapy significantly improved locoregional recurrence and overall survival compared to radiotherapy alone for patients with locoregionally advanced HNSCC. The five years survival rate for treatment with cetuximab combined with radiation was 45.6% compared to 36.4% after radiation treatment alone [32]. However, also simultaneous radiochemotherapy improves survival compared to radiotherapy alone to a similar extent (33.7% *vs.* 27.2%) [4], and a direct comparison has never been performed prospectively. Thus, radiotherapy combined with cetuximab can be seen as alternative treatment option for specific cases but seems not superior to standard radiochemotherapy [33–35]. Some studies showed moderate improvements of local control and long-term survival after treatment with cetuximab plus radiotherapy [36,37]. Results of triple combination in randomized trials have preliminarily been reported and do also not support superiority over radiochemotherapy [38,39]. Concerning toxicity, combination of radiotherapy with cetuximab induces higher rates of mucositis, skin reactions and anaphylactic reactions, whereas radiochemotherapy leads to nephrotoxicity and myelosuppression [40].

To improve treatment outcome by pre-selection of patient subgroups that are expected to benefit from combined radiotherapy and cetuximab, mechanistic as well as functional pre-clinical *in vivo* studies are essential. In different HNSCC models simultaneous radiotherapy and cetuximab leads to heterogeneous effects on local tumor control, potentially correlating with genetic EGFR amplification [41] but not with EGFR expression [42]. Further, potential reasons for cetuximab resistance include the most frequently detected EGFR mutation class III variant (EGFR**v**III) [43], or mutation of the EGFR tyrosine kinase domain [44], or mutation of the oncogene KRAS, BRAF or NRAS that can activate the EGFR even during EGFR inhibition [45–47]. However, these molecular features are rare or not existent in head and neck squamous cell carcinoma, so that the mechanisms of the functional heterogeneity of tumor response are still not well understood.

Recently, the combination of targeted diagnostic and therapeutic applications (theranostics) is developing. The corresponding noninvasive imaging methods like SPECT or PET are appropriate methods to characterize the status of EGFR expressing tissue [48]. According to the application appropriate radionuclides are required. Since the majority of applied radionuclides are metals (Table 1), a rather extensive chelation chemistry has been developed to couple them to mAbs like cetuximab.

3. Radiolabeled Cetuximab

In order to estimate the status of EGFR expression, cetuximab was labeled with different radionuclides. Since EGFR is overexpressed in a variety of tumors, the accumulation of radiolabeled cetuximab in the tumor cells could serve as complementary diagnostic tool. Table 1 summarizes diagnostic and therapeutic radionuclides used for labeling of cetuximab conjugates.

Due to the size of the mAb its pharmacokinetics is slow with a biological half-life of 63 to 230 h [51]. The biological half-life of a substance in a biological organism is exclusively mediated by biological processes and represents the time during which the amount of the respective substance decreases to half of its original value. Moreover, of special importance is the effective half-life, the time during which the amount of a radiopharmaceutical is decreased to half of its value; that is altogether determined by the combination of the biological half-life of the substance and the physical half-life of the used radionuclide. The effective half-life for radiopharmaceuticals is predominantly influenced by the physical half-life of the radionuclide, which is suitable either for imaging or therapy. Accordingly radiolabeled cetuximab requires longer-lived radionuclides for monitoring. Furthermore, immunogenicity for diagnosis is unwanted, but concentrations of radiolabeled cetuximab with high specific activity are usually below nanomolarity (picomolar level) and do not show physiological effects.

Table 1. Diagnostic and therapeutic radionuclides for labeling of cetuximab conjugates [a].

Radionuclide	**Half-life**	**Main types of decay (probability)** [b]	**E_{max} (MeV)**	**Production**
Radionuclides for imaging				
^{64}Cu	12.7 h	β^+ (17.5%) β^- (38.5%) EC (43.5%)	0.653 0.579 1.675	cyclotron ^{64}Ni(p,n)^{64}Cu
^{68}Ga	1.13 h	β^+ (87.7%) EC (8.9%) γ (3.2%)	1.899 2.921 1.077	^{68}Ge/^{68}Ga generator
^{86}Y[c]	14.7 h	β^+ (11.9/5.6%) γ (83/32.6%)	1.221/1.545 1.077/0.628	cyclotron ^{86}Sr(p,n)^{86}Y
^{89}Zr[c]	3.3 dβ^+ (22.7%)	γ(100%)	0.902 0.909	cyclotron ^{89}Y(p,n)^{89}Zr
^{99m}Tc	6 h	γ (99%)	0.141	^{99}Mo/^{99m}Tc generator
^{111}In	2.8 d	γ (100%) EC (99.99%)	0.245 0.417	cyclotron ^{111}Cd(p,n)^{111}In
^{124}I[c]	4.2 d	β^+ (11.7/10.8%) γ (63/10.9%)	1.535/2.135 0.603/1.691	cyclotron ^{124}Te(p,n)^{124}I
^{125}I	59.4 d	γ (100%) EC (100%)	0.035 0.150	nuclear reactor ^{124}Xe(n,γ)^{125}Xe$\rightarrow$^{125}I
^{90}Y	2.67 d	β^-(99.98%)	2.279	^{90}Sr/^{90}Y generator
^{131}I	8 d	β^-(89.4/7.4%) γ (83.1/7.3%)	0.606/0.334 0.364/0.637	nuclear reactor ^{130}Te(n,γ)^{131}Te$\rightarrow$^{131}I
^{177}Lu	6.65 d	β^- (79.3/11.6%) γ (20.3/11%)	0.498/0.177 0.113/0.208	nuclear reactor ^{176}Yb(n,γ)^{177}Yb$\rightarrow$^{177}Lu
^{213}Bi	45.6 min	α (1.9%) β^- (66.2/30.8%)	5.981 1.423/0.983	^{225}Ac/^{213}Bi generator

[a] data from LNHB: http://www.nucleide.org/DDEP_WG/DDEPdata.htm [49]; [b] specification of the main transitions; [c] data from Lubberink Herzog 2011 [50]; EC electron capture; IC internal conversion.

3.1. Radionuclides

The selection of appropriate radionuclides with regard to their requested application is a crucial issue. It is necessary to consider different characteristics of radiation according to the requirements, like decay characteristics, particle range and physical half-life of the radionuclide. Anyhow, radionuclide selection is often done in terms of economic aspects [52]. The preferred approach for treatment of bulky tumors is the application of beta-emitting radionuclides and in future even of alpha emitters. For eradication of small clusters of cancer cells radionuclides that emit auger electrons are considered to be advantageous [53].

3.1.1. Radionuclides for C225 Conjugates Used as Imaging Probes

^{64}Cu. As important positron-emitting radionuclide ^{64}Cu has the potential for application in diagnostic imaging and, to some extent, also for targeted radiotherapy [54] because it additionally emits β^- particles. By the nuclear (p,n) reaction on enriched ^{64}Ni high specific activity of ^{64}Cu can be achieved [55,56] to apply for labeling of biomolecules. Since the positron-energy of ^{64}Cu is rather low, comparable with that of ^{18}F (0.633 MeV), ^{64}Cu PET images exhibit good resolution of high quality. Copper per se is participating in certain metabolic processes like binding on a series of enzymes such as superoxide dismutase, cytochrome c oxidase, or dopamine hydroxylase [57]. Therefore, copper ions should form complexes with high kinetic and thermodynamic stability. Cu(II) is forming stable chelate complexes, thus, in the last years there has been an active research development in this area. In particular, the chelators 1,4,7,10-tetraazacyclododecane-1,4,7,10-tetraacetic acid (DOTA), 1,4,8,11-tetraazacyclotetradecan-1,4,8,11-tetraacetic acid (TETA) and 1,4,7-triazacyclononane-1,4,7-triacetic acid (NOTA) have been studied. ^{64}Cu-TETA complexes are more stable than ^{64}Cu-DOTA complexes, however, it has been shown, that ^{64}Cu-TETA-octreotide is subjected to transchelation [58]. Several studies have been published with ^{64}Cu-labeled cetuximab using exclusively the DOTA chelator [45,59–62]. Recently, investigations of a mAb conjugated both with DOTA and NOTA, and labeled with ^{64}Cu, suggested that the NOTA conjugate was superior to the DOTA conjugate by showing better *in vivo* stability [63].

^{68}Ga. ^{68}Ga is a short-lived positron emitter and can be easily and relatively cheap generated with a ^{68}Ge/^{68}Ga generator. Similar to ^{64}Cu ^{68}Ga forms stable complexes with DOTA and NOTA. The label of ^{68}Ga is more appropriate for smaller molecules with faster biokinetics and bioavailability than for mAb with the aim to diagnose and localize tumors. To target the EGFR ^{68}Ga-labeled peptides [64], Fab fragments [65], affibodies [66] or nanobodies [67] have been applied. ^{68}Ga might also be applied in pretargeting approaches, where conjugates of e.g., hapten peptide [68,69], oligonucleotide [70] or peptide nucleic acid [71], after achieving high accumulation in the target tissue, would bind the ^{68}Ga-labeled complementary parts. Furthermore, ^{68}Ga can be replaced with the gamma emitter ^{67}Ga having a longer physical half-life of 3.26 d, appropriate for SPECT, and thus can be applied for investigations on longer circulating biomolecules like antibodies. In the study of Engle *et al.* [72] the positron emitter ^{66}Ga with a half-life of 9.4 h could be achieved with sufficient specific activity and was recommended as surrogate for ^{68}Ga or ^{67}Ga. Exploiting the longer half-life compared to ^{68}Ga, ^{66}Ga as label for NOTA-cetuximab was investigated in breast tumor bearing mice. However, the resolution of the images due to high energy positrons as well as accumulation in the tumor appeared to be not optimal.

^{86}Y. ^{86}Y is a positron emitter generally produced via the nuclear (p,n) reaction from enriched [^{86}Sr]$SrCO_3$ [73]. ^{86}Y/^{90}Y (and ^{177}Lu) form a matched-pair, thus the same chelators can be used. However, the half-life, presumably good for imaging of smaller molecules like mAb fragments and peptides, seems, similar to ^{64}Cu, short for imaging of large mAbs, and, compared to ^{89}Zr, also short concerning logistic aspects like transport [74]. Furthermore, ^{86}Y emits high energy γ-photons, which together with the annihilation photons might result in false coincidences and thus in quantification artifacts [75,76] affecting the spatial resolution and imaging quality [77]. But emitting positrons abundantly, almost twice as much as ^{64}Cu, the activity of ^{86}Y required for quantitative immuno-PET can be kept rather low. Anyhow, with ^{86}Y promising PET studies using tumor mouse models have been performed [78–82] among others also with cetuximab, that was conjugated to the bifunctional chelator (BFC) CHX-A″-DTPA [83,84] under mild conditions [85]. As PET/RIT pair ^{86}Y as surrogate for ^{90}Y seems to be convenient. It might to be more suitable than the pair ^{89}Zr/^{90}Y since the uptake of

^{89}Zr-labeled cetuximab particular in bone was higher than that of ^{88}Y-labeled cetuximab (^{88}Y as surrogate for ^{90}Y) [74]. Also the PET/RIT surrogate pair ^{86}Y and ^{177}Lu can be of interest.

^{89}Zr. ^{89}Zr is a long-lived positron emitter. The production of choice is the (p,n) reaction on ^{89}Y, an element that does not require enrichment due to its natural abundance of 100% [86]. Since cetuximab has a rather long biological half-live of 63 to 230 h [87] ^{89}Zr is an appropriate radionuclide for application in so-called immuno-PET and offers high sensitivity, resolution and precise quantification. Although it emits also γ photons those do not interfere with the PET image quality and accurate quantification [88]. In PET ^{89}Zr might be used as surrogate to predict biodistribution and dosimetry of ^{177}Lu- and ^{90}Y-labeled mAb conjugates [74,89]. It is coupled to cetuximab via N-succinyl desferrioxamine B. Biodistribution was comparable with that of ^{86}Y- and ^{177}Lu-radiolabeled cetuximab conjugates. Differences can occur due to coupling with other chelators that change the pharmacokinetics and *in vivo* stability [74], but basically ^{89}Zr and ^{90}Y as well as ^{89}Zr and ^{177}Lu appear to be good PET/RIT pairs.

^{99m}Tc. Since the gamma emitter ^{99m}Tc has favorable physical properties for scintigraphic imaging and can be produced with low costs by the ^{99}Mo/^{99m}Tc generator, this radionuclide has been used widely for labeling of radiopharmaceuticals. As stable complex with ethylenedicysteine [90] a conjugate to cetuximab has been formulated [91]. The uptake of this cetuximab conjugate in tumor tissue was still higher than the uptake of ^{99m}Tc complex only, but not convincingly high for analyzable imaging to achieve. Besides, an unexpected high kidney uptake was observed in human breast tumor-bearing rats [92]. The half-life of 6 h for ^{99m}Tc is too short for imaging of mAb like cetuximab when the highest accumulation of the antibody in the tumor is expected after 2 to 3 days. Moreover, in patient studies to visualize head and neck cancer correlations of the imaging results with clinical findings are missing. Furthermore, high liver uptake was observed compared with an uptake in HNSCC [92] that was not sufficiently high. As already discussed for ^{68}Ga Ab conjugates with ^{99m}Tc are not convenient for *in vivo* applications. It would be more adequate to couple ^{99m}Tc complexes to smaller molecules which reach their target faster than mAbs.

^{111}In. ^{111}In is a cyclotron-produced radiometal, and one of the most commonly used radionuclides for SPECT [93] especially as label for mAb due to its adequate physical half-life (2.8 d). Even it emits Auger and internal conversion electrons with low energy that might be interesting for therapeutic approaches [94], primarily γ radiation is used for diagnostic imaging. ^{111}In-labeled mAb conjugates with the chelators DOTA or DTPA have been investigated in small animals [85,95,96] and human [97,98].

^{124}I. ^{124}I is a positron emitter with a complex decay scheme [99]. In addition to two positron emitting transitions, ^{124}I emits γ rays at more than 90 transitions resulting in increased random coincidences in PET. The so-called true-coincidence γ ray background may disturb the PET imaging. And the high energy of the emitted positrons from ^{124}I also contributes to a declined resolution. Furthermore, iodine has been described for the tendency to separate from mAb after injection, because of metabolic degradation, and so it might accumulate in different organs and the interpretation of PET images turns out to be difficult [100]. However, radioiodine can be used for direct labeling without a chelator. In many cases this facilitates the labeling of biomolecules. In this regard, ^{124}I has been used as an imaging nuclide surrogate for ^{131}I [101]. Moreover, the relatively long half-life justifies the use of ^{124}I-labeled mAbs [102,103]. Recently an anti-EGFR antibody has been ^{124}I-labeled and studied successfully *in vitro* and *in vivo* in mice bearing glioma xenografts [104].

^{125}I. Since ^{125}I has a long half-life of 60 d and emits low-energy γ radiation, it can be detected by a gamma-counter. This radionuclide is often coupled to antibodies for application in radioimmunoassays (RIA), and also in preclinical EGFR investigations [105–107]. Furthermore, ^{125}I-labeled cetuximab was applied in tumor bearing mice and showed in general lower uptake in the tumor compared with radiometal labeled cetuximab [74,108,109]. Due to the long half-life and its tendency to degrade faster than radiometal-antibody-conjugates ^{125}I will not be introduced as label for antibodies in clinical trials.

3.1.2. Radionuclides for Cetuximab Conjugates Used as Therapeutics

^{90}Y. The therapeutic β^- emitter ^{90}Y is of particular interest for medical applications due to its suitability for irradiating primary tumor lesions. It is available at moderate costs via ^{90}Sr/^{90}Y-generators, has an appropriate half-life for RIT and a high β^- emission energy with a tissue penetration range of up to 12 mm [110]. Thus, it is more suitable for RIT of large bulky solid tumors. Caution and good biodosimetry is necessary when a tumor is located adjacent to critical organs, especially if combined with EBRT. Yttrium in general should be applied within a stable chelate complex since in free condition it deposits in the bone [111]. The absence of γ emission by ^{90}Y makes it not trivial for *in vivo* imaging [112,113]. Alternatively, for ^{90}Y the longer lived ^{88}Y (half-life 106.6 d, β^+ 0.2%, $E_{\beta\text{-max}}$ 0.76 MeV; γ 99%, E_γ 1.836 MeV) has been used as substitute to estimate biochemical properties [74,114,115]. However, its γ energy is too high for imaging, and the low amount of positrons might be reasonable only for small animal PET to prevent significant scatter of the prompt γ rays into the PET energy window [116]. Recently, ^{90}Y-labeled cetuximab conjugates have been applied in RIT [117], also in combination with external radiation [118,119] (see Section 3.5.).

^{131}I. ^{131}I is a β^- emitter with concomitant γ radiation. The β^--radiation is used for internal radiotherapy of hyperthyroidism [120] and different tumor types, like neuroblastoma, pheochromocytoma [121], and thyroid cancer [122], whereby the γ radiation part is often applied for SPECT imaging [123]. A crucial advantage is the low cost of the radionuclide production, but a disadvantage the low stability resulting in corresponding deiodination reactions *in vivo*. Recently, ^{131}I-labeled cetuximab treatment has been applied in combination with irradiation on epidermoid cancer cells (A431). In result the combination of ^{131}I-cetuximab with external radiation inhibited cell proliferation *in vitro* [124].

^{177}Lu. ^{177}Lu is the more favorable therapeutic radionuclide for treatment of small tumors due to its low energy and tissue penetration of about 1.5 mm [110]. The physical half-life is sufficient for preparation, transport and delivery of therapeutic doses to tumors applied as immunoconjugates like mAbs. Due to its low energy γ-lines it is possible to perform imaging. The chemistry of ^{177}Lu resembles the metallic radionuclide ^{90}Y forming also stable complexes with DOTA and cysteine-based DTPA. Several ^{177}Lu-labeled Ab conjugates have been studied [125–127], including cetuximab conjugates [74,109,128].

^{213}Bi. Recently, mAb have also been labeled with α emitters like ^{213}Bi that as therapeutic radionuclide might be more efficient in killing tumor cells with less damage in the surrounded healthy tissue in targeted therapy [129,130]. The production with a $^{225}Ac/^{213}Bi$ generator has been developed even for application in clinical use [131]. The range of α-particles is rather short in tissue in comparison to beta particles (50–80 μm *vs.* 0.8–12 mm); they have a much higher linear energy transfer (100 keV/μm *vs.* 0.2 keV/μm) [129]. Currently, there are clinical trials for different types of cancer with targeted high potent α-emitters [132–134]. In an *in vitro* study ^{213}Bi-labeled CHX-A″DTPA-cetuximab showed effective double-strand breaks on different human breast cancer cells, but for an approach in patients the safety of targeted α-emitter-labeled radioconjugates has to be evaluated [135]. However, due to the short half-life of only 46 min an application of ^{213}Bi-labeled to CHX-A″DTPA-cetuximab would be rather questionable and likely will not enter the clinics.

3.2. Linking Chelating Units

Almost all radionuclides for diagnostics and therapy of different types of cancer coupled to antibodies, antibody fragments or peptides are radiometals. That requires chelation chemistry for the attachment to the ligands. Several chelators have been conjugated to cetuximab. Hereby it is necessary to find the balance between the required coupling conditions to obtain a stable conjugate preferably without degradation, loss of affinity and immunoreactivity. For stable coupling of radiometals to antibodies and preservation of their special features, mild conjugation procedures have to be established. The chelating agents of choice should form stable metal complexes as well as provide specific functional groups to enable the conjugation to a protein. Such bifunctional chelators (BFC) have to be characterized for several properties: thermodynamic and kinetic stability, pH-dependent dissociation and serum stability [136]. To determine *in vivo* stability of any labeled conjugate only suitable *in vivo* models can provide such information. Figure 1 illustrates the bifunctional chelators used in cetuximab conjugates.

One of the first used bifunctional chelating agents was desferrioxamine B that, conjugated to an antibody, has been radiolabeled with ^{111}In [137]. Derivatives of desferrioxamine, originally developed as chelators for Fe(III), form stable complexes with In(III), Ga(III) and Zr(IV). Thus, desferrioxamine antibody conjugates labeled with ^{67}Ga have earlier been investigated [138]. Recently, desferrioxamine derivatives were conjugated to mAb [86,139,140]. Labeled with ^{89}Zr the conjugates showed promising results with regard to radiochemical purity, integrity, preservation of immunoreactivity and stability [86]. Moreover, with ^{89}Zr-desferrioxamine-cetuximab-conjugates small animal PET studies revealed convincing results with good resolution showing high accumulation in different tumors [141,142]. Particularly, high uptake was demonstrated in FaDu tumors, a model for HNSCC [140].

Starting from DTPA several bifunctional derivatives have been developed and investigated [143,144]. Recently, CHX-A″-DTPA (correct: *p*-SCN-Bn-CHX-A″-DTPA) has been used for conjugation with antibodies to form sufficiently stable ^{86}Y, ^{90}Y, and ^{111}In immunoconjugates, which could successfully be applied *in vivo* [83,145–147]. Among the backbone-substituted DTPA derivatives CHX-A″-DTPA showed very good *in vitro* and *in vivo* stability [143,144] and it can be conjugated and radiolabeled under mild conditions to preserve the immunoreactivity of the resulting conjugate.

Figure 1. Bifunctional chelators (BFC) used in cetuximab conjugates: succinylated desferoxamine (*N*-sucDf, **1a**), desferoxamine-p-SCN (Df–Bz–NCS, **1b**), p-SCN-Bn-DTPA (**2a**), CHX-A″-DTPA (**2b**), DOTA-NHS-ester (**3a**), p-SCN-Bn-DOTA (**3b**), p-SCN-Bn-NOTA (**4**).

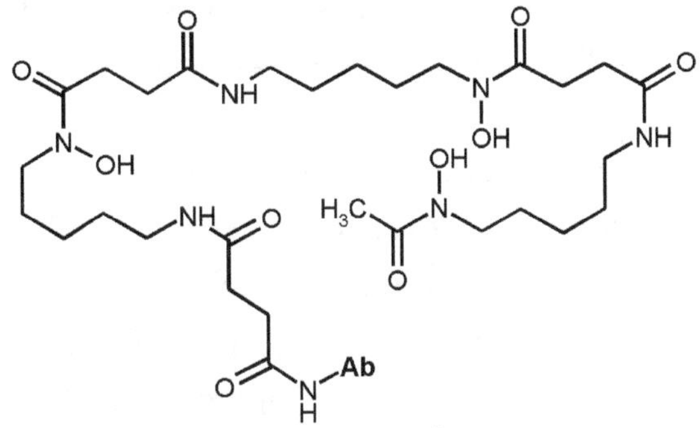

1a

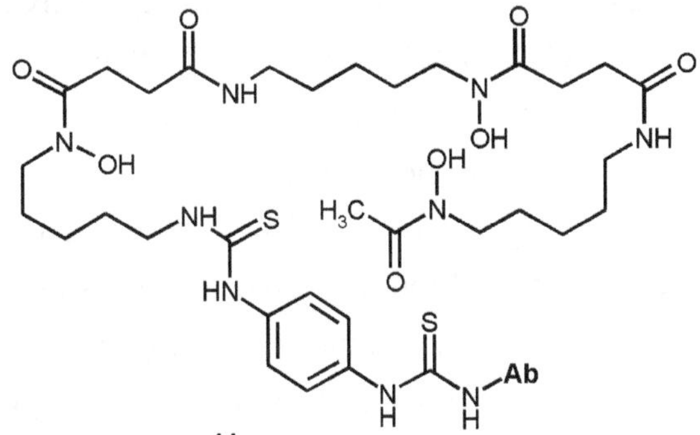

1b

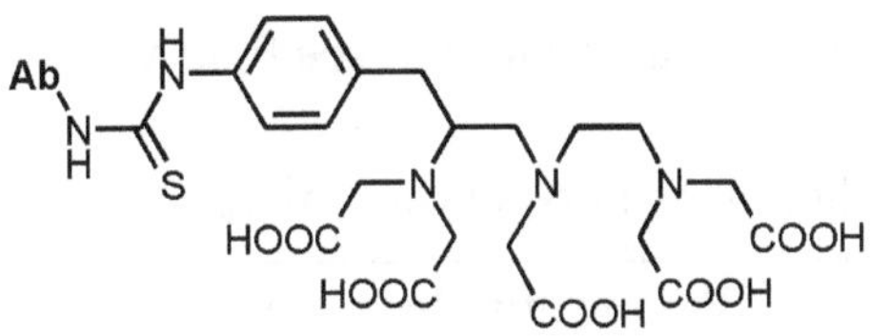

2a

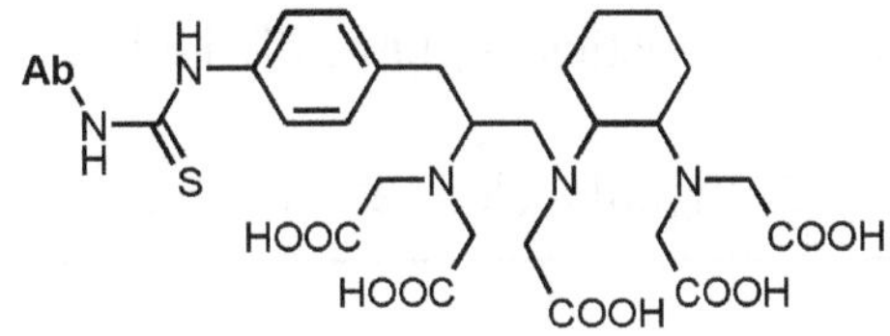

2b

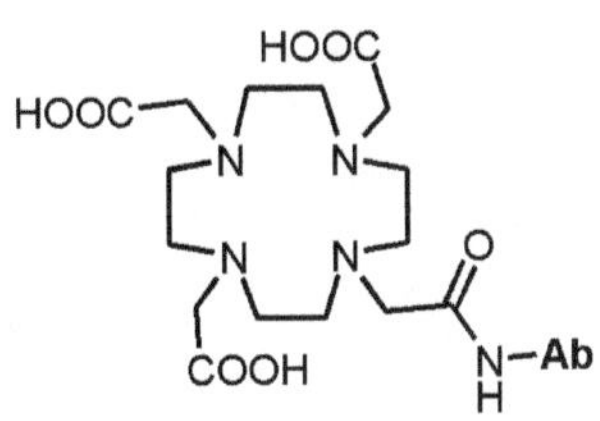

3a

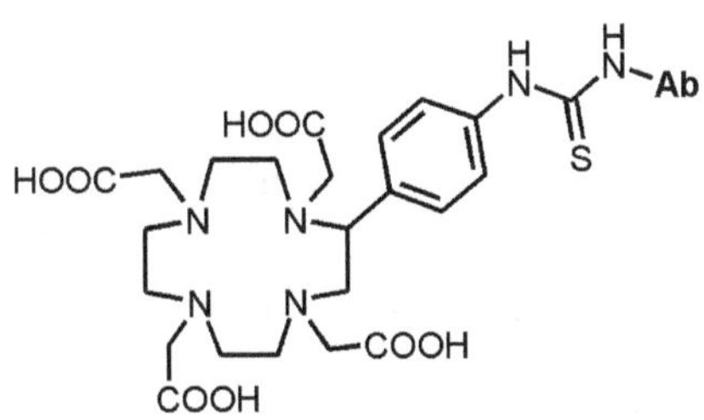

3b

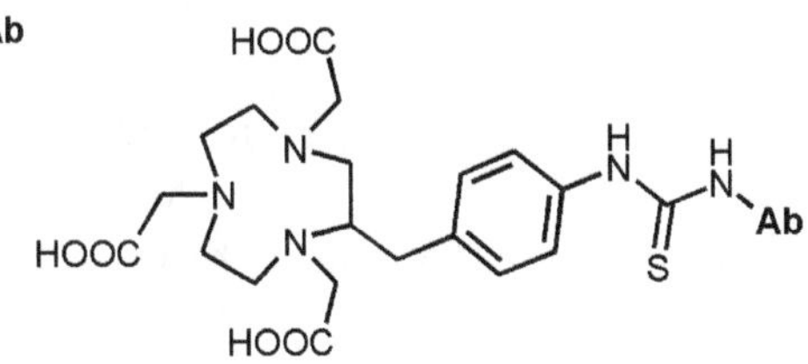

4

The kinetic stability of a radiometal complex plays a more important role for *in vivo* stability than the thermodynamic stability [148], but still, possible predictions can be just assumed. For example the complex [^{111}In-DOTA]$^-$ is kinetically more stable than [^{111}In-DTPA]$^{2-}$, but thermodynamic stability of In(III)-DTPA is about 5 orders higher than the appropriate In(III)-DOTA complex [96].

It was shown that CHX-A″-DTPA, conjugated to a HER2-specific affibody, provides better cellular retention of the radiolabeled Ab, better tumor accumulation and better tumor-to-organ dose ratios in comparison with DOTA [149]. DTPA antibody conjugates have a satisfactory labeling efficiency [150].

Bifunctional chelating units based on DOTA are the chelators of choice for yttrium isotopes and ^{177}Lu [74,125]. DOTA derivatives are also often used for chelating ^{64}Cu [59,151], although it has been claimed that DOTA is not the optimal chelator for ^{64}Cu, because ^{64}Cu-DOTA shows a certain instability *in vivo* [58,148]. However, stability constants measured in an *in vitro* chemical system [152] cannot represent *in vivo* conditions. For instance, it has been described that transchelation for a ^{64}Cu-DOTA antibody was much higher than for the same ^{64}Cu-NOTA antibody [63]. Cross-bridged macrocycles show greater stability with ^{64}Cu. However, there is the need for harsh labeling conditions (95 °C for 2 h) [153] which are incompatible for protein labeling. But still, the tumor uptake of ^{64}Cu-DOTA-cetuximab is relatively high [59–61,117,151].

Particular importance has attained the preservation of the immunoreactivity of the antibody after conjugation reactions. A flow cytometry study showed still high binding capacity after conjugation of CHX-A″-DTPA to cetuximab [154]. Other studies present a preserved immunoreactivity [83,85], and the high affinity of cetuximab to EGFR was kept [119].

The uptake of radiolabeled cetuximab in EGFR expressing model tumors in mice was, in general, significantly higher compared with the uptake in the main body parts, except the liver (Table 2). The decline from the blood appeared to be faster than from the tumor and, unfortunately, also from the liver. Anyhow, the outcome was a high tumor-to-muscle or tumor-to-background ratio. Of note, the data were comparable for most conjugates applied, excepting those using non-appropriate chelating units [91] or those using non-appropriate radionuclides [72]. These are data from rodent models naturally not expressing human EGFR. Therefore, an extrapolation of the biodistribution to human pharmacological characteristics might be difficult, reflecting not the true relations (see below).

Table 2. Radiolabeled cetuximab conjugates studied in tumor-bearing mice.

Radionuclide	Chelator	Tumor type	Application	Tumor uptake	Tumor/muscle ratio	Liver uptake	Reference
				(%ID/g, 24 h post-injection)			
^{64}Cu	DOTA	h GB	i.v.	12.5	5	15	[59]
		h PC		11	4.5	6 (rat)	
		h CRC		~5		2	
		m CRC		10		4	
		h M					
^{64}Cu	DOTA	h CC	i.v.	14	3.5	16	[60]
^{64}Cu	DOTA	PC-3	i.v.	15	15	17	[151]
^{64}Cu	DOTA	A431	i.v.	18.5	8.5	13	[61]
		h M		2.6	1.3	10	
^{64}Cu	DOTA	h HNSCC (UMSCC22B)	i.v.	19	6	11	[117] [a]
^{64}Cu	DOTA	h HNSCC (UMSCC1)	i.v.	6	2.5	13	[117] [a]
^{64}Cu	NOTA	m BC	i.v.	4	4	19	[155]
^{64}Cu	NOTA	m BC	i.v.	20	10	19	[54]
^{66}Ga	NOTA	h BC	i.v.	4	5	6	[72] [b]
^{86}Y	DTPA	h CRC	i.v.	21	11	10	[83]
^{88}Y	DTPA	A431	i.p.	21	14	11	[74]
^{88}Y	DOTA	A431	i.p.	17	11	10	[74]
^{89}Zr	Df	h GB	i.v.	15	15	10-12	[141]
		h CRC		10		10	
		A431		8		8	
		h BC		3		3	
^{89}Zr	Df	A431	i.v.	3.5[c]	10[d]	11[c]	[142]
^{89}Zr	Df	A431	i.p.	21	17	10	[74]
^{89}Zr	Df	A431	i.v.	15	8	9	[139]

Table 2. *Cont.*

Radionuclide	Chelator	Tumor type	Application	Tumor uptake	Tumor/muscle ratio	Liver uptake	Reference
				(%ID/g, 24 h post-injection)			
^{89}Zr +	Df	A431	i.v.	22	19	20	[156]
^{89}Zr + ½ dye [e]	Df			20	19	22	
^{89}Zr + 1 dye	Df			20	19	25	
^{89}Zr + 2 dye	Df			13	16	40	
^{99m}Tc	EC	h BC	i.v.	0.3	8.5	0.6	[91]
^{86}Y	DTPA	h CRC	i.v.	21	11	10	[83]
^{88}Y	DTPA	A431	i.p.	21	14	11	[74]
^{88}Y	DOTA	A431	i.p.	17	11	10	[74]
^{90}Y	DOTA	normal rats	i.v.			2	[157]
^{177}Lu	DOTA	A431	i.p.	18	12	13	[109]
^{177}Lu	DOTA	A431	i.p.	17.5	12	8-13	[74]
^{177}Lu	DTPA	A431	i.p.	17.5	12	7	[74]
^{111}In	DTPA	A431	i.v.	11	29	47	[158] [f]
	DTPA-PEG	A431		8.7	13	25	
^{111}In	DTPA	h OC	i.v.	8.8	11	4	[95] [f]
^{111}In	DTPA	h CRC	i.v.	28/24 [g]	28/24 [g]	9/16 [g]	[85]
		h PC		16	16	6	
		h PancC		10	10	10	
		h OC		13	13	10	
		h M		3	3	9	
^{111}In	DTPA	h HNSCC	i.v.	20	14	11	[108]
^{111}In	DTPA	h BC	i.v.	18/40 [f]	13	11/15 [f]	[135]
^{111}In	DTPA	h HNSCC (FaDu)	i.v.	27	13	8	[159]
^{125}I		h HNSCC	i.v.	11	8	7	[108]
^{125}I		A431	i.p.	8.4	5.6	4	[109]
^{125}I		A431	i.p.	8	5	4	[74]

Df desferrioxamine chelating unit; EC ethylenedicysteine; h human; m murine; GB glioblastoma; CRC colorectal carcinoma; A431 human epidermoid carcinoma; BC breast carcinoma; PC prostate carcinoma; CRC colorectal carcinoma; CC cervical cancer; M melanoma (MDA-MB-435); HNSCC head and neck squamous cell carcinoma; UMSCC22B cells of the lymph node the oropharynx; UMSCC1 cells of the oral cavity; OC ovarian carcinoma; PancC pancreas carcinoma; FaDu hypopharyngeal carcinoma cell line; [a] 20 h after radiotracer injection; [b] 36 h after radiotracer injection; [c] %ID/mL tumor PET analysis; [d] tumor to background (pelvic); [e] different equivalents of the dye IRDye800CW; [f] 48 h after radiotracer injection; [g] value from two different types of h CRC xenografts.

3.3. Liver Accumulation

Liver accumulation appears to be a general problem using mAb-based immunoimaging and immunotherapeutics in animal studies, Table 2. Overall, the liver uptake of ^{90}Y-DOTA- and ^{64}Cu-DOTA cetuximab in rats appears to be proportionally lower as compared to mice. Biodistribution studies revealed that cetuximab is eliminated partly via the reticuloendothelial system, binding on fc receptors of lymphocytes, macrophages *etc.* passing sinusoid capillaries especially into the liver. Thus, a considerable part is accumulating in this organ. Table 2 shows only the values for 24 h post injection, since the accumulation in the liver did not increase after 24 h and declined only slowly thereafter, whereas the highest tumor uptake of a cetuximab conjugate was measured after 72 h. In an ^{89}Zr-labeled cetuximab study a multimodal imaging approach was investigated where a dye, emitting fluorescence in the near-infrared region, was conjugated additionally to the Ab [156]. In this study, the more dye units the Ab received the lower was the tumor uptake and the higher the liver uptake.

In general, accumulation of ^{125}I-labeled cetuximab in the liver was lower compared to the radiometal-labeled cetuximab studies, but also in tumor this conjugate accumulated considerably less. Thus, the question arises to what extent metal chelate complexes influence the uptake of the conjugates. As noted above, radioiodine labeled antibodies are subject to degradation and deiodination due to their *in vivo* instability to proteolysis. A faster degradation of iodine labeled antibodies after internalization causes faster clearance from the target cells and results in images with lower tumor contrast, thus not reflecting the real distribution of the Ab [160]. Moreover, the risk of radioiodine accumulation in the thyroid contributes to the inappropriateness of radioiodine as a therapeutic tracer outside the thyroid.

A dimension independent from the weight of the organs and the body weight is the standard uptake value (SUV). Considering the SUV of 1.6 for liver and 4.2 for FaDu tumor in the biodistribution with ^{90}Y-CHX-A″-DTPA-cetuximab, liver accumulation appears to be justifiable. PET studies with ^{86}Y-CHX-A″-DTPA-cetuximab using FaDu bearing mice showed similar accumulation distribution [83]. With ^{111}In-labeled CHX-A″-DTPA-cetuximab in tumor bearing mice higher liver uptake was observed [85,108,158]. The liver accumulation might partly be due to nonspecific uptake of labeled yttrium caused by transchelation [161]. Since applications with radiolabeled mAbs have been limited by liver uptake, an approach for reduction was the modification of the conjugate with PEG, or also the pretreatment with cetuximab [158]. Recently, the biodistribution of ^{111}In-DTPA-cetuximab-fragments have been compared with ^{111}In-DTPA-cetuximab in FaDu tumor bearing mice. In this study the fragments showed significantly lower uptake in the tumor, but lower uptake in the liver could not be observed, it was even higher within the first 4 h after administration. In addition, more radioactivity was measured in the kidney [159]. In a first clinical imaging study in patients with lung squamous cell carcinoma ^{111}In-DTPA-MAb225, the murine forerunner of cetuximab, also showed a high liver accumulation [98]. The uptake of DTPA-cetuximab conjugates in the liver appears to be somewhat lower compared to the liver uptake of ^{64}Cu-DOTA-cetuximab. ^{89}Zr-desferrioxamine-cetuximab conjugates revealed a similar liver uptake as the yttrium-labeled conjugates. Histological assays of liver tissue have been performed after RIT, whereby no changes were observed [118]. However, a conclusion on potential normal organ toxicity is restricted to the experimental animals [162], because the antibody cetuximab is specific to human EGFR and thus is expected to show a differential organ distribution in humans compared to animals.

Specifically for cetuximab no binding to EGFR in frozen liver sections of mice and rats could be detected, whereas strong cross-reactivity was observed with EGFR expressed on the cell surface of various types of human tissue including skin, lung, and liver [163]. Thus, it is important to consider that the elimination of cetuximab, also in the radiolabeled state, needs to be evaluated separately in humans and cannot be extrapolated from rodent studies.

3.4. The Enhanced Permeability and Retention Effect

Non-specific tumor uptake of radiolabeled Ab often is caused by the enhanced permeability and retention (EPR) effect. Aberrant defective membrane formations of tumor blood vessels with wide fenestrations are leading to an enhanced vascular permeability. Besides, a malfunction of lymphatic vessels in tumor tissue impairs the clearance of macromolecules and lipids, so that they remain in the tumor interstitium for longer time. The EPR effect [164,165] has also been described when labeled antibodies have been used in studies for tumor diagnostics or treatment [166,167]. In a phase I imaging trial with ^{111}In-labeled murine DTPA-MAb225 in patients with lung cancer several patients received the isotope-matched ^{111}In-labeled control mAb [98]. Presumably, due to the EPR effect half of this control group did not show significant differences to the specific Ab. A number of studies used this labeled isotype of IgG1 as negative control to determine nonspecific tumor uptake [54,151,168,169]. Vascular endothelium in tumors also can be perturbed by hypoxic areas [170]. Thus, beside aberrant vessels in the tumor tissue also hypoxia seems to contribute to the EPR effect.

3.5. Therapeutic Approaches with Labeled Cetuximab

Combination of radioimmunotherapeutic approaches, e.g., radiolabeled cetuximab, with curatively intended radio(chemo)therapy are a promising research strategy to improve locoregional tumor control in head and neck or other cancer entities. The therapeutic success depends on the radioligand concentration in the tumor which, in addition to the target expression, seems to depend on tumor microenvironmental parameters [118].

After binding to the EGFR, radiolabeled cetuximab internalizes into the cell [60,107,108] and can cause there, additional damage of the cell as well as to neighbor cells. The combination of ^{90}Y-labeled cetuximab (^{90}Y-CHX-A″-DTPA) treatment with subsequent irradiation reduced clonogenic cell survival more compared to external irradiation alone [119]. Unlabeled cetuximab caused a radiosensitizing effect [171,172] in one out of three cell lines [119]. Recently, an EGFR expression depending number of DNA double strand breaks (DSB) caused by ^{90}Y-CHX-A″-DTPA was demonstrated *in vitro* [173]. Furthermore, also in different breast cancer cells, which were sensitized with an inhibitor of DNA-dependent-protein-kinase, DNA DSB have been assessed after treatment of ^{213}Bi-labeled cetuximab [135]. Rades *et al.* [124] showed that the highest antiproliferative effect in epidermoid cancer cells (A431) occurred after combined treatment with therapeutic ^{131}I-labeled cetuximab and irradiation. These data suggest that higher radiation dose promotes and increases the uptake of the radiolabeled conjugate into the tumor cells.

In vivo, three different human squamous cell carcinoma models have been evaluated in nude mice. Two to 4 days after external beam single dose irradiation either unlabeled or ^{90}Y-labeled cetuximab was applied. While one out of three tumor models did not respond, tumor growth delay could significantly be prolonged in two other HNSCC xenograft models [118]. Permanent local tumor control was evaluated for the non-responder and one responder-model, confirming non-response in UT-SCC5 but a significant improvement of local tumor control in FaDu, the latter being a non- or minimal-responder to radiotherapy with unlabeled cetuximab [41,118,174]. A combined parameter on tumor micromilieu, specifically perfusion, and EGFR expression, appeared as a candidate biomarker for tumor response—this parameter can be measured using PET imaging with ^{86}Y-cetuximab as a tracer. In another study colon tumor-bearing mice showed higher survival after treatment combination of the cytostatic drug cisplatin followed by ^{64}Cu-DOTA-cetuximab and suggested a role of the tumor suppressor protein p53 for the transport of ^{64}Cu into the cell nucleus [175]. Here, even a KRAS mutated cetuximab-resistant tumor model was responding [54]. In a recent case report a patient with brain metastases from non-small cell lung cancer was treated with low concentrations of ^{131}I-labeled cetuximab in addition to therapeutic cetuximab treatment and whole brain irradiation. SPECT was applied to monitor the treatment and showed accumulation of ^{131}I-labeled cetuximab in the brain metastases which showed a decrease in size during the treatment. It remains to be elucidated whether cetuximab generally passes the blood-brain-barrier or only in specific patients [176].

4. Conclusions

Radiolabeled cetuximab derivatives in combination with external radiotherapy or established chemotherapy appear to be a promising theranostic approach for treatment of epithelial tumors, thus fostering more individualized treatment strategies. Since considerable heterogeneity of the functional response to labeled or unlabeled targeted treatments is obvious also within one histological tumor type, there is a clear need to establish predictive biomarkers for the curative effect of such treatments. One good candidate that needs to be validated in patients is PET imaging using labeled cetuximab as a diagnostic tracer. So far, treatment of patients with therapeutic radionuclide-labeled cetuximab has not yet entered into the clinics. Important open questions include the distribution and accumulation of the tracer in healthy organs in humans as well as the feasibility of the combined high-dose EBRT and RIT approach in patients.

Acknowledgments

This work was supported in part by the Bundesministerium für Umwelt, Naturschutz und Reaktorsicherheit via the project “Kompetenzverbund Strahlenforschung” (grant 02NUK006A-E). The excellent assistance of the employees at the Institutes of Radiopharmaceutical Cancer Research and Radiation Oncology, Helmholtz-Zentrum Dresden-Rossendorf, and the Department of Radiation Oncology, University Hospital Carl Gustav Carus, who have contributed to this project is greatly acknowleged.

Author Contributions

W.S. and H.-J.P. initiated the topic and organized the manuscript; W.S., J.P., J.S. and H.-J.P. contributed to literature searches and writing; M.K. and M.B. contributed the clinical background; all authors, W.S., J.P., M.K., M.B., J.S. and H.-J.P. were involved in data interpretation and participated in proofreading and editing of the manuscript.

References

1. Gunderson, L.L.; Ashman, J.B.; Haddock, M.G.; Petersen, I.A.; Moss, A.; Heppell, J.; Gray, R.J.; Pockaj, B.A.; Nelson, H.; Beauchamp, C. Integration of radiation oncology with surgery as combined-modality treatment. *Surg. Oncol. Clin. N. Am.* **2013**, *22*, 405–432.
2. Galaal, K.; van der Heijden, E.; Godfrey, K.; Naik, R.; Kucukmetin, A.; Bryant, A.; Das, N.; Lopes, A.D. Adjuvant radiotherapy and/or chemotherapy after surgery for uterine carcinosarcoma. *Cochrane Database Syst. Rev.* **2013**, *2*, CD006812.
3. Yang, H.; Diao, L.Q.; Shi, M.; Ma, R.; Wang, J.H.; Li, J.P.; Xiao, F.; Xue, Y.; Xu, M.; Zhou, B. Efficacy of intensity-modulated radiotherapy combined with chemotherapy or surgery in locally advanced squamous cell carcinoma of the head-and-neck. *Biologics* **2013**, *7*, 223–229.
4. Pignon, J.P.; le Maître, A.; Maillard, E.; Bourhis, J.; MACH-NC Collaborative Group. Meta-analysis of chemotherapy in head and neck cancer (MACH-NC): An update on 93 randomised trials and 17,346 patients. *Radiother. Oncol.* **2009**, *92*, 4–14.
5. Bourhis, J.; Overgaard, J.; Audry, H.; Ang, K.K.; Saunders, M.; Bernier, J.; Horiot, J.C.; le Maître, A.; Pajak, T.F.; Poulsen, M.G.; *et al.* Meta-Analysis of Radiotherapy in Carcinomas of Head and neck (MARCH) Hyperfractionated or accelerated radiotherapy in head and neck cancer: A meta-analysis. *Lancet* **2006**, *368*, 843–854.
6. Marquardt, H.; Hunkapiller, M.W; Hood L.E.; Twardzik, D.R.; De Larco, J.E.; Stephenson J.R., Todaro, G.J. Transforming growth factors produced by retrovirus-transformed rodent fibroblasts and human melanoma cells: Amino acid sequence homology with epidermal growth factor. *Proc. Natl. Acad. Sci. USA* **1983**, *80*, 4684–4688.
7. Higashiyama, S.; Abraham, J.A.; Miller, J.; Fiddes, J.C.; Klagsbrun, M. A heparin-binding growth factor secreted by macrophage-like cells that is related to EGF. *Science* **1991**, *251*, 936–939.
8. Ciardiello, F.; Kim, N.; Saeki, T.; Dono, R.; Persico, M.G.; Plowman, G.D.; Garrigues, J.; Radke, S.; Todaro, G.J.; Salomon, D.S. Differential expression of epidermal growth factor-related proteins in human colorectal tumors. *Proc. Natl. Acad. Sci. USA* **1991**, *88*, 7792–7796.
9. Sasada, R.; Ono, Y.; Taniyama, Y.; Shing, Y.; Folkman, J.; Igarashi, K. Cloning and expression of cDNA encoding human betacellulin, a new member of the EGF family. *Biochem. Biophys. Res. Commun.* **1993**, *190*, 1173–1179.
10. Olayioye, M.A.; Neve, R.M.; Lane, H.A.; Hynes, N.E. The ErbB signaling network: Receptor heterodimerization in development and cancer. *EMBO J.* **2000**, *19*, 3159–3167.
11. Alroy, I.; Yarden, Y. The ErbB signaling network in embryogenesis and oncogenesis: Signal diversification through combinatorial ligand-receptor interactions. *FEBS Lett.* **1997**, *410*, 83–86.
12. Lewis, T.S.; Shapiro, P.S.; Ahn, N.G. Signal transduction through MAP kinase cascades. *Adv. Cancer Res.* **1998**, *74*, 49–139.
13. Hennessy, B.T.; Smith, D.L.; Ram, P.T.; Lu, Y.; Mills, G.B. Exploiting the PI3K/AKT pathway for cancer drug discovery. *Nat. Rev. Drug Discov.* **2005**, *4*, 988–1004.
14. Silva, C.M. Role of STATs as downstream signal transducers in Src family kinase-mediated tumorigenesis. *Oncogene* **2004**, *23*, 8017–8023.

15. Pensa, S.; Regis, G.; Boselli, D.; Novelli, G.; Poli, V. STAT1 and STAT3 in Tumorigenesis: Two sides of the same coin? In *Madame Curie Bioscience Database*; 2009; Chapter 8, pp. 100–121. Available online: http://www.ncbi.nlm.nih.gov/books/NBK6568/ (accessed on 27 February 2014).
16. Salomon, D.S.; Brandt, R.; Ciardiello, F.; Normanno, N. Epidermal growth factor-related peptides and their receptors in human malignancies. *Crit. Rev. Oncol. Hematol.* **1995**, *19*, 183–232.
17. Humblet, Y. Cetuximab: An IgG(1) monoclonal antibody for the treatment of epidermal growth factor receptor-expressing tumours. *Expert Opin. Pharmacother.* **2004**, *5*, 1621–1633.
18. Harding, J.; Burtness, B. Cetuximab: An epidermal growth factor receptor chemeric human-murine monoclonal antibody. *Drugs Today* **2005**, *41*, 107–127.
19. Santiago, A.; Eicheler, W.; Bussink, J.; Rijken, P.; Yaromina, A.; Beuthien-Baumann, B.; van der Kogel, A.J.; Baumann, M.; Krause, M. Effect of cetuximab and fractionated irradiation on tumour micro-environment. *Radiother. Oncol.* **2010**, *97*, 322–329.
20. Naramura, M.; Gillies, SD.; Mendelsohn, J.; Reisfeld, R.A.; Mueller, B.M. Therapeutic potential of chimeric and murine anti-(epidermal growth factor receptor) antibodies in a metastasis model for human melanoma. *Cancer Immunol. Immunother.* **1993**, *37*, 343–349.
21. Goldstein, N.I.; Prewett, M.; Zuklys, K.; Rockwell, P.; Mendelsohn, J. Biological efficacy of a chimeric antibody to the epidermal growth factor receptor in a human tumor xenograft model. *Clin. Cancer Res.* **1995**, *1*, 1311–1318.
22. De Bono, J.S.; Rowinsky, E.K. The ErbB receptor family: A therapeutic target for cancer. *Trends Mol. Med.* **2002**, *8*, S19–S26.
23. Wu, X.; Rubin, M.; Fan, Z.; DeBlasio, T.; Soos, T.; Koff, A.; Mendelsohn, J. Involvement of p27KIP1 in G1 arrest mediated by an anti-epidermal growth factor receptor monoclonal antibody. *Oncogene* **1996**, *12*, 1397–1403.
24. Peng, D.; Fan, Z.; Lu, Y.; De Blasio, T.; Scher, H.; Mendelsohn, J. Anti-epidermal growth factor receptor monoclonal antibody 225 up-regulates p27KIP1 and induces G1 arrest in prostatic cancer cell line DU145. *Cancer Res.* **1996**, *56*, 3666–3669.
25. Huang, S.M.; Bock, J.M.; Harari, P.M. Epidermal growth factor receptor blockade with C225 modulates proliferation, apoptosis, and radiosensitivity in squamous cell carcinomas of the head and neck. *Cancer Res.* **1999**, *59*, 1935–1940.
26. Baumann, M.; Krause, M.; Dikomey, E.; Dittmann, K.; Dörr, W.; Kasten-Pisula, U.; Rodemann, H.P. EGFR-targeted anti-cancer drugs in radiotherapy: Preclinical evaluation of mechanisms. *Radiother. Oncol.* **2007**, *83*, 238–248.
27. Vermorken, J.B.; Mesia, R.; Rivera, F.; Remenar, E.; Kawecki, A.; Rottey, S.; Erfan, J.; Zabolotnyy, D.; Kienzer, H.R.; Cupissol, D.; *et al.* Platinum-based chemotherapy plus cetuximab in head and neck cancer. *N. Engl. J. Med.* **2008**, *359*, 1116–1127.
28. Van Cutsem, E.; Köhne, C.H.; Hitre, E.; Zaluski, J.; Chang Chien, C.R.; Makhson, A.; D'Haens, G.; Pintér, T.; Lim, R.; Bodoky, G.; *et al.* Cetuximab and chemotherapy as initial treatment for metastatic colorectal cancer. *N. Engl. J. Med.* **2009**, *360*, 1408–1417.
29. Pan, Q.; Gorin, M.A.; Teknos, T.N. Pharmacotherapy of head and neck squamous cell carcinoma. *Expert. Opin. Pharmacother.* **2009**, *10*, 2291–302.

30. Socinski, M.A.; Evans, T.; Gettinger, S.; Hensing, T.A.; Sequist, L.V.; Ireland, B.; Stinchcombe, T.E. Treatment of stage IV non-small cell lung cancer: Diagnosis and management of lung cancer, 3rd ed; American College of Chest Physicians evidence-based clinical practice guidelines. *Chest* **2013**, *143*, e341S–e368S.
31. Faloppi, L.; Andrikou, K.; Cascinu, S. Cetuximab: Still an option in the treatment of pancreatic cancer? *Expert Opin. Biol. Ther.* **2013**, *13*, 791–801.
32. Bonner, J.A.; Harari, P.M.; Giralt, J.; Cohen, R.B.; Jones, C.U.; Sur, R.K.; Raben, D.; Baselga, J.; Spencer, S.A.; Zhu, J.; *et al.* Radiotherapy plus cetuximab for locoregionally advanced head and neck cancer: 5-year survival data from a phase 3 randomised trial, and relation between cetuximab-induced rash and survival. *Lancet Oncol.* **2010**, *11*, 21–28.
33. Bernier, J.; Schneider, D. Cetuximab combined with radiotherapy: An alternative to chemoradiotherapy for patients with locally advanced squamous cell carcinomas of the head and neck? *Eur. J. Cancer* **2007**, *43*, 35–45.
34. Caudell, J.J.; Sawrie, S.M.; Spencer, S.A.; Desmond, R.A.; Carroll, W.R.; Peters, G.E.; Nabell, L.M.; Meredith, R.F.; Bonner, J.A. Locoregionally advanced head and neck cancer treated with primary radiotherapy: A comparison of the addition of cetuximab or chemotherapy and the impact of protocol treatment. *Int. J. Radiat. Oncol. Biol. Phys.* **2008**, *71*, 676–681.
35. Agulnik, M. New approaches to EGFR inhibition for locally advanced or metastatic squamous cell carcinoma of the head and neck (SCCHN). *Med. Oncol.* **2012**, *29*, 2481–2491.
36. Robert, F.; Ezekiel, M.P.; Spencer, S.A.; Meredith, R.F.; Bonner, J.A.; Khazaeli, M.B.; Saleh, M.N.; Carey, D.; LoBuglio, A.F.; Wheeler, R.H.; *et al.* Phase I study of anti-epidermal growth factor receptor antibody cetuximab in combination with radiation therapy in patients with advanced head and neck cancer. *J. Clin. Oncol.* **2001**, *19*, 3234–3243.
37. Dattatreya, S.; Goswami, C. Cetuximab plus radiotherapy in patients with unresectable locally advanced squamous cell carcinoma of head and neck region—A open labelled single arm phase II study. *Indian J. Cancer* **2011**, *48*, 154–157.
38. Ang, K.K.; Zhang, Q.E.; Rosenthal, D.I.; Nguyen-Tan, P.; Sherman, E.J.; Weber, R.S.; Galvin, J.M.; Schwartz, D.L.; El-Naggar, A.K.; Gillison, M.L.; *et al.* A randomized phase III trial (RTOG 0522) of concurrent accelerated radiation plus cisplatin with or without cetuximab for stage III-IV head and neck squamous cell carcinomas (HNC). *J. Clin. Oncol.* **2011**, *29*, 5500.
39. Eriksen, J.G.; Maare, C.; Johansen, J.; Primdahl, H.; Evensen, J.; Kristensen, C.A.; Andersen, L.J.; Overgaard, J. A randomized phase III study of primary curative (chemo)-radiotherapy and the egfr-inhibitor zalutumumab for squamous cell carcinoma of the head and neck (HNSCC). *ESMO*, **2013**, *12*, 5–6.
40. Walsh, L.; Gillham, C.; Dunne, M.; Fraser, I.; Hollywood, D.; Armstrong, J.; Thirion, P. Toxicity of cetuximab versus cisplatin concurrent with radiotherapy in locally advanced head and neck squamous cell cancer (LAHNSCC). *Radiother. Oncol.* **2011**, *98*, 38–41.
41. Gurtner, K.; Deuse, Y.; Bütof, R.; Schaal, K.; Eicheler, W.; Oertel, R.; Grenman, R.; Thames, H.; Yaromina, A.; Baumann, M.; *et al.* Diverse effects of combined radiotherapy and EGFR inhibition with antibodies or TK inhibitors on local tumour control and correlation with EGFR gene expression. *Radiother. Oncol.* **2011**, *99*, 323–330.

42. Stegeman, H.; Kaanders, J.H.; van der Kogel, A.J.; Iida, M.; Wheeler, D.L.; Span, P.N.; Bussink, J. Predictive value of hypoxia, proliferation and tyrosine kinase receptors for EGFR-inhibition and radiotherapy sensitivity in head and neck cancer models. *Radiother. Oncol.* **2013**, *106*, 383–389.
43. Sok, J.C.; Coppelli, F.M.; Thomas, S.M.; Lango, M.N.; Xi, S.; Hunt, J.L.; Freilino, M.L.; Graner, M.W.; Wikstrand, C.J.; Bigner, D.D.; *et al*. Mutant epidermal growth factor receptor (EGFRvIII) contributes to head and neck cancer growth and resistance to EGFR targeting. *Clin. Cancer Res.* **2006**, *12*, 5064–5073.
44. Chen, L.F.; Cohen, E.E.; Grandis, J.R. New strategies in head and neck cancer: Understanding resistance to epidermal growth factor receptor inhibitors. *Clin. Cancer Res.* **2010**, *16*, 2489–2495.
45. Hubbard, J.M.; Alberts, S.R. Alternate dosing of cetuximab for patients with metastatic colorectal cancer. *Gastrointest. Cancer Res.* **2013**, *6*, 47–55.
46. Smilek, P.; Neuwirthova, J.; Jarkovsky, J.; Dusek, L.; Rottenberg, J.; Kostrica, R.; Srovnal, J.; Hajduch, M.; Drabek, J.; Klozar, J. Epidermal growth factor receptor (EGFR) expression and mutations in the EGFR signaling pathway in correlation with anti-EGFR therapy in head and neck squamous cell carcinomas. *Neoplasma* **2012**, *59*, 508–515.
47. Bardelli, A.; Jänne, P.A. The road to resistance: EGFR mutation and cetuximab. *Nat. Med.* **2012**, *18*, 199–200.
48. Corcoran, E.B.; Hanson, R.N. Imaging EGFR and HER2 by PET and SPECT: A Review. *Med. Res. Rev.* **2013**, doi: 10.1002/med.21299.
49. LNHB. Available onlime: http://www.nucleide.org/DDEP_WG/DDEPdata.htm (accessed on 25 February 2014).
50. Lubberink, M.; Herzog, H. Quantitative imaging of ^{124}I and ^{86}Y with PET. *Eur. J. Nucl. Med. Mol. Imaging.* **2011**, *38*, S10–S18.
51. FDA Data Specification. Available online: http://www.accessdata.fda.gov/drugsatfda_docs/label/2009/125084s 168lbl.pdf (accessed on 25 February 2014).
52. Milenic, D.E.; Brady, E.D.; Brechbiel, M.W. Antibody-targeted radiation cancer therapy. *Nat. Rev. Drug Discov.* **2004**, *3*, 488–499.
53. Srivastava, S.; Dadachova, E. Recent advances in radionuclide therapy. *Semin. Nucl. Med.* **2001**, *31*, 330–341.
54. Guo, Y.; Parry, J.J.; Laforest, R.; Rogers, B.E.; Anderson, C.J. The role of p53 in combination radioimmunotherapy with ^{64}Cu-DOTA-cetuximab and cisplatin in a mouse model of colorectal cancer. *J. Nucl. Med.* **2013**, *54*, 1621–1629.
55. Szelecsenyi, F.; Blessing, G.; Qaim, S.M. Excitation function of proton induced nuclear reactions on enriched ^{61}Ni and ^{64}Ni: Possibility of production of no-carrier-added ^{61}Cu and ^{64}Cu at a small cyclotron. *Appl. Radiat. Isot.* **1993**, *44*, 575–580.
56. McCarthy, D.W.; Shefer, R.E.; Klinkowstein, R.E.; Bass, L.A.; Margeneau, W.H.; Cutler, C.S.; Anderson, C.J.; Welch, M.J. Efficient production of high specific activity ^{64}Cu using a biomedical cyclotron. *Nucl. Med. Biol.* **1997**, *24*, 35–2443.
57. Linder, M.C.; Hazegh-Azam, M. Copper biochemistry and molecular biology. *Am. J. Clin. Nutr.* **1996**, *63*, 797S–811S.
58. Anderson, C.J.; Ferdani, R. Copper-64 radiopharmaceuticals for PET imaging of cancer: Advances in preclinical and clinical research. *Cancer Biother. Radiopharm.* **2009**, *24*, 379–393.

59. Cai, W.; Chen, K.; He, L.; Cao, Q.; Koong, A.; Chen, X. Quantitative PET of EGFR expression in xenograft-bearing mice using ^{64}Cu-labeled cetuximab, a chimeric anti-EGFR monoclonal antibody. *Eur. J. Nucl. Med. Mol. Imaging* **2007**, *34*, 850–858.
60. Eiblmaier, M.; Meyer, L.A.; Watson, M.A.; Fracasso, P.M.; Pike, L.J.; Anderson, C.J. Correlating EGFR expression with receptor-binding properties and internalization of ^{64}Cu-DOTA-cetuximab in 5 cervical cancer cell lines. *J. Nucl. Med.* 2008, *49*, 1472–1479.
61. Ping Li, W.; Meyer, L.A.; Capretto, D.A.; Sherman, C.D.; Anderson, C.J. Receptor-binding, biodistribution, and metabolism studies of ^{64}Cu-DOTA-cetuximab, a PET-imaging agent for epidermal growth-factor receptor-positive tumors. *Cancer Biother. Radiopharm.* **2008**, *23*, 158–171.
62. Niu, G.; Li, Z.; Xie, J.; Le, Q.T.; Chen, X. PET of EGFR antibody distribution in head and neck squamous cell carcinoma models. *J. Nucl. Med.* **2009**, *50*, 1116–1123.
63. Zhang, Y.; Hong, H.; Engle, J.W.; Bean, J.; Yang, Y.; Leigh, B.R.; Barnhart, T.E.; Cai, W. Positron emission tomography imaging of CD105 expression with a ^{64}Cu-labeled monoclonal antibody: NOTA is superior to DOTA. *PLoS One* **2011**, *6*, e28005.
64. Velikyan, I.; Sundberg, A.L.; Lindhe, O.; Höglund, A.U.; Eriksson, O.; Werner, E.; Carlsson, J.; Bergström, M.; Långström, B.; Tolmachev, V. Preparation and evaluation of ^{68}Ga-DOTA-hEGF for visualization of EGFR expression in malignant tumors. *J. Nucl. Med.* **2005**, *46*, 1881–1888.
65. Liu, Z.; Cui, L.; Liu, X.; Wang, F. Noninvasive small-animal PET of trastuzumab-mediated EGFR down-regulation with ^{68}Ga-Vec(Fab')2. *J. Nucl. Med.* **2012**, *53*, 342.
66. Strand, J.; Honarvar, H.; Perols, A.; Orlova, A.; Selvaraju, R.K.; Karlström, A.E.; Tolmachev, V. Influence of macrocyclic chelators on the targeting properties of ^{68}Ga-labeled synthetic affibody molecules: Comparison with ^{111}In-labeled counterparts. *PLoS One* **2013**, *8*, e70028.
67. Vosjan, M.J.; Perk, L.R.; Roovers, R.C.; Visser, G.W.; Stigter-van Walsum, M.; van Bergen, E.; Henegouwen, P.M.; van Dongen, G.A. Facile labelling of an anti-epidermal growth factor receptor Nanobody with ^{68}Ga via a novel bifunctional desferal chelate for immuno-PET. *Eur. J. Nucl. Med. Mol. Imaging* **2011**, *38*, 753–763.
68. Griffiths, G.L.; Chang, C.H.; McBride, W.J.; Rossi, E.A.; Sheerin, A.; Tejada, G.R.; Karacay, H.; Sharkey, R.M.; Horak, I.D.; Hansen, H.J.; *et al.* Reagents and methods for PET using bispecific antibody pretargeting and 68Ga-radiolabeled bivalent hapten-peptide-chelate conjugates. *J. Nucl. Med.* **2004**, *45*, 30–39.
69. Schuhmacher, J.; Klivényi, G.; Kaul, S.; Henze, M.; Matys, R.; Hauser, H.; Clorius, J. Pretargeting of human mammary carcinoma xenografts with bispecific anti-MUC1/anti-Ga chelate antibodies and immunoscintigraphy with PET. *Nucl. Med. Biol.* **2001**, *28*, 821–828.
70. Kuijpers, W.H.; Bos, E.S.; Kaspersen, F.M.; Veeneman, G.H.; van Boeckel, C.A. Specific recognition of antibody-oligonucleotide conjugates by radiolabeled antisense nucleotides: A novel approach for two-step radioimmunotherapy of cancer. *Bioconjug. Chem.* **1993**, *4*, 94–102.
71. Rusckowski, M.; Qu, T.; Chang, F.; Hnatowich, D.J. Pretargeting using peptide nucleic acid. *Cancer* **1997**, *80*, 2699–2705.
72. Engle, J.W.; Hong, H.; Zhang, Y.; Valdovinos, H.F.; Myklejord, D.V.; Barnhart, T.E.; Theuer, C.P.; Nickles, R.J.; Cai, W. Positron Emission Tomography Imaging of Tumor Angiogenesis with a ^{66}Ga-Labeled Monoclonal Antibody. *Mol. Pharm.* **2012**, *9*, 1441–1448.

73. Garmestani, K.; Milenic, D.E.; Plascjak, P.S.; Brechbiel, M.W. A new and convenient method for purification of ^{86}Y using a Sr(II) selective resin and comparison of biodistribution of ^{86}Y and ^{111}In labeled Herceptin. *Nucl. Med. Biol.* **2002**, *29*, 599–606.
74. Perk, L.R.; Visser, G.W.; Vosjan, M.J.; Stigter-van Walsum, M.; Tijink, B.M.; Leemans, C.R.; van Dongen, G.A. ^{89}Zr as a PET surrogate radioisotope for scouting biodistribution of the therapeutic radiometals ^{90}Y and ^{177}Lu in tumor-bearing nude mice after coupling to the internalizing antibody cetuximab. *J. Nucl. Med.* **2005**, *46*, 1898–1906.
75. Pentlow, K.S.; Finn, R.D.; Larson, S.M.; Erdi, Y.E.; Beattie, B.J.; Humm, J.L. Quantitative Imaging of Yttrium-86 with PET. The Occurrence and Correction of Anomalous Apparent Activity in High Density Regions. *Clin. Positron Imaging* **2000**, *3*, 85–90.
76. Walrand, S.; Jamar, F.; Mathieu, I.; de camps, j.; Lonneux, M.; Sibomana, M.; Labar, D.; Michel, C.; Pauwels, S. Quantitation in PET using isotopes emitting prompt single gammas: Application to yttrium-86. *Eur. J. Nucl. Med. Mol. Imaging* **2003**, *30*, 354–361.
77. Nayak, T.K.; Brechbiel, M.W. Radioimmunoimaging with longer-lived positron-emitting radionuclides: Potentials and challenges. *Bioconjug Chem.* **2009**, *20*, 825–841.
78. Lövqvist, A.; Humm, J.L.; Sheikh, A.; Finn, R.D.; Koziorowski, J.; Ruan, S.; Pentlow, K.S.; Jungbluth, A.; Welt, S.; Lee, F.T.; *et al.* PET imaging of ^{86}Y-labe.led anti-Lewis Y monoclonal antibodies in a nude mouse model: Comparison between ^{86}Y and (111)In radiolabels. *J. Nucl. Med.* **2001**, *42*, 1281–1287.
79. Palm, S.; Enmon, R.M., Jr.; Matei, C.; Kolbert, K.S.; Xu, S.; Zanzonico, P.B.; Finn, R.L.; Koutcher, J.A.; Larson, S.M.; Sgouros, G. Pharmacokinetics and Biodistribution of ^{86}Y-Trastuzumab for ^{90}Y dosimetry in an ovarian carcinoma model: Correlative MicroPET and MRI. *J. Nucl. Med.* **2003**, *44*, 1148–1155.
80. Schneider, D.W.; Heitner, T.; Alicke, B.; Light, D.R.; McLean, K.; Satozawa, N.; Parry, G.; Yoo, J.; Lewis, J.S.; Parry, R. *In vivo* biodistribution, PET imaging, and tumor accumulation of ^{86}Y- and ^{111}In-antimindin/RG-1, engineered antibody fragments in LNCaP tumor-bearing nude mice. *J. Nucl. Med.* **2009**, *50*, 435–443.
81. Nayak, T.K.; Garmestani, K.; Baidoo, K.E.; Milenic, D.E.; Brechbiel, M.W. Preparation, biological evaluation, and pharmacokinetics of the human anti-HER1 monoclonal antibody panitumumab labeled with ^{86}Y for quantitative PET of carcinoma. *J. Nucl. Med.* **2010**, *51*, 942–950.
82. Wong, K.J.; Baidoo, K.E; Nayak, T.K.; Garmestani, K.; Brechbiel, M.W.; Milenic, D.E. *In Vitro* and *In Vivo* Pre-Clinical Analysis of a F(ab')(2) Fragment of Panitumumab for Molecular Imaging and Therapy of HER1 Positive Cancers. *EJNMMI Res.* **2011**, *1*, 1.
83. Nayak, T.K.; Regino, C.A.; Wong, K.J.; Milenic, D.E.; Garmestani, K.; Baidoo, K.E.; Szajek, L.P.; Brechbiel, M.W. PET imaging of HER1-expressing xenografts in mice with ^{86}Y-CHX-A″-DTPA-cetuximab. *Eur. J. Nucl. Med. Mol. Imaging* **2010**, *37*, 1368–1376.
84. Nayak, T.K.; Garmestani, K.; Milenic, D.E.; Baidoo, K.E.; Brechbiel, M.W. HER1-targeted ^{86}Y-panitumumab possesses superior targeting characteristics than ^{86}Y-cetuximab for PET imaging of human malignant mesothelioma tumors xenografts. *PLoS One* **2011**, *6*, e18198.

85. Milenic, D.E.; Wong, K.J.; Baidoo, K.E.; Ray, G.L.; Garmestani, K.; Williams, M.; Brechbiel, M.W. Cetuximab: Preclinical evaluation of a monoclonal antibody targeting EGFR for radioimmunodiagnostic and radioimmunotherapeutic applications. *Cancer Biother Radiopharm.* **2008**, *23*, 619–631.

86. Verel, I.; Visser, G.W.; Boellaard, R.; Stigter-van Walsum, M.; Snow, G.B.; van Dongen, G.A. ^{89}Zr immuno-PET: Comprehensive procedures for the production of ^{89}Zr-labeled monoclonal antibodies. *J. Nucl. Med.* **2003**, *44*, 1271–1281.

87. FDA-Specification. Available online: http://www.accessdata.fda.gov/drugsatfda_docs/label/2012/125084s225lbl.pdf (accessed on 25 February 2014).

88. Börjesson, P.K.; Jauw, Y.W.; de Bree, R.; Roos, J.C.; Castelijns, J.A.; Leemans, C.R.; van Dongen, G.A.; Boellaard, R. Radiation dosimetry of ^{89}Zr-labeled chimeric monoclonal antibody U36 as used for immuno-PET in head and neck cancer patients. *J. Nucl. Med.* **2009**, *50*, 1828–1836.

89. Perk, L.R.; Visser, O.J.; Stigter-van Walsum, M.; Vosjan, M.J.; Visser, G.W.; Zijlstra, J.M.; Huijgens, P.C.; van Dongen, G.A. Preparation and evaluation of ^{89}Zr-Zevalin for monitoring of ^{90}Y-Zevalin biodistribution with positron emission tomography. *Eur. J. Nucl. Med. Mol. Imaging* **2006**, *33*, 1337–1345.

90. Van Nerom, C.G.; Bormans, G.M.; de Roo, M.J.; Verbruggen, A.M. First experience in healthy volunteers with technetium-99m L,L-ethylenedicysteine, a new renal imaging agent. *Eur. J. Nucl. Med.* **1993**, *20*, 738–746.

91. Schechter, N.R.; Yang, D.J.; Azhdarinia, A.; Kohanim, S.; Wendt, R.; Oh, C.S.; Hu, M.; Yu, D.F.; Bryant, J.; Ang, K.K.; *et al.* Assessment of epidermal growth factor receptor with ^{99m}Tc-ethylenedicysteine-C225 monoclonal antibody. *Anticancer Drugs* **2003**, *14*, 49–56.

92. Schechter, N.R.; Wendt, R.E.; Yang, D.J.; Azhdarinia, A.; Erwin, W.D.; Stachowiak, A.M.; Broemeling, L.D.; Kim, E.E.; Cox, J.D.; Podoloff, D.A.; *et al.* Radiation dosimetry of ^{99m}Tc-labeled C225 in patients with squamous cell carcinoma of the head and neck. *J. Nucl. Med.* **2004**, *45*, 1683–1687.

93. Kaur, S.; Venktaraman, G.; Jain, M.; Senapati, S.; Garg, P.K.; Batra, S.K. Recent trends in antibody-based oncologic imaging. *Cancer Lett.* **2012**, *31*, 97–111.

94. Capello, A.; Krenning, E.P.; Breeman, W.A.; Bernard, B.F.; de Jong, M. Peptide receptor radionuclide therapy *in vitro* using [^{111}In-DTPA0]octreotide. *J. Nucl. Med.* **2003**, *44*, 98–104.

95. Huhtala, T.; Laakkonen, P.; Sallinen, H.; Ylä-Herttuala, S.; Närvänen, A. *In vivo* SPECT/CT imaging of human orthotopic ovarian carcinoma xenografts with 111In-labeled monoclonal antibodies. *Nucl. Med. Biol.* **2010**, *37*, 957–964.

96. Price, E.W.; Zeglis, B.M.; Cawthray, J.F.; Ramogida, C.F.; Ramos, N.; Lewis, J.S.; Adam, M.J.; Orvig, C. H(4)octapa-trastuzumab: Versatile acyclic chelate system for ^{111}In and ^{177}Lu imaging and therapy. *J. Am. Chem. Soc.* **2013**, *135*, 12707–12721.

97. Yoshida, H.; Mochizuki, M.; Kainouchi, M.; Ishida, T.; Sakata, K.; Yokoyama, S.; Hoshino, T.; Takezawa, M.; Matsumoto, Y.; Miyamoto, T.; *et al.* Clinical application of indium-111 antimyosin antibody and thallium-201 dual nuclide single photon emission computed tomography in acute myocardial infarction. *Ann. Nucl. Med.* **1991**, *5*, 41–46.

98. Divgi, C.R.; Welt, S.; Kris, M.; Real, F.X.; Yeh, S.D.; Gralla, R.; Merchant, B.; Schweighart, S.; Unger, M.; Larson, S.M.; *et al.* Phase I and imaging trial of indium-111 labeled anti-epidermal growth factor receptor monoclonal antibody 225 in patients with squamous cell lung carcinoma. *J. Natl. Cancer Inst.* **1991**, *83*, 97–104.
99. Dillman, L.T.; von der Lage, F.C. NM/MIRD Pamphlet No. 10: Radionuclide Decay Schemes and Nuclear Parameters for Use in Radiation-Dose Estimation. New York. *Soc. Nucl. Med.* **1975**, *69*, 54.
100. Bading, J.R.; Hörling, M.; Williams, L.E.; Colcher, D.; Raubitschek, A.; Strand, S.E. Quantitative serial imaging of an 124I anti-CEA monoclonal antibody in tumor-bearing mice. *Cancer Biother. Radiopharm.* **2008**, *23*, 399–409.
101. Yao, M.; Faulhaber, P.F. PET imaging of the head and neck. *PET Clinics* **2012**, *7*, 450.
102. Lee, F.T.; Hall, C.; Rigopoulos, A.; Zweit, J.; Pathmaraj, K.; O'Keefe, G.J.; Smyth, F.E.; Welt, S.; Old, L.J.; Scott, A.M. Immuno-PET of human colon xenograft- bearing BALB/c nude mice using ^{124}I-CDR-grafted humanized A33 monoclonal antibody. *J. Nucl. Med.* **2001**, *42*, 764–769.
103. Fortin, M.A.; Salnikov, A.V.; Nestor, M.; Heldin, N.E.; Rubin, K.; Lundqvist, H. Immuno-PET of undifferentiated thyroid carcinoma with radioiodine-labelled antibody cMAb U36: Application to antibody tumour uptake studies. *Eur. J. Nucl. Med. Mol. Imaging* **2007**, *34*, 1376–1387.
104. Lee, F.T.; O'Keefe, G.J.; Gan, H.K.; Mountain, A.J.; Jones, G.R.; Saunder, T.H.; Sagona, J.; Rigopoulos, A.; Smyth, F.E.; Johns, T.G.; *et al.* Immuno-PET quantitation of de2-7 epidermal growth factor receptor expression in glioma using ^{124}I-IMP-R4-labeled antibody ch806. *J. Nucl. Med.* **2010**, *51*, 967–972.
105. Tijink, B.M.; Neri, D.; Leemans, C.R.; Budde, M.; Dinkelborg, L.M.; Stigter-van Walsum, M,; Zardi, L.; van Dongen, G.A. Radioimmunotherapy of head and neck cancer xenografts using ^{131}I-labeled antibody L19-SIP for selective targeting of tumor vasculature. *J. Nucl. Med.* **2006**, *47*, 1127–1135.
106. Nestor, M.; Ekberg, T.; Dring, J.; van Dongen, G.A.; Wester, K.; Tolmachev, V.; Anniko, M. Quantification of CD44v6 and EGFR expression in head and neck squamous cell carcinomas using a single-dose radioimmunoassay. *Tumour Biol.* **2007**, *28*, 253–263.
107. Nordberg, E.; Friedman, M.; Göstring, L.; Adams, G.P.; Brismar, H.; Nilsson, F.Y.; Ståhl, S.; Glimelius, B.; Carlsson, J. Cellular studies of binding, internalization and retention of a radiolabeled EGFR-binding affibody molecule. *Nucl. Med. Biol.* **2007**, *34*, 609–618.
108. Hoeben, B.A.; Molkenboer-Kuenen, J.D.; Oyen, W.J.; Peeters, W.J.; Kaanders, J.H., Bussink, J.; Boerman, O.C. Radiolabeled cetuximab: Dose optimization for epidermal growth factor receptor imaging in a head-and-neck squamous cell carcinoma model. *Int. J. Cancer* **2011**, *129*, 870–878.
109. Tijink, B.M.; Laeremans, T.; Budde, M.; Stigter-van Walsum, M.; Dreier, T.; de Haard, H.J.; Leemans, C.R.; van Dongen, G.A. Improved tumor targeting of anti-epidermal growth factor receptor Nanobodies through albumin binding: Taking advantage of modular Nanobody technology. *Mol. Cancer Ther.* **2008**, *7*, 2288–2297.
110. Börjesson, P.K.; Postema, E.J.; de Bree, R.; Roos, J.C.; Leemans, C.R.; Kairemo, K.J.; van Dongen, G.A. Radioimmunodetection and radioimmunotherapy of head and neck cancer. *Oral. Oncol.* **2004**, *40*, 761–772.

111. Jowsey, J.; Rowland, R.E.; Marshall, J.H. The deposition of the rare earths in bone. *Radiat. Res.* **1958**, *8*, 490–501.

112. Minarik, D.; Ljungberg, M.; Segars, P.; Gleisner, K.S. Evaluation of quantitative planar 90Y bremsstrahlung whole-body imaging. *Phys. Med. Biol.* **2009**, *54*, 5873–5883.

113. Elschot, M.; Vermolen, B.J.; Lam, M.G.; de Keizer, B.; van den Bosch, M.A.; de Jong, H.W. Quantitative comparison of PET and Bremsstrahlung SPECT for imaging the *in vivo* yttrium-90 microsphere distribution after liver radioembolization. *PLoS One* **2013**, *8*, e55742.

114. Goodwin, D.A.; Meares, C.F.; Watanabe, N.; McTigue, M.; Chaovapong, W.; Ransone, C.M.; Renn, O.; Greiner, D.P.; Kukis D.L.; Kronenberger, S.I. Pharmacokinetics of pretargeted monoclonal antibody 2D12.5 and ^{88}Y-Janus-2-(p-nitrobenzyl)-1,4,7,10-tetraazacyclododecanetetraacetic acid (DOTA) in BALB/c mice with KHJJ mouse adenocarcinoma: A model for ^{90}Y radioimmunotherapy. *Cancer Res.* **1994**, *54*, 5937–5946.

115. Postema, E.J.; Frielink, C.; Oyen, W.J.; Raemaekers, J.M.; Goldenberg, D.M.; Corstens, F.H.; Boerman, O.C. Biodistribution of ^{131}I-, ^{186}Re-, ^{177}Lu-, and ^{88}Y-labeled hLL2 (Epratuzumab) in nude mice with CD22-positive lymphoma. *Cancer Biother. Radiopharm.* **2003**, *18*, 525–533.

116. 116. Walrand, S.; Flux, G.D.; Konijnenberg, M.W.; Valkema, R.; Krenning, E.P.; Lhommel, R.; Pauwels, S.; Jamar, F. Dosimetry of yttrium-labelled radiopharmaceuticals for internal therapy: ^{86}Y or ^{90}Y imaging? *Eur. J. Nucl. Med. Mol. Imaging* **2011**, *38*, S57–S68.

117. Niu, G.; Sun, X.; Cao, Q.; Courter, D.; Koong, A.; Le, Q.T.; Gambhir, S.S.; Chen, X. Cetuximab-based immunotherapy and radioimmunotherapy of head and neck squamous cell carcinoma. *Clin. Cancer Res.* **2010**, *16*, 2095–2105.

118. Koi, L.; Bergmann, R.; Brüchner, K.; Pietzsch, H.J.; Krause, M.; Steinbach, J.; Zips, D.; Baumann, M. Theragnostic radiolabeled EGFR-antibody improves local tumor control after external radiotherapy. *Radiother. Oncol.* **2014**, in press.

119. Saki, M.; Toulany, M.; Sihver, W.; Zenker, M.; Heldt, J.M.; Mosch, B.; Pietzsch, H.J.; Baumann, M.; Steinbach, J.; Rodemann, H.P. Cellular and molecular properties of ^{90}Y-labeled cetuximab in combination with radiotherapy on human tumor cells *in vitro*. *Strahlenther. Onkol.* **2012**, *188*, 823–832.

120. Verburg, F.A.; Luster, M.; Lassmann, M.; Reiners, C. ^{131}I therapy in patients with benign thyroid disease does not conclusively lead to a higher risk of subsequent malignancies. *Nuklearmedizin* **2011**, *50*, 93–99.

121. Grünwald, F.; Ezziddin, S. ^{131}I-metaiodobenzylguanidine therapy of neuroblastoma and other neuroendocrine tumors. *Semin. Nuc. Med.* **2010**, *40*, 153–163.

122. Sisson, J.C.; Carey, J.E. Thyroid carcinoma with high levels of function: Treatment with ^{131}I. *J. Nucl. Med.* **2001**, *42*, 975–983.

123. Xue, Y.L.; Qiu, Z.L.; Song, H.J.; Luo, Q.Y. Value of ^{131}I SPECT/CT for the evaluation of differentiated thyroid cancer: A systematic review of the literature. *Eur. J. Nucl. Med. Mol. Imaging* **2013**, *40*, 768–778.

124. Rades, D.; Wolff, C.; Nadrowitz, R.; Breunig, C.; Schild, S.E.; Baehre, M.; Meller, B. Radioactive EGFR antibody cetuximab in multimodal cancer treatment: Stability and synergistic effects with radiotherapy. *Int. J. Radiat. Oncol. Biol. Phys.* **2009**, *75*, 1226–1231.

125. Schlom, J.; Siler, K.; Milenic, D.E.; Eggensperger, D.; Colcher, D.; Miller, L.S.; Houchens, D.; Cheng, R.; Kaplan, D.; Goeckeler, W. Monoclonal antibody-based therapy of a human tumor xenograft with a ^{177}lutetium-labeled im munoconjugate. *Cancer Res.* **1991**, *51*, 2889–2896.
126. Mulligan, T.; Carrasquillo, J.A.; Chung, Y.; Milenic, D.E.; Schlom, J.; Feuerstein, I.; Paik, C.; Perentesis, P.; Reynolds, J.; Curt, G.; *et al.* Phase I study of intravenous Lu-labeled CC49 murine monoclonal antibody in patients with advanced adenocarcinoma. *J. Clin. Cancer Res.* **1995**, *1*, 1447–1454.
127. Stein, R.; Govindan, S.V.; Chen, S.; Reed, L.; Richel, H.; Griffiths, G.L.; Hansen, H.J.; Goldenberg, D.M. Radioimmunotherapy of a human lung cancer xenograft with monoclonal antibody RS7: Evaluation of ^{177}Lu and comparison of its efficacy with that of ^{90}Y and residualizing ^{131}I. *J. Nucl. Med.* **2001**, *42*, 967–974.
128. Lee, S.Y.; Hong, Y.D.; Kim, H.S.; Choi, S.J. Synthesis and application of a novel cysteine-based DTPA-NCS for targeted radioimmunotherapy. *Nucl. Med. Biol.* **2013**, *40*, 424–429.
129. Jurcic, J.G.; Larson, S.M.; Sgouros, G.; McDevitt, M.R.; Finn, R.D.; Divgi, C.R.; Ballangrud, A.M.; Hamacher, K.A.; Ma, D.; Humm, J.L.; *et al.* Targeted alpha particle immunotherapy for myeloid leukemia. *Blood* **2002**, *100*, 1233–1239.
130. Song, H.; Shahverdi, K.; Huso, D.L.; Esaias, C.; Fox, J.; Liedy, A.; Zhang, Z.; Reilly, R.T.; Apostolidis, C.; Morgenstern, A.; *et al.* ^{213}Bi (alpha-emitter)-antibody targeting of breast cancer metastases in the neu-N transgenic mouse model. *Cancer Res.* **2008**, *68*, 3873–3880.
131. Ma, D.; McDevitt, M.R.; Finn, R.D.; Scheinberg, D.A. Breakthrough of ^{225}Ac and its radionuclide daughters from an ^{225}Ac/^{21}3Bi generator: Development of new methods, quantitative characterization, and implications for clinical use. *Appl. Radiat. Isot.* **2001**, *55*, 667–678.
132. Rosenblat, T.L.; McDevitt, M.R.; Mulford, D.A.; Pandit-Taskar, N.; Divgi, C.R.; Panageas, K.S.; Heaney, M.L.; Chanel, S.; Morgenstern, A.; Sgouros, G.; *et al.* Sequential cytarabine and alpha-particle immunotherapy with bismuth-213-lintuzumab (HuM195) for acute myeloid leukemia. *Clin. Cancer Res.* **2010**, *16*, 5303–5311.
133. Andersson, H.; Cederkrantz, E.; Bäck, T.; Divgi, C.; Elgqvist, J.; Himmelman, J.; Horvath, G.; Jacobsson, L.; Jensen, H.; Lindegren, S.; *et al.* Intraperitoneal alpha-particle radioimmunotherapy of ovarian cancer patients: Pharmacokinetics and dosimetry of ^{211}At-MX35 F(ab')2—A phase I study. *J. Nucl. Med.* **2009**, *50*, 1153–1160.
134. Allen, B.J.; Singla, A.A.; Rizvi, S.M.; Graham, P.; Bruchertseifer, F.; Apostolidis, C.; Morgenstern, A. Analysis of patient survival in a Phase I trial of systemic targeted α-therapy for metastatic melanoma. *Immunotherapy* **2011**, *3*, 1041–1050.
135. Song, H.; Hedayati, M.; Hobbs, R.F.; Shao, C.; Bruchertseifer, F.; Morgenstern, A.; Deweese, T.L.; Sgouros, G. Targeting aberrant DNA double strand break repair in triple negative breast cancer with alpha particle emitter radiolabeled anti-EGFR antibody. *Mol. Cancer Ther.* **2013**, *12*, 2043–2054.
136. Brechbiel, M.W. Bifunctional chelates for metal nuclides. *Q. J. Nucl. Med. Mol. Imaging* **2008**, *52*, 166–173.
137. Pritchard, J.H.; Ackerman, M.; Tubis, M.; Blahd, W.H. Indium-111-labeled antibody heavy metal chelate conjugates: A potential alternative to radioiodination. *Proc. Soc. Exp. Biol. Med.* **1976**, *151*, 297–302.

138. Ward, M.C.; Roberts, K.R.; Babich, J.W.; Bukhari, M.A.; Coghlan, G.; Westwood, J.H.; McCready, V.R.; Ott, R.J. An antibody-desferrioxamine conjugate labelled with ^{67}Ga. *Int. J. Rad. Appl. Instrum. B* **1986**, *13*, 505–307.

139. Perk, L.R.; Vosjan, M.J.; Visser, G.W.; Budde, M.; Jurek, P.; Kiefer, G.E.; van Dongen, G.A. p-Isothiocyanatobenzyl-desferrioxamine: A new bifunctional chelate for facile radiolabeling of monoclonal antibodies with zirconium-89 for immuno-PET imaging. *Eur. J. Nucl. Med. Mol. Imaging* **2010**, *37*, 250–259.

140. Chang, A.J.; de Silva, R.A.; Lapi, S.E. Development and characterization of ^{89}Zr-labeled panitumumab for immuno-positron emission tomographic imaging of the epidermal growth factor receptor. *Mol. Imaging* **2013**, *12*, 17–27.

141. Aerts, H.J.; Dubois, L.; Perk, L.; Vermaelen, P.; van Dongen, G.A.; Wouters, B.G.; Lambin, P. Disparity between *in vivo* EGFR expression and ^{89}Zr-labeled cetuximab uptake assessed with PET. *J. Nucl. Med.* **2009**, *50*, 123–131.

142. Karmani, L.; Labar, D.; Valembois, V.; Bouchat, V.; Nagaswaran, P.G.; Bol, A.; Gillart, J.; Levêque, P.; Bouzin, C.; Bonifazi, D.; *et al.* Antibody-functionalized nanoparticles for imaging cancer: Influence of conjugation to gold nanoparticles on the biodistribution of ^{89}Zr-labeled cetuximab in mice. *Contrast Media Mol. Imaging* **2013**, *8*, 402–408.

143. McMurry, T.J.; Pippin, C.G.; Wu, C.; Deal, K.A.; Brechbiel, M.W.; Mirzadeh, S.; Gansow, O.A. Physical parameters and biological stability of yttrium(III) diethylenetriaminepentaacetic acid derivative conjugates. *J. Med. Chem.* **1998**, *41*, 3546–3549.

144. Kobayashi, H.; Wu, C.; Yoo, T.M.; Sun, B.F.; Drumm, D.; Pastan, I.; Paik, C.H.; Gansow, O.A.; Carrasquillo, J.A.; Brechbiel, M.W. Evaluation of the *in vivo* biodistribution of yttrium-labeled isomers of CHX-DTPA-conjugated monoclonal antibodies. *J. Nucl. Med.* **1998**, *39*, 829–836.

145. Lee, F.T.; Mountain, A.J.; Kelly, M.P.; Hall, C.; Rigopoulos, A.; Johns, T.G.; Smyth, F.E.; Brechbiel, M.W.; Nice, E.C.; Burgess, A.W.; *et al.* Enhanced efficacy of radioimmunotherapy with ^{90}Y-CHX-A″-DTPA-hu3S193 by inhibition of epidermal growth factor receptor (EGFR) signaling with EGFR tyrosine kinase inhibitor AG1478. *Clin. Cancer Res.* **2005**, *11*, 7080s–7086s.

146. Fani, M.; Bouziotis, P.; Harris, A.L.; Psimadas, D.; Gourni, E.; Loudos, G.; Varvarigou, A.D.; Maecke, H.R. ^{177}Lu-labeled-VG76e monoclonal antibody in tumor angiogenesis: A comparative study using DOTA and DTPA chelating systems. *Radiochim. Acta* **2007**, *95*, 351–357.

147. Ray, G.L.; Baidoo, K.E.; Wong, K.J.; Williams, M.; Garmestani, K.; Brechbiel, M.W.; Milenic, D.E. Preclinical evaluation of a monoclonal antibody targeting the epidermal growth factor receptor as a radioimmunodiagnostic and radioimmunotherapeutic agent. *Br. J. Pharmacol.* **2009**, *157*, 1541–1548.

148. Boswell, C.A.; Sun, X.; Niu, W.; Weisman, G.R.; Wong, E.H.; Rheingold, A.L.; Anderson, C.J. Comparative *in vivo* stability of copper-64-labeled cross-bridged and conventional tetraazamacrocyclic complexes. *J. Med. Chem.* **2004**, *47*, 1465–1474.

149. Tolmachev, V.; Wållberg, H.; Andersson, K.; Wennborg, A.; Lundqvist, H.; Orlova, A. The influence of Bz-DOTA and CHX-A″-DTPA on the biodistribution of ABD-fused anti-HER2 Affibody molecules: implications for ^{114m}In-mediated targeting therapy. *Eur. J. Nucl. Med. Mol. Imaging.* **2009**, *36*, 1460–1468.

150. Milenic, D.E.; Garmestani, K.; Chappell, L.L.; Dadachova, E.; Yordanov, A.; Ma, D.; Schlom, J.; Brechbiel, M.W. *In vivo* comparison of macrocyclic and acyclic ligands for radiolabeling of monoclonal antibodies with ^{177}Lu for radioimmunotherapeutic applications. *Nucl. Med. Biol.* **2002**, *29*, 431–442.
151. Niu, G.; Cai, W.; Chen, K.; Chen, X. Non-invasive PET imaging of EGFR degradation induced by a heat shock protein 90 inhibitor. *Mol. Imaging Biol.* **2008**, *10*, 99–106.
152. Delgado, R.; Sun, Y.; Motekaitis, R.J.; Martell, A.E. Stabilities of divalent and trivalent metal ion complexes of macrocyclic triazatriacetic acids. *Inorg. Chem.* **1993**, *32*, 3320–3326.
153. Sprague, J.E.; Peng, Y.; Sun, X.; Weisman, G.R.; Wong, E.H.; Achilefu, S.; Anderson, C.J. Preparation and biological evaluation of copper-64-labeled Tyr3-Octreotate using a cross-bridged macrocyclic cheator. *Clin. Cancer Res.* **2004**, *10*, 8674–8682.
154. Ingargiola, M.; Dittfeld, C.; Runge, R.; Zenker, M.; Heldt, J.M.; Steinbach, J.; Cordes, N.; Baumann, M.; Kotzerke, J.; Kunz-Schughart, L.A. Flow cytometric cell-based assay to preselect antibody constructs for radionuclide conjugation. *Cytometry A* **2012**, *81*, 865–873.
155. Zhang, Y.; Hong, H.; Engle, J.W.; Yang, Y.; Theuer, C.P.; Barnhart, T.E.; Cai, W. Positron Emission Tomography and Optical Imaging of Tumor CD105 Expression with a Dual-Labeled Monoclonal Antibody. *Mol. Pharm.* **2012**, *9*, 645–653.
156. Cohen, R.; Stammes, M.A.; de Roos, I.H.; Stigter-van Walsum, M.; Visser, G.W.; van Dongen, G.A. Inert coupling of IRDye800CW to monoclonal antibodies for clinical optical imaging of tumor targets. *EJNMMI Res.* **2011**, *1*, 31.
157. Vakili, A.; Jalilian, A.R.; Yavari, K.; Shirvani-Arani, S.; Khanchi, A. Bahrami-Samani, A.; Salimi, B.; Khorrami-Moghadam, A. Preparation and quality control and biodistribution studies of [^{90}Y]-DOTA-cetuximab for radioimmunotherapy. *J. Radioanal. Nucl. Chem.* **2013**, *296*, 1287–1294.
158. Wen, X.; Wu, Q.P.; Ke, S.; Ellis, L.; Charnsangavej, C.; Delpassand, A.S.; Wallace, S.; Li, C. Conjugation with ^{111}In-DTPA-poly(ethylene glycol) improves imaging of anti-EGF receptor antibody C225. *J. Nucl. Med.* **2001**, *42*, 1530–1537.
159. Van Dijk, L.K.; Hoeben, B.A.; Stegeman, H.; Kaanders, J.H.; Franssen, G.M.; Boerman, O.C.; Bussink, J. ^{111}In-cetuximab-F(ab')2 SPECT imaging for quantification of accessible epidermal growth factor receptors (EGFR) in HNSCC xenografts. *Radiother. Oncol.* **2013**, *108*, 484–488.
160. Van Dongen, G.A.; Visser, G.W.; Lub-de Hooge, M.N.; de Vries, E.G.; Perk, L.R. Immuno-PET: A navigator in monoclonal antibody development and applications. *Oncologist* **2007**, *12*, 1379–1389.
161. Walrand, S.; Barone, R.; Pauwels, S.; Jamar, F. Experimental facts supporting a red marrow uptake due to radiometal transchelation in ^{90}Y-DOTATOC therapy and relationship to the decrease of platelet counts. *Eur. J. Nucl. Med. Mol. Imaging* **2011**, *38*, 1270–1280.
162. Vakili, A.; Jalilian, A.R.; Moghadam, A.K.; Ghazi-Zahedi, M.; Salimi, B. Evaluation and comparison of human absorbed dose of ^{90}Y-DOTA-Cetuximab in various age groups based on distribution data in rats. *J. Med. Phys.* **2012**, *37*, 226–234.
163. Pilaro, A.M. Pharmacology/toxicology review and evaluation. Erbitux. Accessdata FDA Application number STN/BLA 125084. *Cent. Drug Eval. Res.* **2003**, *1*, 1–32.

164. Matsumura, Y.; Maeda, H. A new concept for macromolecular therapeutics in cancer chemotherapy: Mechanism of tumoritropic accumulation of proteins and the antitumor agent smancs. *Cancer Res.* **1986**, *46*, 6387–6392.
165. Maeda, H.; Nakamura, H.; Fang, J. The EPR effect for macromolecular drug delivery to solid tumors: Improvement of tumor uptake, lowering of systemic toxicity, and distinct tumor imaging *in vivo*. *Adv. Drug. Deliv. Rev.* **2013**, *65*, 71–79.
166. Ogawa, M.; Regino, C.A.; Choyke, P.L.; Kobayashi, H. *In vivo* target-specific activatable near-infrared optical labeling of humanized monoclonal antibodies. *Mol. Cancer Ther.* **2009**, *8*, 232–239.
167. Maeda, H.; Bharate, G.Y.; Daruwalla, J. Polymeric drugs for efficient tumor-targeted drug delivery based on EPR-effect. *Eur. J. Pharm. Biopharm.* **2009**, *71*, 409–419.
168. Perera, R.M.; Zoncu, R.; Johns, T.G.; Pypaert, M.; Lee, F.T.; Mellman, I.; Old, L.J.; Toomre, D.K.; Scott, A.M. Internalization, intracellular trafficking, and biodistribution of monoclonal antibody 806: A novel anti-epidermal growth factor receptor antibody. *Neoplasia* **2007**, *9*, 1099–1110.
169. Oude Munnink, T.H.; Tamas, K.R.; Lub-de Hooge, M.N.; Vedelaar, S.R.; Timmer-Bosscha, H.; Walenkamp, A.M.; Weidner, K.M.; Herting, F.; Tessier, J.; de Vries, E.G. Placental growth factor (PlGF)-specific uptake in tumor microenvironment of ^{89}Zr-labeled PlGF antibody RO5323441. *J. Nucl. Med.* **2013**, *54*, 929–935.
170. Danhier, F.; Feron, O.; Préat, V. To exploit the tumor microenvironment: Passive and active tumor targeting of nanocarriers for anti-cancer drug delivery. *J. Control Release* **2010**, *148*, 135–146.
171. Dittmann, K.; Mayer, C.; Rodemann, H.P. Inhibition of radiation-induced EGFR nuclear import by C225 (Cetuximab) suppresses DNA-PK activity. *Radiother. Oncol.* **2005**, *76*, 157–161.
172. Karar, J.; Maity, A. Modulating the tumor microenvironment to increase radiation responsiveness. *Cancer Biol. Ther.* **2009**, *8*, 1994–2001.
173. Saker, J.; Kriegs, M.; Zenker, M.; Heldt, J.M.; Eke, I.; Pietzsch, H.J.; Grénman, R.; Cordes, N.; Petersen, C.; Baumann, M.; *et al.* Inactivation of HNSCC cells by ^{90}Y-labeled cetuximab strictly depends on the number of induced DNA double-strand breaks. *J. Nucl. Med.* **2013**, *54*, 416–423.
174. Krause, M.; Ostermann, G.; Petersen, C.; Yaromina, A.; Hessel, F.; Harstrick, A.; van der Kogel, A.J.; Thames, H.D.; Baumann, M. Decreased repopulation as well as increased reoxygenation contribute to the improvement in local control after targeting of the EGFR by C225 during fractionated irradiation. *Radiother. Oncol.* **2005**, *76*, 162–167.
175. Eiblmaier, M; Meyer, L.A.; Anderson, C.J. The role of p53 in the trafficking of copper-64 to tumor cell nuclei. *Cancer Biol. Ther.* **2008**, *7*, 63–69.
176. Rades, D.; Nadrowitz, R.; Buchmann, I.; Hunold, P.; Noack, F.; Schild, S.E.; Meller, B. Radiolabeled cetuximab plus whole-brain irradiation (WBI) for the treatment of brain metastases from non-small cell lung cancer (NSCLC). *Strahlenther. Onkol.* **2010**, *186*, 458–462.

Permissions

All chapters in this book were first published by MDPI; hereby published with permission under the Creative Commons Attribution License or equivalent. Every chapter published in this book has been scrutinized by our experts. Their significance has been extensively debated. The topics covered herein carry significant findings which will fuel the growth of the discipline. They may even be implemented as practical applications or may be referred to as a beginning point for another development.

The contributors of this book come from diverse backgrounds, making this book a truly international effort. This book will bring forth new frontiers with its revolutionizing research information and detailed analysis of the nascent developments around the world.

We would like to thank all the contributing authors for lending their expertise to make the book truly unique. They have played a crucial role in the development of this book. Without their invaluable contributions this book wouldn't have been possible. They have made vital efforts to compile up to date information on the varied aspects of this subject to make this book a valuable addition to the collection of many professionals and students.

This book was conceptualized with the vision of imparting up-to-date information and advanced data in this field. To ensure the same, a matchless editorial board was set up. Every individual on the board went through rigorous rounds of assessment to prove their worth. After which they invested a large part of their time researching and compiling the most relevant data for our readers.

The editorial board has been involved in producing this book since its inception. They have spent rigorous hours researching and exploring the diverse topics which have resulted in the successful publishing of this book. They have passed on their knowledge of decades through this book. To expedite this challenging task, the publisher supported the team at every step. A small team of assistant editors was also appointed to further simplify the editing procedure and attain best results for the readers.

Apart from the editorial board, the designing team has also invested a significant amount of their time in understanding the subject and creating the most relevant covers. They scrutinized every image to scout for the most suitable representation of the subject and create an appropriate cover for the book.

The publishing team has been an ardent support to the editorial, designing and production team. Their endless efforts to recruit the best for this project, has resulted in the accomplishment of this book. They are a veteran in the field of academics and their pool of knowledge is as vast as their experience in printing. Their expertise and guidance has proved useful at every step. Their uncompromising quality standards have made this book an exceptional effort. Their encouragement from time to time has been an inspiration for everyone.

The publisher and the editorial board hope that this book will prove to be a valuable piece of knowledge for researchers, students, practitioners and scholars across the globe.

List of Contributors

Irina Velikyan
Section of Nuclear Medicine and PET, Department of Surgical Sciences, Uppsala University, Uppsala SE-751 85, Sweden
PET Center, Center for Medical Imaging, Uppsala University Hospital, Uppsala SE-751 85, Sweden

Benjamin Baur, Christoph Solbach, Gordon Winter, Hans-Jürgen Machulla and Sven N. Reske
Clinic for Nuclear Medicine, University of Ulm, Albert-Einstein-Allee, 89081 Ulm, Germany

Elena Andreolli
Clinic for Nuclear Medicine, University of Ulm, Albert-Einstein-Allee, 89081 Ulm, Germany
Department of Health Sciences, University of Milano-Bicocca, Milan 20900, Italy

Cristina Müller, Josefine Reber and Stephanie Haller
Center for Radiopharmaceutical Sciences ETH-PSIUSZ, Paul Scherrer Institute, 5232 Villigen-PSI, Switzerland

Konstantin Zhernosekov
Laboratory of Radiochemistry and Environmental Chemistry, Paul Scherrer Institute, 5232 Villigen-PSI, Switzerland

Andreas Türler and Holger Dorrer
Laboratory of Radiochemistry and Environmental Chemistry, Paul Scherrer Institute, 5232 Villigen-PSI, Switzerland
Laboratory of Radiochemistry and Environmental Chemistry, Department of Chemistry and Biochemistry University of Bern, 3012 Berne, Switzerland

Ulli Köster
Institut Laue-Langevin, 38000 Grenoble, France

Karl Johnston
Physics Department, ISOLDE/CERN, 1211 Geneva, Switzerland

Roger Schibli
Center for Radiopharmaceutical Sciences ETH-PSIUSZ, Paul Scherrer Institute, 5232 Villigen-PSI, Switzerland
Center for Radiopharmaceutical Sciences of ETH-PSIUSZ, Department of Nuclear Medicine, University Hospital Zürich, CH-8091 Zürich, Switzerland
Center for Radiopharmaceutical Sciences of ETH-PSIUSZ, Institute of Pharmaceutical Sciences, Department of Chemistry and Applied Biosciences, ETH Zurich, CH-8093 Zürich, Switzerland

Christiane A. Fischer, Sandra Vomstein and Thomas L. Mindt
University of Basel Hospital, Clinic of Radiology and Nuclear Medicine, Division of Radiopharmaceutical Chemistry, Petersgraben 4, 4031 Basel, Switzerland

Matthias Kuntzsch, Denis Lamparter, Nils Brüggener, Gabriele J. Kienzle and Gerald Reischl
Department of Preclinical Imaging and Radiopharmacy, Eberhard Karls University Tübingen, Röntgenweg 15, Tübingen D-72076, Germany

Marco Müller
Department of Radiochemistry, ABX GmbH, Heinrich-Gläser-Straße 10, Radeberg D-01454, Germany

Linjing Mu and Kasim Popaj
Center for Radiopharmaceutical Sciences of ETH-PSIUSZ, Department of Nuclear Medicine, University Hospital Zürich, CH-8091 Zürich, Switzerland

Roger Slavik, Adrienne Müller, Stefanie D. Krämer, Stjepko Čermak and Simon M. Ametamey
Center for Radiopharmaceutical Sciences of ETH-PSIUSZ, Institute of Pharmaceutical Sciences, Department of Chemistry and Applied Biosciences, ETH Zurich, CH-8093 Zürich, Switzerland
Neuromuscular Diseases Unit/ALS Clinic, Kantonsspital St. Gallen, CH-9007 St. Gallen, Switzerland

Markus Weber
Neuromuscular Diseases Unit/ALS Clinic, Kantonsspital St. Gallen, CH-9007 St. Gallen, Switzerland

Simone Maschauer, Tina Ruckdeschel, Philipp Tripal, Torsten Kuwert and Olaf Prante
Department of Nuclear Medicine, Laboratory of Molecular Imaging and Radiochemistry, Friedrich Alexander University, Schwabachanlage 6, 91054 Erlangen, Germany

Roland Haubner
Department of Nuclear Medicine, Innsbruck Medical University, Anichstr. 35, 6020 Innsbruck, Austria

Jürgen Einsiedel, Harald Hübner and Peter Gmeiner
Department of Chemistry and Pharmacy, Medicinal Chemistry, Emil Fischer Center, Friedrich Alexander University, Schuhstraße 19, 91052 Erlangen, Germany

Roger Slavik, Adrienne Müller, Stefanie D. Krämer, Stjepko Čermak and Simon M. Ametamey
Center for Radiopharmaceutical Sciences of ETH-PSI-USZ, Institute of Pharmaceutical Sciences, Department of Chemistry and Applied Biosciences, ETH Zurich, CH-8093 Zürich, Switzerland
Neuromuscular Diseases Unit/ ALS Clinic, Kantonsspital St. Gallen, CH-9007 St. Gallen, Switzerland

Markus Mitterhauser and Wolfgang Wadsak
Radiochemistry and Biomarker Development Unit, Department of Biomedical Imaging and Image-guided Therapy, Division of Nuclear Medicine, Medical University of Vienna, A-1090 Vienna, Austria

Katharina Holl, Dirk Schepmann and Bernhard Wünsch
Institut für Pharmazeutische und Medizinische Chemie der Westfälischen Wilhelms-Universität Münster, Correnssstraße 48, Münster D-48149, Germany

Christiane A. Fischer, Sandra Vomstein and Thomas L. Mindt
University of Basel Hospital, Clinic of Radiology and Nuclear Medicine, Division of Radiopharmaceutical Chemistry, Petersgraben 4, 4031 Basel, Switzerland

Linjing Mu and Kasim Popaj
Center for Radiopharmaceutical Sciences of ETH-PSI-USZ, Department of Nuclear Medicine, University Hospital Zürich, CH-8091 Zürich, Switzerland

Katharina Stockhofe, Johannes M. Postema, Hanno Schieferstein and Tobias L. Ross
Institute of Nuclear Chemistry, Johannes Gutenberg-University Mainz, Fritz-Strassmann-Weg 2, 55128 Mainz, Germany

Marco Müller
Department of Radiochemistry, ABX GmbH, Heinrich-Gläser-Straße 10, Radeberg D-01454, Germany

Steffen Fischer, Friedrich-Alexander Ludwig, Achim Hiller, Cornelius K. Donat, Winnie Deuther-Conrad and Peter Brust
Helmholtz-Zentrum Dresden-Rossendorf, Institut für Radiopharmazeutische Krebsforschung, Forschungsstelle Leipzig, Abteilung Neuroradiopharmaka, Permoserstraße 15, Leipzig D-04318, Germany

Wiebke Sihver and Hans-Jürgen Pietzsch
Helmholtz-Zentrum Dresden-Rossendorf (HZDR), Institute of Radiopharmaceutical Cancer Research, Bautzner Landstraße 400, Dresden 01328, Germany

Mechthild Krause and Michael Baumann
Department of Radiation Oncology and OncoRay, Medical Faculty and University Hospital Carl Gustav Carus, Technische Universität Dresden, Dresden 01307, Germany
OncoRay—National Center for Radiation Research in Oncology, Medical Faculty and University Hospital Carl Gustav Carus, Technische Universität Dresden, Dresden 01307, Germany
German Cancer Consortium (DKTK) Dresden and German Cancer Research Center (DKFZ), Heidelberg 69120, Germany
HZDR, Institute of Radiation Oncology, Bautzner Landstraße 400, Dresden 01328, Germany

Jens Pietzsch and Jörg Steinbach
Helmholtz-Zentrum Dresden-Rossendorf (HZDR), Institute of Radiopharmaceutical Cancer Research, Bautzner Landstraße 400, Dresden 01328, Germany
Department of Chemistry and Food Chemistry, Technische Universität Dresden, Dresden 01062, Germany

Index

www.ingramcontent.com/pod-product-compliance
Lightning Source LLC
LaVergne TN
LVHW082138200926
848484LV00008B/2071